David Ip

Orthopedic Traumatc

Second Edition

To the

Most

awesome

orthopedics

Surgeon

in the

making.

Lots of
Love.

Mandeep.

About the Author

Dr. David Ip is a fellow of various professional organizations, including the Royal College of Surgeons and the Hong Kong College of Orthopedic Surgeons, and is a member of the American Academy of Orthopedic Surgeons and the American Association of Academic Physiatrists, among many others, such as the International Association for the Study of Pain and various Gait Analysis societies. His biography is included in *Marquis Who's Who in Science & Engineering*, *Who's Who in Medicine and Healthcare*, *Sterling's Who's Who in NY*, and the *International Who's Who Historical Society*. In his capacity as Director General (Asia) of the International Biographical Association of the UK and as Clinical Governor of the American Biographical Institute he has contributed significantly to peer-reviewed journal articles and has written several books on orthopedics, which have received positive reviews from the Royal College of Surgeons and the *Journal of Bone and Joint Surgery*. He is also the reviewer of selected orthopedic journals published in Europe, and holds honorary consultancy positions for various companies like the Lehrman Gerson group, Brand's Institute, Medacorp, among many others.

Preface to the Second Edition

The author and the publisher would like to take this opportunity to thank the medical community for the utmost warm welcome given to the first edition of this book. A second edition is deemed necessary not only because of the extreme popularity of the first edition such that the international stock of the book was sold out in less than a year, but also because, as mentioned in the first edition, orthopaedic traumatology is a rapidly expanding field.

In this second edition, some important chapters like those on computer-aided surgery and surgical navigation have been completely revised, as well as the chapter on fracture fixation principles, while many new chapters have been added to keep front-line workers in trauma abreast of the rapidly changing paradigm shift in fragility fracture management. That a much more positive attitude should be taken by orthopods with regard to their role in concomitant osteoporosis management is echoed by the recent policy statement of the AAOS, and is reflected in the contents of the "blue book" or official publication of the British Orthopaedic Association. Such changes come about thanks partly to the great efforts of leaders in this field such as Drs Gallacher and McLellan from Glasgow, who successfully pioneered the "Fragility Fracture Liaison Service", which is now used in many general hospitals across Europe, as well as in parts of Asia. However, in order for a programme that tackles secondary prevention of hip fractures to be successful, there is a strong need for an evidence-based fracture hip protocol that incorporates the latest research findings in biophysics, neurophysiology, fall prevention, physiotherapy, gait analysis and orthopaedics. To this end, a new chapter on this subject has been added.

There is also a need for a brand new user-friendly "Fall Scale" that can be used by general practitioners, volunteers, community nurses, paramedics and other medical staff to monitor the patient's progress after physiotherapy training to act as an early warning system in case of de-conditioning. To this end, the author has described a new fall scale known as the "Simplified Fall Scale", which meets the requirements of being easy to perform in less than a minute, with no need for special equipment apart from a standard high-chair with arms, and it can easily be remembered and taught by staff with little orthopaedic experience such as volunteer teams and family doctors who are not frequently exposed to orthopaedic fracture conditions.

Finally, as this book is mainly written for front-line workers, the author has deemed it necessary to include another new chapter on orthopaedic emergencies.

Lastly, the author wishes to thank again Professor Court-Brown, Edinburgh, and Professor John Wedge of the Toronto Hospital for Sick Children for their kindness in writing the forewords for the first edition of this book, which proved to be a major success. For those readers using this book in preparation for professional exams, I wish them the best of luck and happy reading!

David Ip
Hong Kong, November 2007

Foreword to the First Edition

Doctor Ip is to be congratulated for writing such a useful book on orthopaedic trauma. This is a rapidly expanding field and many disciplines now treat fractures, dislocations and soft tissue injuries and their sequelae. There is a need for a book to help educate trainees in orthopaedic surgery, nursing, physiotherapy and rehabilitation medicine as well as medical students, and this book fulfils that need. It is succinct, but contains a great deal of information important to these and other paramedical disciplines.

There are 15 chapters dealing with all aspects of orthopaedic trauma and its management. It is to Doctor Ip's credit that he has not forgotten the future of orthopaedic trauma, and there are chapters on minimally invasive and computer-aided surgery and fall prevention in the elderly. In addition, the book has chapters on high energy trauma, bone healing, the principles of fracture management and the management of different fractures

The format is user-friendly and it will appeal to all paramedical disciplines, senior medical students and surgeons-in-training. I have no doubt that they will find it useful and I hope they enjoy reading it.

Charles Court-Brown, Edinburgh

Foreword to the First Edition

David Ip has written a remarkable book for orthopaedic residents that reduces the complexity of modern traumatology to basic concepts, principles and guidelines, providing the learner with a practical approach to trauma management. Each of the 15 chapters easily stands alone and may be consumed in a single study session. The organisation of this concise treatise is consistent from chapter to chapter and has numerous "tips" and "pearls", building on a sound conceptual framework.

This is not intended to be a technical manual or comprehensive textbook – the resident already has many of these to choose from – but rather a compendium of essential information to be enhanced by clinical experience and detailed literature review. More than 200 illustrations nicely complement the text, providing excellent examples of both common and less common serious injuries.

I believe this book meets the author's very important objective of a reasonably brief, yet comprehensive, survey of trauma management that fulfils the resident's need for core information. The chapters on normal and abnormal bone healing and on the principles of fracture fixation are particularly clear and informative.

My compliments to the author for writing a much-needed concise and excellent guide to trauma management.

John H. Wedge

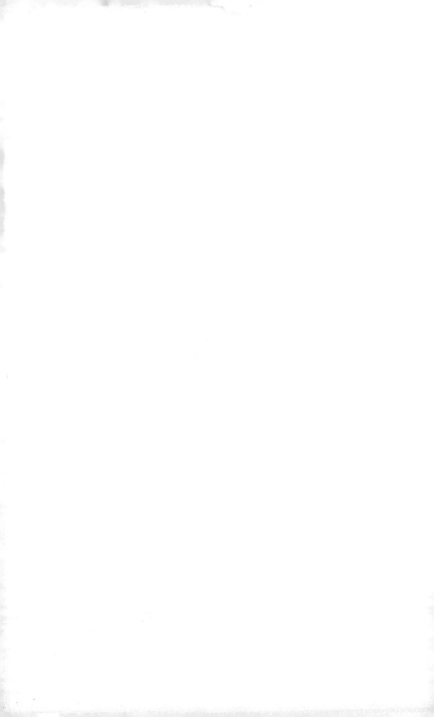

Preface to the First Edition

Like its popular companion volume, *Orthopaedic Principles – A Resident's Guide*, which was well received by the medical community, *Orthopaedic Traumatology – A Resident's Guide* was written to stimulate interest in modern orthopaedic traumatology, which is a very dynamic and rapidly changing field. This book aims at a very wide readership. From the resident preparing for professional examinations, to the physical and occupational therapists and nurses involved in the daily care of fracture patients, since fractures form the bulk of emergency orthopaedic admissions in many major hospitals. Also, surgeons requiring re-certification as well as surgeons in developing or under-developed countries will find the volume useful in their daily practice. Finally, this book is structured in such a way as to facilitate review of the subject matter before board exams and quickens the process of information retrieval of both classic and recent references. Happy reading!

David Ip
Hong Kong, November 2005

Contents

Ten Questions for Residents

Introductory Comment

- This is a very short chapter
- It serves as a brainstorming session for our young surgeons-in-training, urging them to think about some critical issues relating to modern orthopaedic trauma
- Most of the answers to the 10 questions can be found in the ensuing 14 chapters of this book

1.1   High Energy Trauma: Are We Doing Enough to Keep It in Check?

- The study of the management of patients suffering from high energy poly-trauma is vital, since many of these are young patients in the prime of their life. High energy trauma is in fact the main cause of death in young people in many countries (leading cause of death in the <40-year-olds)
- Poor management can create significant morbidity and mortality. Prevention is always the best strategy. However, this can only be achieved by the concerted efforts of the legislators, vehicle engineers, highway architects, proper trauma triage, and development of trauma centres, as well as having good orthopaedic traumatologists
- The prevention and management of this problem will be discussed in Chap. 2

1.2   Medico-Legal Corner: Why Are Fractures Being Missed?

1.2.1   The Two Faces of a Fracture

- The commonest cause of missing a fracture is depending on only one X-ray view of human bones, which are essentially three-dimensional structures
- It is recommended that at least two X-ray views 90° to each other be taken for any anatomical region to be assessed

1.2.2   Other Causes of a Missed Fracture in the Stable Patient

- Bones with a complex shape frequently require more than two X-ray views for proper assessment of any fracture. A common example is the scaphoid fracture (Fig. 1.1)
- Fractures can be missed in bones that are obscured by other structures on the X-ray. An example is missing a fractured sacrum due to the anatomical details being obscured by bowel gas
- We may sometimes opt to perform more sophisticated investigations such as a computed tomography (CT) scan for more complex fractures like the acetabulum; even CT can miss the fracture if the plane of the fracture line lies in the same plane as the CT cut
- Some fractures simply do not reveal themselves in the acute X-ray film. These difficult cases can only be diagnosed given time either by serial X-rays, or special investigations such as bone scanning or MRI. Examples can be found in some stress fractures, which are discussed in Chap. 5

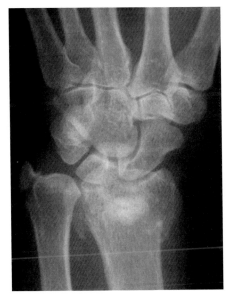

Fig. 1.1 The scaphoid fracture was not noted preoperatively, as attention was drawn to the obviously fractured distal radius, until fluoroscopic screening in theatre in multiple planes

1.2.3   Reasons for Missing Fractures in the Poly-traumatised Patient

- Recent literature revealed that missing injuries including fractures is common even in this day and age, amounting to around 22 %, and up to 75 % of the missed injuries in a recent study were musculoskeletal (Brooks et al. 2004)

- This highlights the importance of repeated clinical examination in these frequently obtunded patients. The concept of tertiary survey was first emphasised by Enderson et al. in 1990, but in fact the concept originated from the ideas of Prof. Gissane

- In particular, missing cervical spine injuries can be devastating to both the surgeon and the patient. Any poly-traumatised patient coming to the accident service should be assumed to have a cervical spine injury until proven otherwise; and the cervical spine of the patient should be assumed unstable until proven otherwise. Poorly taken lateral views of the cervical spine is of little help and give a false sense of security; be liberal in the use of CT scanning to assess the cervical spine region. Having said that, do not miss concomitant spinal injury elsewhere, which can occur in up to 7 % of cases

1.3   Why Does the Postoperative X-ray Not Always Look as Good as It Should?

- We often hear expressions from residents like: "I am positive the fracture was reduced intraoperatively, why is it that I have come up with a horrible looking postoperative X-ray?"

1.3.1   Answer: The Two Faces of a Fracture Reduction

- Just as looking at a bone with a suspected fracture using one X-ray view may miss the fracture, the same is true of an intraoperative fracture reduction

- The reduction or alignment may look perfect in one plane, but much displaced in another (Figs. 1.2, 1.3). Thus, to prevent any postopera-

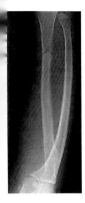

Fig. 1.2 One X-ray view of this forearm fracture, or in fact any fracture, is far from adequate in judging alignment and can be most deceiving

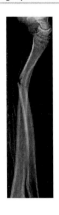

Fig. 1.3 The lateral radiograph gives away the true degree of malalignment and angulation of the fracture

tive surprises, it is essential to screen our intraoperative fracture reduction using at least two views, preferably 90° to each other

1.4 Is There a Rigid Guideline for All Intra-articular Fracture Reductions?

- The likely answer is in the negative
- This is because the effect of articular incongruity on a joint varies depending on the articular cartilage thickness, the modulus of the articular cartilage, and the geometry of the joint, as well as its global congruity
- Example: greater leeway can be given to articular step-offs at the lateral tibial plateau, while very little compromise can be given to step-offs at the weight-bearing dome of the acetabulum

1.5 What Importance Do We Give to a Perfect-Looking Postoperative X-ray?

- In the past, patients and surgeons paid much attention to a good-looking X-ray. This is best exemplified by the traditional AO concept of perfect anatomical reduction and fixation of fractures

- However, although perfect anatomical reduction is still required for intra-articular fractures (though not always predictive of outcome: see Sect. 1.7.1); the same perfect anatomical reduction and rigid fixation is not always needed or preferable in meta-diaphyseal fractures. This will be discussed in Chap. 4, when we discuss the concept of relative stability

1.6   Relative Stability (in Meta-diaphyseal Fractures): How Much Is Enough?

- The key here is the concept of elasticity or "elastic flexible fixation"
- This implies that displacement of the fracture ends under load must be reversible. Locked internal fixator technique (such as locking compression plate [LCP]) takes advantage of the elastic properties of metals, especially that of pure titanium, in fixing bones of limited strength like osteoporotic bones, by dint of the deformability of the implant, enabling the use of the elastic flexible fixation concept
- In short, this new concept of elasticity in fixation has the advantage that the implant–bone construct or anchorage is less likely to fail in the event of a single sudden high loading challenge to the construct or a traumatic event
- Exactly how much elasticity is enough for a given fracture is difficult to quantify, but this concept is very likely to be a move in the right direction, especially for the rising number of osteoporotic fractures. Osteoporotic fracture management will be discussed in detail in Chaps. 5 and 6

1.7   Radiological and Clinical Outcome: Do They Correlate?

- The fact that a good fracture outcome (of, say, intra-articular fractures) is not always predicted by a good- or perfect-looking postoperative X-ray is well known and reported in the literature

1.7.1   Reasons for the Discrepancy

- Diffuse injury to the cartilage can severely affect the outcome. This may not be reviewed by postoperative radiographs. This is because much of the injury to the cartilage was done at the time of the high energy injury
- Articular step-offs of the articular cartilage are not an uncommon finding; despite a seemingly good postoperative X-ray, this relative incongruity can cause maldistribution of contact pressure on impact loading, especially in lower limb joints
- Some recent studies have shown that using X-ray as the tool for assessing the degree of accuracy of articular fragment reconstruction in intra-articular fractures is rather low. (These studies have shown that frequently CT or arthroscopy is better in this respect)
- Some other well-known factors that may complicate the issue of fracture outcome, despite a perfect-looking postoperative X-ray include: worker's compensation issues and psychological make-up of the patient. These issues will be brought up and discussed in detail in Chap. 10
- Using intra-articular fractures as an example, there are many factors that determine outcome *besides* mere articular surface reconstruction. According to the ideas of Joseph Schatzker, the important factors include:
  - Correction of meta- and diaphyseal deformity
  - Restoration of joint stability
  - Restoration of range of motion (ROM)

1.8   Soft Tissue Injury in a Fracture Patient: Does It Matter?

- Assessment and documentation of soft tissue injury is so important that we often hear the common saying: "fractures are essentially soft tissue injuries in which the bone happens to break"
- The degree of soft tissue injury affects the fracture in many ways as the following discussion will show

1.8.1   Importance of Assessment of Soft Tissues in Fracture Patients

- Assessment is important because:
  - Nature of soft tissue injury affects the timing of surgery. This is especially true for regions with a thinner soft tissue envelope such as the tibia, the ankle, etc.
  - Soft tissue complications can affect healing of fractures. Example: Court-Brown and McQueen of Edinburgh demonstrated delay in healing of tibial fractures if the patient developed compartment syndrome
  - Neurovascular injuries are important as their presence affects the decision-making process of the orthopaedist, such as Holstein fracture with radial nerve palsy. Occasional cases of acute ischaemia also need early revascularisation
  - In open fractures, the degree of soft tissue injury affects the healing as the vascularity is affected to different extents. This can be seen by the different healing times of open fractures with different Gustilo's grades. This will be discussed in Chap. 5
  - Management of soft tissue injuries in high energy trauma and soft tissue coverage problems will be dealt with in Chap. 2

1.9   Computer-Aided Surgery: Are We on the Right Track?

- Substantiating evidence to say that we are on the right track on this score includes:
  - The use of computer guidance in the performance of highly accurate tasks is not new. This is already a well-developed field in neurosurgery: e.g. use of stereotactic surgery in tackling strategic brain lesions. The same is true of using this new technological know-how in for instance fixing pelvic/acetabular fractures, like administration of iliosacral screws where the margin of safety is small
  - There has been a general move towards minimally invasive techniques to minimise surgical trauma to the patient in all fields of surgery in recent decades. Techniques like virtual fluoroscopy

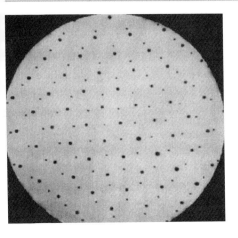

Fig. 1.4 The dots shown are in fact markers appearing on the fluoroscopic images and are used for image calibration. The computer has to calibrate the acquired image before virtual fluoroscopy can commence

(Fig. 1.4) can aid performance in this respect. As an example, the starting point for intramedullary (IM) nail insertion can be identified by virtual fluoroscopy, via the trajectory "look-ahead" feature, which can be used to align the drill guide with the femoral canal in two planes in femoral nailing

- Other advantages: good teaching tool for future surgical residents, less exposure to radiation since stored images can be employed to provide surgical guidance and can be readily updated after intraoperative fracture reduction
- We often associate CT-guided navigation and virtual fluoroscopy when we talk about computer-aided surgery. The scope with which the computer can aid the orthopaedic surgeon is much larger, for example:
    - The newly developed Taylor spatial frame: although it resembles an Ilizarov, on entering the correct data into the computer before correction of deformity, simultaneous correction in all planes of freedom can now be achieved for the first time in orthopaedic surgery (cf. if the Ilizarov construct is used, the planes of deformity such as translation and rotation are corrected sequentially)

- The computer is also indispensable in many other fields of orthopaedics, such as analysing not only two-dimensional but also the more recently developed three-dimensional gait analysis results to help plan surgery
- The possible future use of robotics is also highly dependent on computer technology

1.10   Fragility Fractures Rising (Exponentially): What Can Orthopaedists Do?

- There is an exponential increase in incidence of hip and other fragility fractures (Fig. 1.5) as shown by recent epidemiological data
- We expect a soaring incidence of fractured hips, particularly in countries with an aging population
- The best way to circumvent this vast problem is still prevention. This includes both primary and secondary prevention. To this end, the

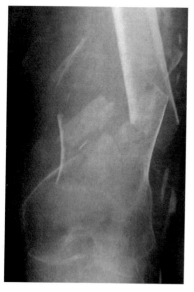

Fig. 1.5 It should be noted that the presence of a fragility fracture is predictive of others. This patient with a fractured distal femur also had bilateral hip fractures in the past

administration of a fall prevention programme is vitally important, as well as treatment and prophylaxis of osteoporosis

It is surprising to note that large scale primary and secondary fall prevention programmes may not be the norm, even in well developed countries. This underscores the urgency of the problem, which will be dealt with in Chap. 15

General Bibliography

1.   Ip D (2005) Orthopedic principles – a resident's guide. Springer, Heidelberg, Berlin New York

Selected Bibliography of Journal Articles

1.   Brooks A, Holroyd B, et al. (2004) Missed injury in major trauma. Injury 35:407–410
2.   Enderson BL, Reath DB, Meadors J, Dallas W, DeBoo JM, Maull KI (1990) The tertiary trauma survey: a prospective study of missed injury. J Trauma 30(6):666–669
3.   Harrop JS, Vaccaro AR, et al. (2005) Failure of standard imaging to detect a cervical spine fracture in a patient with ankylosing spondylitis. Spine 30(14):E417–419
4.   Helm PA, Eckel TS (1998) Accuracy of registration methods in frameless stereotaxis. Comput Aided Surg 3:51–6
5.   Seagger R, Howell J (2004) Prevention of secondary osteoporotic fractures – why are we ignoring the evidence? Injury 35:986–988

High Energy Trauma Management

Contents

2.1   Why Study High Energy Trauma?

- High energy trauma is a major cause of mortality among young citizens of modern society
- One recent study in US revealed that injury is the leading cause of death under the age of 40. The total cost of injury to society approaches $100 billion a year

2.2   Trauma Triage and Scores

2.2.1   What Is Triage?
- Triage comes from a French word meaning "to sort"
- It had its roots initially during wartime in Napoleonic times when they sorted out those less wounded soldiers who could go back into battle
- In modern traumatology, we do the opposite, i.e. sort out those severely injured persons who need the support of a trauma centre

2.2.2   Evolution of Civilian Triage over the Years
- At first, the aim of pre-hospital triage mainly focused on identification of trauma victims who would benefit from the care of specialised trauma centres (see American College of Surgeons [ACS] guidelines to be discussed)
- It soon became obvious that optimal care should also be provided to those victims with somewhat lesser injuries. This forms the concept of "inclusive" care

2.2.3   Main Types of Trauma Triage
- Pre-hospital triage in the field
- Triage of patients after hospital arrival
- Triage during disasters
- Triage during wartime (wartime triage and triage in disasters will not be discussed in this book)

2.2.4   Which Trauma Score to Use?

- There are many different trauma scoring systems available. But it will be advisable only to adhere to those that are user-friendly, do not involve complex calculations, and have a reasonable degree of sensitivity and specificity

2.2.5   Sensitivity and Specificity

- Sensitivity of a trauma score: the higher the sensitivity, the higher the likelihood of detecting the really severely traumatised patients
- Specificity of a trauma score: the higher the specificity, the lesser the likelihood of missing the really severely traumatised patients
- Scores with low sensitivity risk the chance of "over-triage"
- Scores with low specificity risk the chance of "under-triage"

2.2.6   The Spectrum of Trauma Scores

- There are over 50 scoring systems that have been developed for triage and research over the years and yet the task of separating the stable from the unstable patients is still difficult
- Detailed description of each of the scores will not be included here

2.2.7   Which System to Use?

- Besides issues of sensitivity and specificity, the exact trauma score to be used depends on the clinical situation at hand. It is thus difficult to comment on the best trauma scoring system
- For example, the director of an Intensive Care unit may be more interested in scores that can predict the likelihood of survival of his patients, but the same may not be the focus of concern of the cost-conscious hospital administrator

2.3   Mortality in High Energy Trauma

2.3.1   Timing and Mortality

- There are three main phases:
  - Mortality before arrival in hospital: from major destructive injury of organ system(s)

- Early day 1 mortality: common causes include severe head injury, hypovolaemia and hypoxia
- Late mortality: mostly from multiple organ dysfunction (MODS), – include entities like adult respiratory distress (ARDS) and disseminated intravascular coagulation (DIC)

2.3.2   Key Point

■ Haemorrhage is the major cause of death in the first 3 h (the first 3 h are sometimes called the Golden Hours)

2.3.3   Causes of Pre-hospital Mortality

■ These occur shortly after the injury and are most likely due to severe brain injury or disruptions of the heart or the large vessels

■ Severe injuries like these can cause death within minutes

2.3.4   Ways to Prevent Pre-hospital Mortality

■ Road safety measures, especially on highways
■ Law enforcement, e.g. concerning drink-driving
■ Better vehicle design
■ Swift transport of trauma victims, including helicopters
■ Triage to Trauma Centre
■ Pre-hospital trauma scoring
■ Pre-hospital trauma life support

2.3.5   Importance of Pre-hospital Triage

■ As many as 50% of trauma deaths from severe trauma occur *prior* to hospitalisation (reported in literature from US)

■ A well-developed system of early notification and rapid transport (including helicopter transport) is necessary, especially if the accident occurs in rural areas or less accessible areas

2.3.6   Elements of Pre-hospital Triage

■ There are three main aspects involved in pre-hospital trauma triage:
  - Physiology parameters
  - Anatomical parameters

– Mechanism of injury

(Also of importance may be age and associated medical conditions)

2.3.7   ACS-Recommended Guidelines for Pre-hospital Triage

■ The ACS guidelines (adapted from American College of Surgeons Committee on Trauma, 1999):
  – Physiological parameters:
  – Glasgow Coma Scale (GCS) < 14
  – Systolic blood pressure (SBP) < 90
  – Respiratory rate (RR) < 10 or > 29
  – Revised trauma score < 11

(Admit to trauma centre if any one of above present)

  – Anatomical parameters:
  – Flail chest
  – ≥ Two proximal long bone fractures
  – Penetrating injuries to head/neck/trunk or proximal extremity
  – Fractured pelvis
  – Amputation proximal to ankle and wrist
  – Combined burns and trauma

(If any of above present, admit to trauma centre)

  – Injury mechanism parameters:
  – Death occurring in same passenger compartment of vehicle or major vehicle deformity
  – Time of extrication > 20 min
  – Fall from > 20 feet (6 m)
  – Ejected from vehicle or rolled over or pedestrian thrown away by vehicle

(If any of above present, contact control and assess need for trauma centre)

  – Assessment of age and associated conditions:
  – Age < 5 or > 55
  – Pregnancy
  – Cardiopulmonary disorders
  – Immunosuppressed/insulin-dependent diabetes mellitus (IDDM)/ morbid obesity, etc.

— History of bleeding problems

(If any of above present, contact control and assess need for trauma centre)

2.4   Why Triage to Trauma Centres?

2.4.1   Need for Organised Trauma Centres

- A paper by Trunkey (West et al. 1979) serves as an excellent reference on systems of trauma care. It compares an organised system of trauma delivery in San Francisco with a random arrangement in the LA area of Orange County in USA. Significantly more patients accessed appropriate care in San Francisco
- It should be noted, however, that only an estimated 25 % of the US population currently lives in regions with a designated trauma centre

2.4.2   Mortality Reduction
with Trauma Centre Development

- It has been shown that the setting up of trauma centres can reduce mortality of severely injured trauma victims
- Literature reported that overall roughly 5 – 10% of trauma patients are in need of proper pre-hospital triage to these trauma centres
- The idea of pre-hospital triage of severely injured patients to trauma centres has now been adopted in many countries

2.5   Preventing Mortality in the First 24 Hours

- Advanced trauma life support (ATLS) protocol
- Emergency surgery
- End-points of resuscitation
- Trauma scoring after hospital arrival and definition of severe trauma
- Concept of damage control and damage control orthopaedics

2.5.1   The Injury Severity Score

- The Injury Severity Score (ISS) assigns a score of 1 to 5 (minor to critical) to six organ systems. The three worst organ system scores are squared and the ISS is the sum of those three squares. Imperfect though this may seem, it is one of the best guidelines we have for ranking injury severity
- Example: three organ systems that each score 5 produce a maximum ISS of 75 points – a fairly uniformly fatal measure of injury
- Example: for scoring of orthopaedic trauma under ISS, a femur shaft fracture is also regarded as a severe injury (score = 3). However, ISS is not a perfect score since the difference in score it gives to bilateral femoral shaft fractures is not great, despite the fact that there is $\times 2$ mortality

2.5.2   Revised Trauma Score

- Also a popular scoring system
- Said by some to be the most consistently referenced system in the literature, it is based on respiratory rate, systolic blood pressure and the Glasgow Coma Score. If the sum of these scores is less than 11, treatment of the victim in a comprehensive facility is necessary

2.5.3   Definition of Severe Trauma

- A popular definition of severe trauma involves a patient with an ISS >16 (some reports in literature have mentioned 17 or 18)
- In fact, the ISS is a commonly used trauma score used by traumatologists after the severely traumatised patient has arrived at the trauma centre

2.6   Concepts of Damage Control

2.6.1   Definition

- The principle of damage control works on the principle of limiting the surgical burden (or 2nd hit phenomenon) on the immune response that occurs in poly-trauma patients with an already high risk of adverse outcome. This is based on the finding that prolonged operation on poly-trauma patients can lead to coagulation disturbances and an abnormal immuno-inflammatory state causing remote organ injury

- The concept of damage control has its roots from US Navy, where the idea was to keep the damaged warship afloat and limit fire and flooding. The term "damage control orthopaedics" only came about in 1990s after the observation of ARDS after reamed femoral nailing in the severely injured given early definitive stabilisation by the more traditional concept of early total care (ETC)

- Damage control should be regarded as part of the resuscitation process

2.6.2   Evolution of Concepts of Damage Control

- In late 18th century, tamponade packing of deep bleeding wounds was described
- Also used by Pringle in early 20th century
- In the 1970s therapeutic packing of the liver was found to be effective
- In 1983, Stone reported success in intra-abdominal packing of trauma patients bleeding profusely from associated hypothermia and coagulopathy
- Few decades ago, early fracture stabilisation was not routinely done for patients with multiple traumas. It was believed that poly-trauma patients could not cope physiologically
- It was not until 1980s that studies showed early (usually within 24 h) definitive stabilisation of long bone fractures reduced the incidence of fat embolism. The era of ETC began

2.6.3   ETC Era

- Improvements that allow the performance of ETC: development of trauma centres, rapid rescue facilities, prompt and appropriate resuscitation, availability of intensive care facilities, interventional radiography, improved abdominal packing products/haemostatic agents, advances in re-warming, reversal of coagulopathy, etc.

2.6.4   Problems of ETC and Damage Control Era

- It is now realised that practice of ETC during the *initial* phase of management of multiple trauma, especially those in extremis, had poor outcome
- High incidence of complications, especially seen in those with severe thoracic injuries, haemorrhagic shock, and unstable patients who underwent surgery. On the orthopaedic side, high incidence of complications (Cx) arises from fixation of, say, femoral shaft fractures in a badly traumatised patient, especially in the presence of significant pulmonary injuries

2.6.5   How Does Damage Control Involve Orthopaedists?

- Damage control (DC) involves initial temporary fracture stabilisation in borderline patients with high ISS scores, in order to prevent unexpected post-traumatic Cx
- Results in a new approach in the management of orthopaedic trauma
- DC concepts and protocols began to be used by trauma centres in 1990s

2.6.6   The 2nd Hit Theory

- It is now realised that the timing and quality of any medical intervention (such as a major operation lasting several hours) can cause additional trauma to the patient (known as the second hit) in addition to the initial trauma (or first hit)

2.6.7   Other "Hits"

- These may include:
    - Septic episodes
    - Dehydration or inadequate fluid resuscitation
    - Hypothermia
    - Surgical intervention

2.6.8 Description of Phases of Damage Control from University of Pennsylvania

- Phase 1: recognition
- Phase 2: salvage (from bleeding and contamination)
- Phase 3: intensive care
- Phase 4: definitive repair and reconstruction

2.6.8.1 Details of Phase 1

- Involves Ground Zero recognition
- Involves assessment and decision-making to initiate damage control

2.6.8.2 Details of Phase 2

- Involves control of contamination and control of haemorrhage in the OR
- Intra-abdominal/pelvic packing as needed

2.6.8.3 Details of Phase 3

- Re-warming to reverse hypothermia
- Treatment (Rn) of coagulopathy
- Ventilatory and ICU support
- Then re-examination and further planning

2.6.8.4 Details of Phase 4

- Intra-abdominal/pelvic pack removal
- Definitive corrective/reconstructive surgery
- ± Wound closure

2.6.9 Summary of Key Points

- DC should be regarded as part of the resuscitation process
- Using the DC concept can decrease the resultant inflammatory response, leading to better clinical outcome. Early major operation (when the patient is not yet stabilised) has to be considered as too great a burden for severely poly-traumatised patients. By careful choice of the type and timing of operation; blood loss and tissue trauma can be minimised

2.7   Damage Control for Pelvic Fractures

2.7.1   Aim of Treatment in the Acute Phase
- Prevent early death from bleeding, i.e. save life, rather than getting involved in fancy demanding surgery
- Early recognition and initiation of damage control orthopaedics in acute pelvic ring injuries in unstable patients. In essence, this phase involves concomitant decompression of body cavities like the chest or brain and repair of hollow viscus by general surgeons. The trauma team tries to find and control all bleeding sources, and the orthopaedists need to stabilise central fractures such as pelvic ring disruptions

2.7.2   Mortality After Fractured Pelvis?
- Most of the deaths in the first 24 h are due to uncontrolled bleeding
- Late mortalitics are due to death from sepsis-related multi-organ failure, and from associated injuries

2.7.3   Sources of Bleeding
- Venous plexus – especially pre-sacral plexus
- Arterial bleeding (iliac vessel and its branches, arterial bleeder as culprit in 10 % of cases)
- Cancellous bone surfaces
- Other organs (e.g. abdominal organs)

2.7.4   Classification to Use
- During the resuscitative phase, it is best to use the Young and Burgess Classification system
- Reason: helps predict local and distant associated injuries, resuscitation needs, and expected mortality rate
- Tile's classification is more useful during decision for definitive fracture fixation

2.7.5   Young/Burgess Classification
- APC (anteroposterior compression): 1 = stable, 2 = partially stable, 3 = unstable

- LC (lateral compression): 1 = stable, 2 = partially stable, 3 = unstable
- VS (vertical shear): all unstable
- CMI (combined mechanical injury): unstable

(The classification is based on mechanism and stability)

2.7.6   Tile's Classification

- Tile's A = pelvic ring stable
- Tile's B = partially stable pelvic ring
- Tile's C = complete unstable pelvic ring

(The classification is mainly based on directions of instability)

2.7.7   Types of Fractured Pelvis That Cause Severe Bleeding

- AP compression types II and III
- Vertical shear
- Lateral compression III
- Some CMI cases
  - In one series, it was found that APC Type III injuries required the most blood replacement, followed by vertical shear cases

2.7.7.1 Explanation

- Situations that lead to tearing of the pelvic floor will most likely increase chance of severe bleeding
  - APC thus most likely to bleed (if severe)
  - LC injuries least likely to bleed (unless severe)

2.7.8   Pearls to Control the Bleeding

- Initial recognition and means of arresting bleeding, and managing shock
- Find out the sources of bleeding
- Most need external fixation
- If no response, may consider packing, etc. to control haemorrhage if in extremis
- Correction of hypothermia, acidosis and coagulopathy is imperative

2.7.9 Different Ways to Stop Bleeding

- Pelvic sling
- Pelvic binder
- Anti-shock garment
- External fixation (EF) and pelvic C-clamp
- Arterial in-flow arrest
- Pelvic packing
- Angiography and embolisation
- Internal fixation

2.7.9.1 Pelvic Sling and Binder

- Valuable initial method to arrest bleeding
- Does not require much technical expertise, easy to apply, closes the pelvis
- Applies at both trochanters
- Works by decreasing the volume of the injured pelvic ring (e.g. open book injury)

2.7.9.2 Anti-shock Garment

- Pros: get more blood to the vital organs, splint associated fracture, ease of transport
- Cons: assessment difficult (e.g. of the abdomen, cannot perform per rectum/per vagina examinations), can produce or mask compartment syndrome, lower limb ischaemia, can hinder breathing

2.7.9.3 External Fixator

- Common method of arresting bleeding (if bleeding is from the pelvis)
- Can be used even with concomitant bladder and bowel disruptions
- Works by control of pelvic volume, direct compression at fracture site, provides some stability to bones and/or better alignment to prevent clot from being dislodged
- Does not just work by limiting space for blood loss as it was found that the amount of blood loss can be much greater than space increase in the pelvis

2.7.9.3.1 Where Does the Bleeding Go?

- The administration of EF can aid tamponade by controlling the pelvic volume
- But it should be realised that the retro-peritoneum can contain up to 4 l of blood and bleeding can continue until intravascular pressure is overcome
- In cases in which there is extensive disruption of retroperitoneal muscle compartments, the above may not be true and uncontrolled bleeding can occur. This is because the retroperitoneum is not a closed space and pressure-induced tamponade does not always occur

2.7.9.4 Pelvic C-clamp

- Consists of two pins applied to the posterior ilium in region of sacro-ilial joint (SIJ)
- Offers compression where the area of greatest bleeding usually occurs
- Cx: neurovascular injury, nerve injury from compression of associated sacral fractures
- May not be indicated in fractured ilium, and trans-iliac fracture dislocations

2.7.9.5 Arterial Clamping

- Clamping of internal iliac or even the aorta in cases of exsanguination have been reported
- Aorta occlusion can be by open cross clamping, or percutaneous/open balloon catheter techniques

2.7.9.6 Pelvic Packing

- Used aggressively and more popular in Europe
- May be the only method for patients in extremis
- Packing is applied at paravesical and pre-sacral areas. These regions are packed from posterior to anterior by standard techniques. Beware never to close the abdomen as this will risk abdominal compartment syndrome

■ Change or remove dressing 48 h after injury

2.7.9.7 Angiographic Embolisation

■ Many workers emphasised the importance of the application of EF prior to embolisation
■ Previous studies reported good results if the bleeding is arterial. Even bilateral internal iliac artery embolisation has been reported in the literature
■ There is, however, danger to the patient during transport, and embolisation does not always work for large-bore vessels. It is time-consuming

2.7.9.7.1 Role of Packing Versus Angiographic Embolisation

■ Angiographic embolisation is effective if there is an arterial bleeder (10 % of cases)
■ Since it is time-consuming and may in fact prevent dynamic patient assessment, should be considered as an adjunct in the *more stable* patient with, say, an expanding haematoma
■ Pelvic packing is considered in cases in which ongoing bleeder and shock occurs despite EF stabilisation. In general, patients who require pelvic packing have a much higher mortality and much higher need for transfusions than those who may need embolisation

2.7.9.8 Internal Fixation

■ Little role in the emergency setting
■ Used in elective reconstruction

2.8   Damage Control in Long Bone Fracture of Extremities

2.8.1   Types of Long Bone Injuries That Warrant Damage Control

■ Patients with bilateral femoral shaft fractures in particular have been associated with an increased risk of adverse outcome

- Reason:
  - Femoral shaft is the most frequent long bone fracture in poly-trauma; can be associated with much bleeding if both femurs are fractured
  - Associated with high velocity injury, and *since the femur has a large soft tissue envelope, it is more likely to release more inflammatory mediators and cytokines*
- Result: higher mortality rate reported (up to 16% for isolated femoral injuries in some series)
- In a multicentre study in which > 1,000 femoral fractures received primary stabilisation < 24 h, most developed pulmonary Cx
- Recent studies now recommend that any primary procedure if deemed absolutely necessary should not last > 6 h operating time

2.8.2   Rationale for DC in Multiple Long Bone Fractures

- In view of the fact that patients with long bone fractures who have a large soft tissue envelope (e.g. femoral shaft fracture) tend to have a higher mortality and morbidity than those in areas like the upper extremity, the concept of DC can also be applied to patients with multiple long bone fractures

2.8.3   Phases of DC in Multiple Fractures of Long Bones of Extremities

- First 1 – 2 h (acute phase): for life-saving procedures
- Primary period (day 1): includes Rn of open fractures and dislocations, fracture stabilisation
- Secondary period (days 2 – 3): ± reconstruction surgery
- Tertiary period (> day 3) ± reconstruction surgery

2.8.4   Evidence of Higher Mortality with Early IM Fixation in Fractured Femur if ISS > 15

- Example: Fakhry et al. (1994)
- In this retrospective state-wide study in North Carolina reviewing > 2,800 patients, the mortality rates with different surgical timing are:

- 3.8% mortality with fracture fixed in 1 day
- 1.8% mortality with fracture fixed within 2–4 days
- 1.5% mortality with fracture fixed after the 4th day

2.9   Late Mortality

- MODS
- Related Cx: ARDS, DIC
- Major trauma on individual organ systems in the setting of multiple fractures

2.9.1   Body's Response to Severe Trauma

- When the body is subjected to significant trauma, release of cytokines from cells of damaged tissues produce pro-inflammatory mediators. If severe, this process may lead to SIRS (systemic inflammatory response syndrome)
- The initial systemic inflammatory response may be followed by a period of immunosuppression

2.9.2   Causes of MODS

- Sometimes the SIRS is intense and this overshooting of the inflammatory response may cause organ necrosis, i.e. multi-organ dysfunction syndrome (MODS). Many of these cases present as early MODS
- Despite intense investigations over the years, there is still no uniformly effective therapy to treat MODS
- Late MODS is believed to be related to those cases with very intense immunosuppression. As infection is likely with immunosuppression, infection is a common trigger in late MODS cases. One common source of sepsis in these cases is GI tract bacterial translocation

2.9.3   Significance of MODS

- High mortality
- Much morbidity
- Usually involves prolonged ICU support
- High cost to the hospital administration

2.9.4   Management of MODS

- Mainly supportive
- No effective pharmacotherapy at present
- Most effective treatment is prevention

2.9.5   Ways to Prevent MODS

- Prevent and treat sepsis
- Adequate resuscitation and treatment of shock
- Prevent hypoxia and tissue ischaemia
- Early fracture fixation
- Debridement of devitalised tissues

2.9.6   Patients at High Risk of MODS

- Age > 55
- ISS > 25
- Blood transfusion requirement > 6 units (Arch Surg 1994)
- Lab test: possible use of IL-6 as serum marker of severity

2.9.7   Mainstay of Supportive Therapy for MODS

- Proper oxygenation
- Proper ventilatory support
- Careful fluid resuscitation
- Careful haemodynamic monitoring by pulmonary catheterisation
- Early enteral feeding
- Haemodialysis/haemofiltration for renal failure

2.9.8   Indicators of a Successful Resuscitation (Vincent and Manikis)

- Stable haemodynamics
- No hypovolaemia or hypercapnia
- Lactate < 2 mmol/l

- Normovolaemia
- No need for inotropic support
- Urinary output >1 ml/kg/h

2.9.9   Can the Immune Response Be Quantified?
- Measurements of pro-inflammatory cytokines appear useful
- Tumour necrosis factor and IL-1 have been used in the past, but not reliable due to short plasma half-lives
- IL-6 appears more reliable. Seems to correlate with high ISS and be associated with late adverse outcomes. IL-6 levels in severe injury remain elevated for 5 days. Recent studies claimed that IL-6 assay can detect patients who are likely to develop MODS later. Subsequent increase will correlate with magnitude of operation

2.10   Effects of Trauma to Vital Organs in Patients with Multiple Fractures

2.10.1   Lung Injury and Its Assessment
- CXR: severity may be underestimated at time of initial taking of CXR (e.g. pulmonary oedema may take 2–3 days to develop)
- Spiral CT: mostly used in rapid assessment of suspected lung injuries in most trauma units
- Blood gases
- Others: only in selected cases are the following performed:
  - Bronchoscopy – can be diagnostic and therapeutic, may cause deterioration in blood gas values in poly-trauma patients reported in literature
  - Monitoring of pulmonary arterial pressure
  - V/Q scan in some cases of suspected pulmonary embolism

2.10.1.1   *How Do Multiple Fractures Influence the Pulmonary Injury?*
- The pulmonary pathophysiologic factors include frustrated respiratory effort, increased capillary-alveolar pressure and an embolic shower of debris from fracture sites

- The normal lung clears these materials – but not in ARDS where the result is declining oxygen tension and decreased pulmonary compliance

2.10.1.1.1 Our Goal

- Rapid restoration of oxygen transport by mobilising the patient to an upright posture, leaving them on a ventilator for a while to clear their lungs
- Reamed intramedullary nailing, especially for femoral fractures should be avoided in the presence of significant pulmonary injury or complications in these poly-traumatised patients

2.10.1.2 Evidence of High Mortality in Fracture Fixation with Severe Chest Injury

- Example 1: Fakhry et al. (1994): in this study, it was found that the patient subgroup with severe chest injury had a mortality of 4.6% if operated on the 1st day; but none of the patients died despite the presence of severe chest injury if operated between days 2 and 4 or > day 4
- Example 2: the same view of avoiding early IM fracture fixation in poly-trauma patients with severe lung injury was shared by Pape et al. (1993)

2.10.1.2.1 Opponents to This View: Are Their Arguments Well Founded?

- The retrospective study by Bone et al. (1995) claiming no detrimental effects of early IM nailing in poly-trauma patients with chest injuries should be read with caution
- In this study, the different treatment groups included patients who were not comparable with respect to age and degree of soft tissue and chest trauma. Moreover, fractures in the proximal and distal ends of the femur were included besides femoral shaft fractures

.10.2 Poly-trauma and the Liver

- The coagulation and inflammatory response to injury stimulates phagocytosis and the release of enzymatic by-products. These inflammatory by-products are filtered by the liver
- Unfortunately when these bi-products get to the damaged liver, *the damaged liver itself* will contribute to more mediators, possibly via hepatic macrophages, thereby releasing their products into the lung and causing further problems

2.10.3 Severe Head Injury and Long Bone Fractures

2.10.3.1 What Constitutes Severe Head Injury

- In this context, we refer to those patients with severe head injury (HI) who have GCS ≤8 on arrival at our trauma service

2.10.3.2 Pathophysiology

- CPP (cerebral perfusion pressure) = MAP (mean arterial pressure) – ICP (intracerebral pressure)
- In healthy persons, there is auto-regulation of cerebral blood flow
- In severe head injury, autoregulatory mechanisms may be disrupted
- Consequence is that ICP tends to follow MAP
- Cerebral blood flow is usually lowest in first 24 h after significant head injury, then increases

2.10.3.3 Effect of Head Injury on Bone Healing

- Fractured callus more prominent and abundant commonly, seen in head injury
- This is thought to be mediated by an as yet unknown humoral factor

2.10.3.4 Ways to Prevent Secondary Brain Injury

- Prevent acute lowering of cerebral blood flow causing cerebral ischaemia by (aim CPP > 70):
  - Adequate fluid resuscitation – avoid systolic hypotension <SBP 90 mmHg

- Proper oxygenation – avoid $PaO_2 < 90\%$
- Hyperventilation
- Pharmacological means, e.g. mannitol
- Elevation of the head
- Close ICP monitoring

2.10.3.5 Pearls
- Prolonged operation can cause intraoperative hypotension, hypoxia and coagulopathy in combination with increased blood loss and fluid requirements during and after the orthopaedic surgery
- This will be detrimental to cerebral perfusion and will be an additional insult to the already injured brain (secondary brain injury) thus potentially outweighing the benefits of early fixation

2.10.3.6 Effects of Femoral IM Nailing
- Our main worry being increased pulmonary complications (e.g ARDS) or cerebral complications (e.g. fat emboli can be monitored by transcranial Doppler in the laboratory)

2.10.3.7 Proponents of IM Nailing in Severe Head Injury
- Some previous studies showed detrimental effects with >40-fold increase in pulmonary complications with *delayed* femoral fracture fixation (J Orthop Trauma 1998)
- Other studies did not, however, find detrimental effects of early fixation by reamed IM nailing affecting neurologic outcome (J Trauma 1997)

2.10.3.8 Opponents of Femoral IM Nailing in Severe Head Injury (J Orthop Trauma 1997)
- Some studies (with a small sample group) in the past concluded early fracture fixation may be "detrimental" in severe head injury – but only in terms of involving more crystalloid intraoperative resuscitation

*.10.3.9 Summary

- Early fixation of femoral shaft fractures by reamed nailing does not appear to affect neurological outcome based on recent literature
- There is some evidence that a delay may increase pulmonary complications
- Words of caution:
  - For patients in extremis, the above may not apply
  - Other forms of fixation (e.g. EF) may be considered if the patient has concomitant severe pulmonary injuries on admission to the trauma service

2.11   Limb Salvage Versus Amputation

2.11.1   General Priorities

- Save life then save the limb
- Standard ATLS protocol should be initiated to save life first

2.11.2   Assessment of a Severely Injured Limb (Figs. 2.1, 2.2)

- This should include:
  - Assessment of vascularity

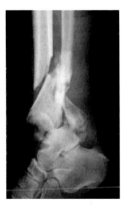

Fig. 2.1 The shattered skeletal elements of a mangled extremity after high energy trauma

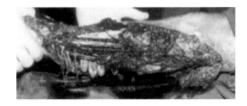

Fig. 2.2 It is often the soft tissue envelope that determines whether the limb is salvageable

- Capillary return
- Haemodynamic status
- Bony fracture patterns
- Skin and soft tissue losses
- If compound fracture, the Gustilo's class
- Any muscle crushing
- Assessment of sensibility
- Any compartment syndrome
- Documentation of nature and extent of open wound and degree of contamination

2.11.3   Other Relevant Investigations

- Bedside Doppler
- Ankle-brachial index
- X-ray to ascertain fracture pattern, and identification of associated injury
- Angiogram (in X-ray department or even intraoperatively) if indicated

2.12   Orthopaedic Emergencies Resulting from Soft Tissue Trauma

- Compartment syndrome
- Vascular injury (complete vs partial)
- Nerve injury

2.12.1   Pearl

- Many traumatologists view limb fractures as soft tissue injury to the limb in which the bone happens to break. This helps to highlight to us the importance of considering the soft tissue status in all fracture cases rather than concentrating on the X-ray

2.12.2   Classification of Soft Tissue Injury in Fracture Surgery

- Tscherne classification is most often used:
  - Grade 0: closed fracture, no soft tissue injury
  - Grade 1: indirect injury, superficial laceration
  - Grade 2: direct injury with significant blistering and oedema, impending compartment syndrome
  - Grade 3: extensive crushing and muscle damage. Vascular injury or compartment syndrome

2.12.3   Decision to Amputate Versus Limb Salvage in Severe Limb Injury

- The decision to adopt amputation vs limb salvage has to be made *early* on after the injury
- Preferably, the decision can be made at the time of admission. If not feasible, the decision should not be prolonged for >24–48 h
- Example: if the surgeon gives an EF to a non-salvageable limb; this will give a false sense of hope of salvage, and the patient may find it difficult to accept amputation later
- One should realise that *amputation is a proper and recognised form of reconstructive procedure*

2.12.4   Use of Scoring Systems

- Mangled extremity severity score (MESS)
- Mangled extremity severity index (MESI)
- Predictive salvage index (PSI)
- However, recent studies have not found these scoring systems to be a reliable indicator (Bonanni et al. 1993), such as the recent LEAP study conducted in the USA

2.12.5   Special Cases
- Traumatic amputation and replantation: the reader is referred to the companion volume to this book: *Orthopaedic Principles – A Resident's Guide*
- Open fracture management – refer to Chap. 5.

2.13   Soft Tissue Reconstruction

2.13.1   Ladder of Reconstruction
- Primary wound closure and healing by secondary intention
- Delayed primary closure
- Management of the marginal wound
- Skin grafting – split and full-thickness skin graft
- Local or regional flap
- Free flap

2.13.1.1   *Primary and Delayed Primary Closure*
- Should be the goal in clean uncomplicated wounds
- If unsure, especially in the face of high-energy trauma, it is better to wait since significant signs like fracture blisters will become apparent within days

2.13.1.1.1   *Timing of Closure*
- Contraindications for closure:
    - Too much tension
    - Actively infected

(In many other cases, the exact timing has to be individualised)

2.13.1.1.2   *Relative Contraindications for Early Wound Closure*
- Associated fracture blisters
- Associated degloving
- X-ray signs suggestive of very high-energy trauma, e.g. segmental fractures, very comminuted fractures

- Increased compartmental pressure that may turn into compartment syndrome
- Lack of time to observe the wound, especially in a patient with high energy trauma – true extent of the soft tissue injury does not reveal itself immediately, but takes time, e.g. 5–7 days

2.13.1.1.3 The Marginal Wound

- Can still consider closure with the help of adjunctive techniques (sometimes need input from plastic surgeon)
  - Pie-crusting
  - Z-plasty
  - Acute stretching
  - Undermining
  - Vacuum-assisted closure

2.13.1.1.4 General Pearls

- Whatever is done, try not to burn any bridges, e.g. if not sure whether a subsequent flap is required, do not sacrifice the local veins for fear of hindering the venous return. Also, some special flap types like the reverse flow flaps require adequate venous anastomosis
- Be proactive. Example: in planning an EF placement in, say, an open Type IIIB fractured tibia, do not place the Schanz pins in a manner that will hinder the plastic surgeon performing flap coverage for the leg

2.13.1.1.5 Other Pearls

- Wounds with important tissues immediately beneath: common examples include bone (especially devoid of periosteum) and tendon (especially devoid of paratenon) require coverage, usually by a flap
- Wounds with an avascular bed – these cases may also eventually need a flap
- If healing is expected to be problematic due to host factors, e.g. host with severe malnutrition (check serum albumen, transferrin, lymphocyte counts, etc.), adequate nutritional support should be given

2.13.1.2 Use of Skin Grafting

- Options: SSG (split skin grafting) and FTSG (full thickness skin grafting)
  - Both require an underlying vascular bed (e.g. covered by muscle in order to take
  - Avoid the use of SSG over joints

2.13.1.3 Local and Regional Flaps

- Refer to the appendix that follows for principles of flap coverage
- In general, local or regional flaps are preferable to free flaps. Free flaps are only used in special situations listed below

2.13.1.4 Free Flaps

- Should be avoided if soft tissue coverage can be achieved with local or regional flaps
- Most commonly used ones: groin flap, parascapular flaps, rectus abdominus flap
- Good indications include:
  - Wide zone of local injury increasing the risk of failure of local or regional flaps
  - Local soft tissue situation requires the use of a composite tissue not available locally, e.g. use of free vascularised bone grafting
  - Surgeon wants to use clean vascular non-infected tissue onto a recently debrided significantly infected bed

2.14   Appendix: Principles of Flap Coverage

2.14.1   Definition of a Flap

- Flaps are transplanted tissues with their own blood supply

2.14.2   Flap Surgery: Introduction

- The dermis of the skin is supplied by a rich network of subdermal vascular plexus (basis of random pattern flap)

- In addition, the skin receives blood from the following feeding vessels:
  - Directly: through a long course artery (i.e. basis of cutaneous flap) or through an interstitial artery such as the septal perforator artery (i.e. basis of fasciocutaneous flap)
  - Indirectly: through, e.g. muscle branches (i.e. basis for myocutaneous flap)

2.14.3 Classification of Flaps

- By utilisation: free, rotation, island
- By vascular pattern: random, pedicled/axial
- By tissue components: e.g. skin, fascia, muscle, bone, or composite

2.14.4 Commonly Used Flaps with Examples

2.14.4.1 *Random Pattern Flap*

- Refers to a local skin flap based on a random pattern. Blood supply from subdermal plexus
- Length:width ratio should not exceed 1:1 in this flap type

2.14.4.2 *Transposition/Rotation*

- Examples:
  - Z-plasty
  - Rotation flap
  - Limberg flap

2.14.4.3 *Based on True Axial Artery*

- Example: groin flap
- Based on true axial artery of skin, which perforates deep fascia and runs obliquely in subcutaneous plane

2.14.4.4 *Neurocutaneous Flap*

- Dissection studies showed that vessels that follow and supply nerves also send out small branches to supply the nearby skin

- Along their courses are also numerous anastomoses with deep vasculature
- Example: neurocutaneous sural flap

2.14.4.5 Fasciocutaneous Flap
- Usually an axial artery running in the space between two muscles in the limbs
- It sends out septal branches called perforators along its course to supply skin and sometimes muscles
- An example of the use of fasciocutaneous flaps is in the leg to cover soft tissue defects after an open fracture

2.14.4.6 Principles of Reverse Flow Flaps
- Unlike in the case of raising a cutaneous flap, in raising for instance a fasciocutaneous flap, provided that there exists anastomosis with a deep or parallel axis, the feeding vessel may receive a retrograde flow of blood if ligated proximally
- This is made possible by the various inter-connections between the veins so much so that despite the presence of valves in veins, retrograde flow is possible
- Example: retrograde radial forearm flap or Chinese flap

2.14.4.7 Muscle Flaps
- Vascular patterns found in muscles include:
  - Type 1: one vascular pedicle, e.g. gastrocnemius
  - Type 2: one dominant, many minor, e.g. gracilis
  - Type 3: two dominant, e.g. serratus anterior
  - Type 4: segmental, e.g. sartorius
  - Type 5: one dominant and secondary segmental, e.g. latissimus dorsi. Example of muscle flap: use of gastrocnemius flap to cover soft tissue defects of the knee

General Bibliography

.. American College of Surgeons Committee on Trauma (1999) Resources for the optimal care of the injured patient. American College of Surgeons, Chicago
?. Royal College of Surgeons of England/British Orthopaedic Association (2000) Working party report on better care for the severely injured. Royal College of Surgeons of England/British Orthopaedic Association, London
3. Masquelet AC, Gilbert A (1995) An atlas of flaps in limb reconstruction. Dunitz, London

Selected Bibliography of Journal Articles

1. American College of Surgeons Committee on Trauma (1986) Hospital and pre-hospital resources for optimal care of the injured patient; Appendix F: field categorization of trauma patients (field triage). Bull Am Coll Surg 71:17–21
2. Bonanni F, Rhodes M, Lucke JF (1993) The futility of predictive scoring of mangled lower extremities. J Trauma 34:99–104
3. Bone LB, Jojnson KD, et al. (1989) Early vs delayed stabilization of femoral fractures. J Bone Joint Surg Am 71(3):336–340
4. Bone LB, Babikian G, Stegemann PM (1995) Femoral canal reaming in the polytrauma patient with chest injury. A clinical perspective. Clin Orthop Relat Res 318:91–94
5. Fakhry SM, Rutledge R, Dahners LE, Kessler D (1994) Incidence, management, and outcome of femoral shaft fracture: a statewide population-based analysis of 2805 adult patients in a rural state. J Trauma 37:255–260
6. Marius K, Otmar T (2005) Pathophysiology of trauma. Injury 36:691–709
7. Odland MD, Gustilo RB, et al. (1990) Combined orthopaedic and vascular injury in the lower extremities: indications for amputation. Surgery 108:660–666
8. Pape HC, Auf'm'kolk M, et al. (1993) Primary intramedullary femur fixation in multiple trauma patients with associated lung contusion – a cause of post-traumatic ARDS? J Trauma 34(4):540–547
9. Pryor JP, Reilly PM (2004) Initial care of the patient with blunt polytrauma. Clin Orthop Relat Res 422:30–36
10. Regel G, Nerlich ML, et al. (1989) Induction of pulmonary injury by polymorphonuclear leukocytes after bone marrow fat injection and endotoxaemia: a sheep model. Theor Surg 4:22
11. Riska EB, Bonsdorff HV, et al. (1976) Prevention of fat embolism by early internal fixation of fractures in patients with multiple injuries. Injury 8:110–116

12. Riska EB, Bonsdorff HV, et al. (1977) Primary operative fixation of long bone frac
     tures in patients with multiple injuries. J Trauma 17(2):111–121
13. Scalea TM, Boswell SA, et al. (2000) External fixation as a bridge to intramedullary
     nailing for patients with multiple injuries with femur fractures: damage control ortho
     paedics. J Trauma 48(4):613–621
14. Sharma BR (2005) Triage in trauma-care system: a forensic view. J Clin Forensic Med
     12:64–73
15. West JG, Trunkey DD, Lim RC (1979) Systems of trauma care: a study of two coun
     ties. Arch Surg 114:455–460

Contents

3.1 The Basics

3.1.1 Normal Protective Mechanisms Against Trauma

- Importance of muscle contractions to counteract the load application to bone and offer a protective effect (fatigue fracture has a greater tendency to occur with muscle fatigue upon prolonged strenuous exercise)
- Ability of normal bone to remodel and repair its defects helps prevent fatigue fracture
- With aging, bones increase their area moment of inertia, distributing even more bone tissue in the periphery away from the central axis by increasing the diameter of the medullary cavity

3.1.2 Definition of a Fracture

- A fracture essentially involves a breach in the continuity of bone, whether on a macroscopic or microscopic scale

3.1.3 Normal Bone Healing

- As will be seen in the following discussion, natural bone healing involves a complex process whereby the body regenerates bone by replacement of the initial cartilage model

3.1.3.1 Stages of Bone Healing

- In the 1700s Hunter from Scotland came up with the concept that there were stages of fracture healing

3.1.3.1.1 Stage of Impact

- The first stage of healing is the impact stage. In fact, fracture healing response begins the moment the injury occurs. A certain amount of energy is impacted on the fracture

3.1.3.1.2 Stage of Induction

- The stage of induction follows the initial impact. Occurs after the fracture, but at first there are no radiological changes, although much activity is going on at the microscopic and molecular levels

Blood Flow Changes
- There is a reduction of blood flow for the first week or so, then at 1–4 weeks it increases several fold, and at 5–8 weeks it starts returning to normal. There is also a change in the way the body autoregulates the blood flow

What Is Happening at the Cellular and Molecular Level?
- There is a commonly asked question regarding the origin of cells that perform the important task of bone healing or regeneration
- There is a good chance that there are some blood-derived primitive cells, endothelial-capillary cells – maybe a real donor source for differentiation of these bone precursors

3.1.3.1.3 The Inflammatory Stage
- There is clinically increased swelling at the fracture site during this stage
- Investigation by ultrasound revealed that there is increased blood flow

3.1.3.1.4 The Stage of Soft Callus
- The inflammatory phase passes to a soft callus phase
- Clinically, some local bony swelling may be felt
- The area of action is called the periosteal reaction. The delta zone is between the areas of periosteal reaction. This delta zone is the area where the key activity is going on
- This cellular activity is the key to callus formation
- The cartilage model appears in this phase
- Notice that *the fracture site is the last place where union takes place.* Thus, do not expect to look at an X-ray and see callus at the fracture site. Bone healing is effected by the peripheral callus
- The new cortex is in the periphery. That ring of new peripheral bone is what gives fractures strength, offering enhanced stiffness to bending by increasing the local diameter of the bone
- The strength of a callus is much greater with a non-immobilised versus immobilised fracture (animal experiments)

3.1.3.1.5 Stage of the Hard Callus

- Next the callus becomes hard and at this stage protected weight-bearing is usually prescribed for the patient
- There is a chondro-osseous change in the osteogenic phase and regeneration. There is a *transformation* of cell types going on

3.1.3.1.6 Remodelling – Cortical Bone

- Cortical bone remodelling is quite complex. The osteoclasts have to drill a hole of about 200 µm in diameter (the typical size of a Haversian system) through the solid bone. Following behind them, there is a layer of osteoblasts with a capillary in the middle
- Osteoclastic cutting cone leaving a wake of osteoblasts, which deposit within the osteoclastic resorption cavity

3.1.3.1.7 Remodelling – Cancellous Bone

- Osteoclasts eat a hole at the surface of the trabeculum, pluripotential cells then follow
- They ultimately differentiate into osteoblasts, which lay down matrix around them

3.1.3.1.8 Nature of Remodelling

- The stiffness of the callus increases with time – sometimes even harder than the nearby bone!
- Another reason the bone gets stronger after it is healed is because there is an increase in the cross-sectional diameter
- It therefore involves a change in the moment of inertia, and the modulus of elasticity because there is formation of material external to the fracture site and there is a change in the cell types from collagen and fibrous tissue to bone respectively

3.1.3.2 Key Concept

- Bone healing is actually bone regeneration. This involves replacement of a damaged cell type with the same cell type as opposed to scarring (Brighton)
- Fracture healing with callus can thus be visualised as the formation of temporary organ of regeneration

■ Orthopaedists should therefore prevent deformity, but should not impair bone healing and avoid interference with this organ of regeneration as far as possible

3.1.3.3 Feature of the Fracture Callus
■ Scientists now believe that this regenerating organ is able to sense bone instability, and changes in cell differentiation can occur with different degree of stability
■ In normal indirect healing by external callus, there will be changes in modulus of elasticity by going through different cell types

3.1.3.4 Anatomy of the Fracture Callus
■ Dissection studies revealed that a multitude of small holes at the point of entrance and exit of the peripheral vessels that heal the fracture can be found in the external callus. This is absent in fractures that healed with rigid fixation
■ These small holes represent vertical vessels from the periphery entering the fracture site to form bone

3.1.4 Concepts of Direct or Indirect Bone Healing
3.1.4.1 Direct Healing
■ Described by Willenegger and Schenk
■ Featured by absence of radiological callus formation

3.1.4.2 Features of Indirect Bone Healing
■ To keep things simple, we can state that indirect bone healing occurs whenever the criteria for direct healing (such as absolute rigidity and interfragmentary compression) are not be being met. When this is the case, neither gap healing nor contact healing can occur (see below)
■ Micro-instability ± macro-instability induces bone resorption at the fracture site – this is one of the hallmarks of indirect bone healing. Periosteal new bone formation predominates as the main method of healing

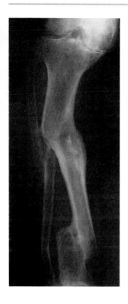

Fig. 3.1 Natural healing is strong, although often malaligned

3.1.4.3 Why Is Direct Bone Healing Not as Strong as Indirect Healing?

- Motion at the fracture site is probably the single most important factor in osteogenesis
- Healing by formation of natural callus (especially the strong callus formed if the fracture is not too rigidly immobilised) is found to be the strongest (Fig. 3.1) (P.S. We often see re-fractures after, say, direct healing by plating, partly due to the stress risers of screw holes, plate-related osteopenia, but also because of the absence of the strong periosteal natural callus)
- Internal fixation per se will not make fractures heal; it only helps with alignment and with the stability and restoration of nearby joints

3.1.4.4 Healing After Plating/IM Nail

- Plating and intramedullary nailing are techniques of fracture care
- It is important to remember that these techniques do not automatically imply, nor do they guarantee a particular type of fracture healing

- The type of bone healing (if any) that occurs (direct or indirect) will depend on the mechanical as well as the biological environment; and not necessarily on the implant used

3.1.4.4.1 Examples
- Indirect healing can occur after plating fractures with rigid fixation especially if the technique is not good enough so that micro-motion occurs
- Furthermore, it should be noted that indirect and direct bone healing can occur within different parts of the same fracture, e.g. when the near cortex is under compression, but the far cortex is not
- In such situations, some resorption of bone may be seen at that part of the fracture site that has micro-motion with a modest amount of new periosteal bone, showing that indirect bone healing is occurring

3.1.4.5 Healing After Properly Performed ORIF
- Properly performed open reduction and internal fixation (ORIF) using AO techniques results in direct bone healing without the formation of callus
- This type of healing is in fact a form of internal remodelling induced by necrosis because there is no mechanical induction of bone formation after attainment of absolute rigidity

3.1.4.5.1 Pre-requisite for This Type of Healing
The requirements for direct bone healing are:
- First, it requires an exact *anatomic reduction* of the fracture
- Secondly, it requires *absolute stability* – that is, no motion at the fracture site and compression of the fracture surfaces
- Finally, it requires existence of *sufficient blood supply* to provide for direct healing of the fracture – this is why stripping of vast amounts of periosteum may not lead to direct bone healing

3.1.4.5.2 Concomitant Contact and Gap Healing in Practice
- Direct bone healing has been segmented into gap healing and contact healing. In any fracture, even one anatomically reduced and compressed, at the microscopic level there are only small areas of

direct contact of the bone ends and large areas of gap. It has been demonstrated that contact areas and gap areas heal through slightly different mechanisms

Contact Healing

- Contact areas are relatively small, even in a compressed and anatomically reduced fracture, but they are very important in that the compression across them protects the gaps by absorbing the stress and preventing micro-motion
- Contact areas heal directly by Haversian remodelling

Gap Healing

- Gap healing will occur only if the gap size is less than or equal to 1 mm. Gaps larger than 1 mm cannot heal via direct bone healing and must heal through some other mechanism
- Gap healing also requires that there is no micro-motion at the site. This means that there must be compression across the contact areas, which then absorb stresses and prevent micro-motion; this can only be achieved with some sort of external device applied to the bone, most often a plate and screws

Stages of Gap Healing

- Gap healing occurs in three stages
- Stage 1: involves rapid filling of the gap with *woven* bone. The time line is usually within a couple of weeks of the fracture
- Stage 2: involves *Haversian remodelling* of the avascular areas right at the margins of the fractured bone ends. Microscopically may be able to see a cutting cone at the fracture's edge, where avascular bone is being remodelled
- Stage 3: involves *remodelling* of the woven bone to lamellar bone and occurs where Haversian systems are formed across the fracture gap and making it lamellar bone, which spans the gap

Clinical Correlation Based on Knowledge of Direct Bone Healing

- First, we must achieve an anatomic reduction of a fracture in order to expect direct healing, achieving gap areas less than 1 mm

- Secondly, we must provide interfragmentary compression across contact areas in order to achieve direct healing
- Thirdly, in order to prevent micro-motion at the fracture site, we must apply a plate with the appropriate number of screws for the bone we are stabilising
- Finally, we must preserve the vascularity of the bone for direct healing to occur

3.1.4.5.3 Summary of Fracture Healing After Plating

- Plating does not universally result in direct bone healing, because not all plating meets the specific requirements for direct bone healing (Figs. 3.2, 3.3)
- Direct bone healing occurs only when the mechanical and biological requirements that were discussed earlier are met
- Direct and indirect bone healing can occur in different parts of the same fracture if the mechanical and/or biological environments differ across a fracture

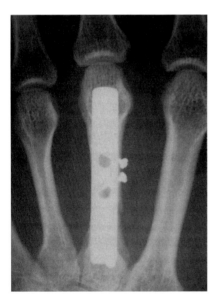

Fig. 3.2 This metacarpal fracture was initially treated with ORIF

- Plating is a technique to provide stability to fractures and will not guarantee a special type of fracture healing

3.1.4.5.4 Complications After Plating

- Interference with the peripheral (periosteal) blood supply can hinder vascularity and delay healing
- Direct bone healing is not as strong a form of healing as by natural external callus. Thus re-fractures are not uncommon after plate removal
- Plating has the effect of stress shielding and it is not uncommon to see decreased bone density in the region of the plated bone
- Sepsis
- Healing problems

3.1.4.5.5 Consequence of Altered Vascularity

- The relative lack of blood supply can induce a cascade of deleterious events within the adjacent living bone. This increases the chance of infection, sequester formation and non-union

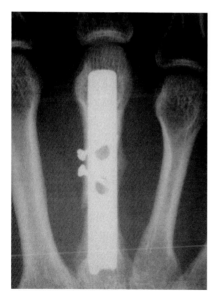

Fig. 3.3 Serial follow-up of the same metacarpal fracture revealed callus healing; there was probably residual micro-motion after the plating

3.1.4.5.6 What Happens in a Poorly Done ORIF?

- Excess soft tissue stripping hinders blood supply and will predispose to infection and union problems as just described
- Poorly internally fixed fractures will not go on to union
- If the near cortex is compressed and the far cortex is not, there will be resorption in the far cortex

3.1.4.6 Bone Healing After IM Nails

- Motion at the fracture site is probably the single most important factor in osteogenesis and this probably explains why fractures properly fixed by intramedullary (IM) nails heal by callus because intramedullary nails do not rigidly immobilise the fracture
- Further discussion on IM nails including the effects of reaming on vascularity will be made in the section on IM nailing in Chap. 4

3.1.4.7 Rationale of Functional Bracing

- Sarmiento taught us that in closed fractures, the initial shortening frequently remains unchanged – regardless of fracture treatment. The ultimate shortening is determined at the time of the initial insult
- Sarmiento found that the strength of the callus is greatest in oblique fractures (Fig. 3.4) that are not rigidly immobilised. The fracture that is rigidly immobilised develops the worst callus. This is another rationale for the early use of functional bracing, e.g. for fractured tibia

3.1.4.7.1 Sarmiento Findings

- In Sarmiento's studies, for axially unstable closed fractures of the tibia that had the potential to shorten, no attempt was made to regain original length if he thought the immediate post-injury shortening was acceptable
- After a week or so in a cast, the fractured limb was fitted with a brace, which permitted knee and ankle motion. The patient was asked to bear weight on the extremity according to symptoms
- This early weight-bearing is very important to stimulate osteogenesis. Measurements were repeated every week until all motion ceased with fracture healing

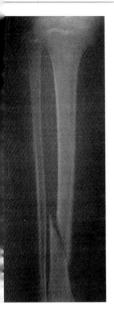

Fig. 3.4 A typical tibial shaft fracture pattern that was included in Sarmiento's famous study. Not every tibial shaft fracture needs a nail

- On closer look at the studies, there was as much as 5 mm of elastic motion in the above sub-group of patients when weight was first borne on the fractured extremity, thus the fracture was subjected to possible macro- instead of micro-motion

3.1.4.7.2 Indications for Sarmiento Bracing
- Sarmiento noticed that closed and low-grade open fractures experience ultimate shortening, usually at the time of the initial insult
- In Sarmiento's experience, the overwhelming majority of closed fractures of the tibia, particularly the axially unstable, i.e. the comminuted, the oblique and the spiral fractures, tended to align very well, in most instances by simple methods

3.1.4.7.3 Contraindications
- It is very difficult to control shortening in severe, open fractures. That is the reason why functional bracing does not have much of a place in the management of open fractures

- Fracture bracing is particularly indicated for closed, low energy fractures

3.1.4.7.4 Finer Points on Sarmiento's Techniques
- Weight-bearing should be regulated by symptoms
- After an initial period of long leg casting with the knee and ankle immobilised, early healing is permitted to begin
- The timing of functional brace fitting: when the acute symptoms subside, which occurs in most instances from 10 days up to 4 weeks
- If angulation increases, an attempt can be made to control it by returning to casting or opting for other methods of internal or external fixation

3.1.4.7.5 Sarmiento's Published Results
- Sarmiento's paper reported the results of over 1,000 fractures treated at the University of Southern California (USC)
- Treatment protocol: patients were treated with braces and graduated weight-bearing after a period of immobilisation in a long leg cast
- Exclusion criteria: patients who had severe and unacceptable initial shortening that required treatment by other methods

3.1.4.7.6 Are There Any Pitfalls?
- There are always worries that the tibial fractures may heal with shortening and malalignment, with possible sequelae such as ankle arthrosis
- However, the exact limits of acceptable varus/valgus alignment may be debated. Also, there is literature stating that a few degrees of angulation might not produce arthritis. According to Kristensen from Denmark, over 15 years, no patients with a tibial angulation of 10–15° sought treatment for arthrosis of the ankle (Acta Orthop Scand 1989). Similar reports were filed by Merchant and Dietz in J Pediatr Orthop

1.4.7.7 The Issue of Compartment Syndrome

- In Sarmiento's series, compartment syndrome was not a problem, partly because the high energy tibial fractures are not included
- Also, the fractures were not braced immediately, but mostly 2–3 weeks afterwards

1.4.7.8 Functional Results

- Ninety percent of the fractures healed with less than 6° of angulation. Of those 322 patients who had a residual varus (the most common deformity), 90% had less than 6° and 95% less than 8°. Such degrees of deformity are acceptable in the overwhelming majority of patients
- 99% of the fractures healed (a 1% non-union rate!)
- 95% of closed fractures in this series healed with less than 12 mm of shortening

3.2   Non-union and Delayed Union

3.2.1   Definition

- Although it is controversial, the most frequently used definition of a delayed union and non-union are if a fracture is not healed after 4 and 6 months respectively. The US Food and Drug Administration (FDA) criteria use 9 months for non-unions
- Pitfall – these cannot explain why a delayed union will heal after a certain time interval, and a non-union will never heal – because it may take many years to make this distinction, it is most practical to use the time criteria mentioned

3.2.2   Categories of Causes of Non-union

- Biological causes, e.g. impaired vascularity
- Mechanical causes, e.g. instability and gaps, over-distraction (Fig. 3.5)
- Infection
- General (miscellaneous) causes

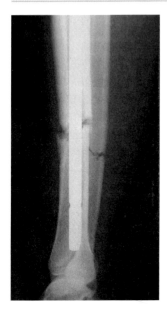

Fig. 3.5 Locked nailing in the presence of distraction may create a "non-union machine"

3.2.3   Classification of Non-union

- Hypertrophic non-unions – instability of fracture usually, but osteogenic response is intact
- Atrophic non-unions – insufficient osteogenic activity at fracture site – in advanced cases, bone ends resorption occurs and produces a pencil-like appearance, mostly due to impaired vascularity

3.2.4   Principles of Treatment

- Hypertrophic non-unions – to restore stability ± avoid heavy external loading, may need revision of a previous osteosynthesis
- Atrophic non-unions – to restore the osteogenic potential of the fracture, resection of fibrous tissue within the non-union gap sometimes needed, and bone grafting (usually autograft). (In both categories, one important key is to avoid nearby joint stiffness, especially in peri-articular non-unions; Fig. 3.6)

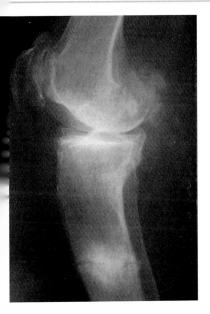

Fig. 3.6 The significance of avoiding nearby joint stiffness in peri-articular non-union is exemplified here. This seemingly benign proximal tibial fracture failed to heal, since motion mainly occurs in the fracture owing to the marked knee stiffness

3.2.5   Categories of Ways to Enhance Bone Healing

3.2.5.1 *Biological Means*

- Bone grafts: autografts (cortical/cancellous/cortico-cancellous), allografts (fresh, frozen, freeze-dried, demineralised bone matrix)
- Autologous bone marrow
- Bone substitutes, e.g. calcium phosphate ceramics
- Growth factors, e.g. bone morphogenetic proteins (BMP), beta-type transforming growth factor (TGF-β)
- Gene therapy, e.g. BMP-producing cells
- Others: composite biosynthetic grafts, and other systemic methodology (e.g. osteogenic growth peptide, progaglandin [PG], parathyroid hormone [PTH])

3.2.5.2 *Mechanical Means*

- Axial micro-movements, e.g. dynamisation (in EF/nails)

- Less rigid metal implants, e.g. titanium
- Revision osteosynthesis to improve stability, e.g. reamed IM nail after plating/EF in selected cases; exchange reamed nailing

3.2.5.3 Biophysical Methods

- Electricity, e.g. direct current, electromagnetic, capacitive coupling
- Ultrasound, e.g. low-intensity pulsed ultrasound

3.2.6　Some Details of the Causes of Non-union

3.2.6.1 Insufficient Vascularity

- Damage to the local vessels: periosteal (e.g. plating, soft tissue [ST] stripping in open fractures); intramedullary – as in reaming
- Pressure (e.g. relation between compartment syndrome and delayed union in tibial shaft fractures reported by Court-Brown

3.2.6.1.1 Prevention Is Important

- Many causes may partly be prevented (e.g. care in ST handling, use of unreamed nails, early detection and Rn of compartment syndrome)

3.2.6.2 Mechanical Causes

- Unstable fracture fixation – too much motion or instability as in some conservatively managed cases, other causes include poor fixation, etc.
- Too much or too premature external loading
- Absence of contact between fracture gaps (e.g. ST interposition, static fixation, but with distraction at fracture site)

3.2.6.3 Infection

- Source of bacteria can be from open fractures, or seeding during operation
- Some predisposing causes: long operation time, ST necrosis, necrotic bony fragments
- Sustained by, e.g. a primarily unstable osteosynthesis, or secondary instability through resorption of bone can sustain the infection

- The problem associated with glycocalyx production in the presence of any implanted device is important

3.2.6.4 Other Predisposing Factors

- General causes: e.g. fracture communition, malnutrition, drinking, smoking, diabetes mellitus (DM), peripheral vascular disease (PVD), poly-trauma, drugs like cytotoxics/steroids
- Pathology in bone itself, e.g. metastases, metabolic bone disease

3.2.7 Comments on Some Special Bone-Stimulating Methods
3.2.7.1 Bone Grafts

- Cancellous autograft remains the gold standard for Rn of bone defects – excellent incorporation into host bone, both osteo-conductive and osteo-inductive with BMPs, there are also cells with osteogenic activity
- Disadvantage: prolonged operation time, and morbidity of the donor site

3.2.7.2 Bone Marrow Injection

- Osteogenic mesenchymal stem cells present that are required for fracture healing
- Relatively simple procedure of harvest, then injection into the fracture site
- Relatively little donor site morbidity
- Cheap

3.2.7.2.1 Disadvantage of BM Injection

- The number of osteoprogenitor cells in fresh marrow is quite small – 0.001% of nucleated cells
- There have been efforts to expand and differentiate these mesenchymal cells in vitro (Clin Orthop Relat Res 1999)

3.2.7.3 Bone Substitutes

- A large number of these are available

- Most popular one among the calcium phosphate ceramics is hydroxyapatite
- Example: prospective randomised trial in bone defects in tibial plateau fractures reported by Bucholtz in CORR
- Note – the first generation of hydroxyapatite-based materials are not resorbable. Recent reports of resorbable calcium phosphate cements now available – shown in animal experiments to be resorbed by osteoclasts as part of the normal bone remodelling process

3.2.7.4 Bone Tissue Engineering
- A promising field full of potential
- Refers in the current setting to: use of growth factors and gene therapy

3.2.7.4.1 Growth Factors
- Definition: the application of growth factors to stimulate new bone formation in the treatment of skeletal injuries is also known as bone tissue engineering
- Two big categories of important growth factors: TGF-β super-family (which includes BMP) and others, e.g. fibroblast growth factors (FGFs)
- Recent reports of various successes obtained in animal models of bone defects, fractures and osteotomies (Boden 1999; Einhorn 1995)

3.2.7.4.2 Gene Therapy
- Gene therapy: this method involves the in vitro transfection of mesenchymal cells with the gene of an osteo-inductive factor (one of the BMPs) and subsequent implantation of these cells into a bone defect or fracture
- Due to transient production of the osteo-inductive factor by these cells, new bone formation occurs and bone healing is stimulated

3.2.7.5 Composite Grafts
- These composite grafts, as the name implies, consist of a carrier material combined with osteogenic cells and/or growth factors

- The "carrier" acts as an osteoconductive matrix and delivery vehicle for cells/growth factors
- Example: segmental bone defect model (Clin Orthop Relat Res 1995), while Chapman used a hydroxyapatite-based bone ceramic (1995)

3.2.7.6 Biophysical Methods

- Pulsed magnetic implanted direct current (DC) provides electrical stimulation. But contraindicated in those with pacemakers and sepsis
- To date, no conceivable explanation for the stimulating effect of electricity on bone repair
- However, the most recent studies seem to indicate that although the initial events in signal transduction were found to be different when capacitive coupling was compared with inductive coupling and with combined electromagnetic fields, the final pathway is the same for all three signals – that is, there is an increase in cytosolic calcium and an increase in activated cytoskeletal calmodulin (Brighton 2001)
- Eletromagnetic stimulation – externally applied coils that produce magnetic fields, which in turn induce bone formation. Non-invasive. The ultimate mechanism of bone stimulation may be similar to DC method
- Mechanism by pulsed ultrasound not known. The biophysical stimuli are probably translated into biochemical signals that modulate tissue regeneration and ossification. It may also have a stimulant effect on the osteoblast
- Low intensity pulsed ultrasound has been demonstrated to accelerate tibial fracture healing (Heckman 1994); but as yet not too many evidence-based reports as reviewed in a recent meta-analysis (Bause 2002), although there is some recent resurgence of interest in its use in treating non-unions (Leung 2004)

3.3   Infection in the Presence of an Implanted Device: General Guidelines (with Infection After Spine Surgery as an Example)

3.3.1   Incidence
- One study concerning infection after Texas Scottish Rite Hospital (TSRH) instrumentation treatment – 6%
- Hong Kong study on infection after TSRH treatment, 2% at 2 years
- But incidence much lower for short segment fusions – 0.2%, (possibly due to shorter operation time)

3.3.2   Mechanism
- Intraoperative seeding – often low virulence microbes
- Blood spread
- Fretting – micro-motion among the components of the implant (predisposing factors – DM, steroids, obesity, chronic sepsis history, smoker, prolonged hospitalisation, longer operation time, high blood loss [definition of high blood loss and long hours – >1,500 cc, >3 h])

3.3.3   Pathology
- Glycocalyx membrane surrounding the germs
- Some say these are mainly soft tissue and not bony infections
- Contribute factor sometimes from dead space (though Harrington rod with less dead space)
- Titanium is believed to have some inhibition on these low virulence organisms
- Can be associated with implant loosening and spine not being fused

3.3.4   Clinical Features
- Back pain
- Fluctuating mass
- Draining sinus

.3.5   Managing Late Infection After Surgery

- Removal of implant (especially if fused)
- Debridement – include glycocalyx
- Primary wound closure

.3.6   Use of Prophylactic Antibiotics

- Most use 2–3 doses for prevention
- Johns Hopkin's experience – an extra dose if long operation (> 4 h) or if more blood loss (> 2,000 cc)

3.3.7   Use of Antibiotics in Definitive Rn

- Six weeks, or until normal erythrocyte sedimentation rate (ESR)
- Can sometimes change to oral after initial intravenous therapy

3.3.8   Common Clinical Scenarios

- Infected open fracture with metallic implant remaining
- Infected total joint implants (discussed in the companion volume of this book). Refer to the works of Gristina
- Spine cases – infection after scoliosis surgery has just been discussed above, but the same principle can be extrapolated to spinal infection after spinal instrumentation for fractures

3.3.9   Conclusions from Studies at Case Western in Clin Orthop Relat Res (Animal Model)

- Establishing infected non-union is of course difficult, but in this study they inject bacteria in an animal (hamster) partial osteotomy model and found that:
    - Highest infection rate in inadequately fixed fractures that are malaligned
    - Poor fixation is worse than no metal – foreign body (FB) affecting host defence; and fracture motion causing more tissue damage
    - Presence of metal did not necessarily increase the infection rate; rigid fixation (not loose implant and properly fixed fractures) can further reduce the infection rate
    - Chance of infection also depends on the bacterial adherence and glycocalyx formation

— In cases of mixed growth: predominant Gram-positive infection
  – can increase the infection rate in the presence of Gram-nega-
  tive organisms, but the reverse seemed to have less effect

3.4   Septic Non-unions

3.4.1   General Principles

- Adequate and thorough debridement to viable and healthy bone.
  Soft tissues also need to be adequately debrided – remove non-viable
  muscles, debris, or scars in chronic cases
- Repeat debridement frequently necessary
- Soft tissue cover brought in early (preferably < 1 week if bed not contaminated, and flap needed). Notice that: muscle flaps preferable as
  help fight infection, better cover for tibia, and good base for later
  split-thickness skin graft (SSG), emergency soft tissue cover sometimes needed – e.g. if joint exposed, bare tendon
- Eliminate dead space and IV antibiotics
- Skeletal stabilisation always, EF useful if large wound since will aid
  in nursing care
- Later treatment of bone defects – vascular BG considered if bone
  defect >6 cm and bed not contaminated. Alternative is the Ilizarov
  procedure

3.4.2   Pearls

- Soft tissue healing very important or infection persists
- Pasteur: the bug is nothing, the environment is everything
- Especially in trauma open fracture wounds, frequently polymicro-
  bial

3.4.3   Cierny-Mader Classes
(Here Referring to Osteomyelitis of the Tibia)

- 1 = Medullary, e.g. IM nail, rule out nail and reaming
- 2 = Superficial, e.g. in presence of plate and screws, i.e. contagious
  focus

- 3 = Local, e.g. local full thickness dead bone, can be removed, but reassess stability
- 4 = Diffuse, e.g. needs intercalary resection and unstable situation
- Host A → normal, Host B divided into BL → local compromise, and BS → systemic compromised, BSL – unfavourable both local and systemic factors → if operating, may make host worse

3.4.4   Systemic Factors
- DM, nutrition, renal failure (RF), hypoxia, immunity, carcinoma (CA), extremes of age

3.4.5   Local Factors
- Lymph drainage affected, venous stasis, vascular insufficiency, arteritis, effect of radiotherapy, fibrosis, smoking, neuropathy

3.4.6   Diagnosis
- Clinical features: pain, swelling, drainage
- Cultures: blood, and bone. More often positive in acute cases
- X-ray: may see non-union, sometimes sclerosis, sometimes sequestrum, periosteum reaction
- Scan: e.g. gallium binds to transferrin; technetium (Tc) scan detects the increased blood flow
- CT: see sequester and areas of increased bone density
- MRI: assess the longitudinal extent of the lesion and soft tissue status

3.4.7   Treatment
- Surgical (adequate debridement, dead space treatment, soft tissue handling, fracture stability), vs amputation
- Antibiotics
- Nutrition
- Smoking should cease

3.4.8   Vascularised Bone Graft Results
- 70% only union if aetiology is infection

- 90% union for the other Dx
- Recent years more success with better wound Rn and local antibiotic beads, early flaps needed
- Vascularised bone grafts (VBG) mostly for >6 cm bone defect, an satisfactory non-contaminated soft tissues
- Three usual steps – debridement, soft tissue management, obliterat dead space, and bone stability → EF, BG after healing of ST
- Sometimes may see VBG hypertrophy – bone scan hot, but some times complicated by Fatique fracture
- Muscle flaps – decrease dead space, bed for SSG, ST cover, fight sep sis and increase chance of wound viability. Example: local flaps lik gastrocnemius flap; free flaps like gracilis, latissimus dorsi, rectu flap

3.4.9   Summary of Key Concepts
- Multiple adequate debridement to healthy bone and assess whethe limb is salvageable
- Maintain stability
- Find and eradicate the microbe – intravenous antibiotics and some times beads to fill dead space
- Soft tissue envelope – get cover early, e.g. as in compound tibial frac tures
- Later reconstruction, e.g. of bone defect.

3.5   Malunion (Fig. 3.7)

3.5.1   Why Tackle Malunions?
- Danger of loss of function, e.g. rotational malunion of digits hinder grasp
- Altered biomechanics/early arthrosis of joints – especially in weight-bearing lower limb (LL) joints
- Decreased motion, e.g. more likely in peri-articular locations of the malunion, the degree that the body can compensate depends on the mobility of the adjacent joint and on the exact plane of the deformity

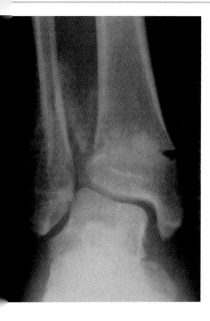

Fig. 3.7 Malunion is common in neglected fractures; it can have far reaching effects if the lower limb mechanical axis is affected

- Soft tissue imbalance, e.g. best illustrated in the hand – the place where function depends on a fine balance between the flexors and extensors
- Any accompanying shortening will also affect the function and mechanics of soft tissue such as tendons
- Cosmesis

3.5.2   Principal Ways to Tackle Malunions
3.5.2.1 Work-up
- Define the deformity:
    - Assess angulation in sagittal plane
    - Assess angulation in coronal plane
    - Assess rotational malalignment
    - Assess mechanical axis
    - Assess degree of shortening
    - Assess any translational deformity

— Assess articular surface
- Check status of nearby joint, which, if stiff, puts a lot of stress on the non-union site and can cause persistent non-union
- Check status of soft tissues
- Check the status of the bone – normal bone stock or pathologic bone

3.5.2.2 Principles of Management
- Pros and cons of tackling deformity right at the original site of mal-union – will be discussed
- Always assess the need for arthroscopic or open release if nearby joints stiffens up to regain function
- The rest will depend on which one of the three major methods we adopted to tackle the malunion; the discussion of which is outside the scope of this book (the three main methods include: the overlay method of Mast vs Paley's method based on finding the centre of rotation of angulation (CORA), vs computer-aided methods)

3.5.2.3 Correction at the Site of Deformity
- Can address complex/combined deformity (e.g. that of angulation, shortening and rotation)
- Correction at a distant level may sometimes create a zig-zag deformity, representing a compensation for the deformity
- But has to address the problem of possible associated joint stiffness if the deformity is peri-articular – this is because otherwise the osteotomy created for deformity correction will be under too much stress. The other reason is that joint release helps restore function

3.5.2.4 Correction Away from the Site of Deformity
- Technically sometimes easier
- Sometimes for a special reason. A typical example of situation after trauma is intra-articular malunion, especially if mature, after trauma (obviously, need to consider joint replacement or fusion in severe articular malunions with arthrosis). Another example in a situation not post-trauma is in correction of Blount's disease – deformity is

at the physeal line, but due to the presence of growth plate and patella tendon, the site of corrective osteotomy is placed distally to the CORA

3.5.3 Role and Use of Acute Corrections Versus Gradual Corrections

3.5.3.1 Advantages of Acute Corrections

- Correction completed upon completion of operation
- No need for postoperative adjustment

3.5.3.2 Order of Correction in Acute Corrections

- Correct rotation first, then correct angulation and translation

3.5.3.3 Disadvantages of Acute Corrections

- As little as 5° of acute correction in the direction that may pose risk to neurovascular bundle can create damage
- Sometimes damage to periosteum
- Complex deformity especially with translation less likely to be correctable by acute correction
- Intraoperative long film to assess alignment more difficult

3.5.3.4 Advantages of Gradual Corrections

- Capable of correcting complex multiplane deformities and correcting any shortening (e.g. by Ilizarov)
- Less chance of causing damage to neurovascular structures and periosteum
- Amount of corrections significantly larger than acute corrections
- Especially in the case of Ilizarov, since not a one-off procedure; can adjust our corrections postoperatively
- Newer frames run by computer software are now being developed with feasibility to effect simultaneous correction of deformity in all planes at the same attempt (Taylor spatial frame)

3.5.3.5 Order of Correction in Gradual Corrections

- If dome osteotomy is used, initially apply some distraction, before planar corrections including rotation

- If we do not plan to use dome-type osteotomy, plan the hinge that acts as rotation axis in, say, the Ilizarov method, such that there will be greater distraction on the side where angular corrections need to be applied

3.5.3.6 Disadvantages of Gradual Corrections

- Frequently more complicated, lengthy, labour-intensive procedures (e.g. circular frame-wearing for a few months)
- In children, may lead to psychological impact
- May cause nearby joint stiffness, even subluxation if concomitant lengthening procedures are undertaken

3.5.3.7 Commonly Used Fixators for Gradual Corrections

- Monolateral frames equipped with facilities for compression and distraction, e.g. Orthofix
- Circular fixators: of which the Ilizarov fixator is the most used (see section on principles of Ilizarov techniques in Chap. 4); equipped with capabilities for multiplane corrections and for lengthening

3.6   Appendix: Management of Bone Defects

3.6.1   Bone Defect Classification

- By Orthopaedic Trauma Association (OTA)

Type 1: involves <50% of diameter

Type 2: > 50% of diameter

Type 3: Complete loss involving a circumferential segment

(NB Gustilo's open fracture classification does not directly address the problem of bone loss)

3.6.1.1 Type 1

- The implant (nail/EF) not unduly stressed because of shared loading
- Soft tissue allowed to heal and autograft done in 4–6 weeks

3.6.1.2 Type 2

- Ensure adequate circulation and assess need for vascular repair; some require fasciotomies
- BG at around 6 weeks usually if good quality soft tissue cover present
- Occasionally, acute shortening used to convert the fracture line to a more stable configuration with better vascularised bone ends (De Bastiani)

3.6.1.3 Type 3

- There are many Rn options for these massive bone defects, which will now be discussed

3.6.2   Method 1: Massive Autograft

- Considered if defect <6 cm (refer to the 6-cm rule according to Harmon (J Bone Joint Surg Am 1965))
- Papineau technique – place cancellous autograft on the anterior surface of the tibia through original wound
  - Must adequately debride the wound, allow complete cover by granulation tissue by keeping wound moist through repeated normal saline (NS) irrigation
  - A second layer of graft is then inserted and procedure repeated until the bone defect completely filled and bony union achieved
  - The skin is then allowed to heal by secondary intention
- Posterolateral grafting of the tibia
  - Reason: anteromedial site of the tibia is usually injured and prone to sepsis. Thus, select site at the posterior compartment of the leg – care in dissection never to enter the anterior compartment as it may be infected. The periosteum of the posterior tibia is elevated 5 cm on each side of the fracture; the bone surface decorticated and graft placed in situ. Deep fascia left open and suction drain
- Marrow injection – Conolly (1991), discussed above
- Percutaneous introduction – only for filling a small defect/the graft is in paste form, and injected into the defect (Ebraheim 1991)
- Christian's method to fill space with gentamicin beads and pack with graft later

- Chapman's method – tackling the femoral defect with IM nail and push BG down using a plastic tube as a guide

3.6.3   Method 2: Muscle Pedicle Graft
- One option for defects > 6 cm
- Here the bone retains intact muscle attachment and therefore its blood supply
- In the tibia, this method can be used if mid-segment of fibula intact
- Preoperative angiogram to show the patency and anatomy of the tibial and peroneal vessels that can be damaged
- With an intact peroneal and anterior tibial muscle attachment, the vascular supply to the fibula is from the nutrient vessel and from rich network of musculoperiosteal vessels
- Disadvantage: lose fibula contribution of mechanical stability; needs added stabilisation procedure, loss of fibula also make the creation of a tibio-fibular synostosis for salvage impossible

3.6.4   Method 3: Vascularised Pedicled Graft
- An important example is in the proximal femur by rotating a pedicled vascular iliac crest graft
- Unlike muscle pedicle graft with short rotation arc, some of these vascular pedicled grafts have long pedicle – e.g. iliac crest graft based on the deep circumflex iliac vessels
- Advantage of the iliac crest graft: combination of both cortical and cancellous bone – provides both enhancement of graft incorporation and mechanical strength. Can also be used as a composite graft to provide both ST and skin coverage
- Note: the length of the iliac crest graft can be half that of the crest since the deep circumflex reaches the mid-point of the crest before anastomosing with the iliolumbar and superior gluteal arteries
- One other example of such a graft: use of distal radius in forearm reconstruction using pedicles of the radial/ulna arteries

3.6.5   Method 4: Free Vascularised Bone Graft
- Advantages include:
  - Survival not dependent on an excellent recipient bed

- Retain blood supply and still viable cells
- Adaptive hypertrophy frequently seen
- Better able to withstand infection
- Can also be used as composite especially in IIIB/C open fractures. Sites: iliac crest, fibula, rib, scapula lateral border, distal radius

3.6.5.1 Example 1: Free Vascularised Iliac Crest

- Up to 15 cm can be harvested
- Advantages: much cancellous bone (c.f. fibula) better incorporation, larger cross-section means better for juxta-articular region; larger diameter vessels higher success rate. Not much donor site morbidity
- Disadvantages: has curvature, not for defects > 15 cm
- Technique: origin of the deep circumflex identified when branch from the external iliac artery just proximal to the inguinal ligament – landmark is the origin of the inferior epigastric vessels on the lateral side of the external iliac artery. The deep circumflex followed to anterior superior iliac spine (ASIS) where it penetrates the transversalis fascia (if used as composite, avoid kinking of musculocutaneous perforators)

3.6.5.1.1 Vascularised Iliac Crest

- In avascular necrosis (AVN) hip
- In tumour/bone defect reconstruction – mainly proximal humerus, sometimes distal radius
- Features:
  - Advantage: besides cortical, cancellous part may increase viability
  - Open trough helps drain the haematoma
  - Long-term results comparable to Urbaniak's vascular fibula grafting
  - No microscopic anastomosis, since has pedicle attached
- Results: 1/3 long lasting, 1/3 slow collapse seen, 1/3 early failure

3.6.5.2 Example 2: Free Vascularised Fibula

- Advantage: long (up to 20 cm), excellent mechanical strength; can use as composite with soleus and skin

- Disadvantage: donor site morbidity and sometimes loss of moto power and even knee laxity, not quite cancellous
- Technique: based on the peroneal artery, which gives the fibular ar tery as the nutrient. Preserve the periosteal branch arising from the muscle branch of the peroneal – take a cuff of nearby muscle. Ente between the peroneus longus and soleus. Peroneal artery seen as i enters the superomedial side of flexor hallucis longus (FHL) – tracee to its origin from the posterior tibial. Incise interosseus membrane (IOM), leaving the tibial nerve intact
- Always take care to include the foramen of the nutrient artery – located 18–22 cm from proximal end of fibula
- Osteotomise fibula anterolaterally distal to the nutrient artery

3.6.5.3 Others: Rib and Distal Radius
- Rib: two sources – anterior/posterior intercostal arteries – not too good since small diameter and curved
- Distal radius: based on the radial artery

3.6.5.4 Miscellaneous Choices
- Allografts: more often used in tumour or limb salvage surgery, revision joint surgery. Seldom used in open fractures since worries of delayed union and sepsis, although may be considered in those cases with articular involvement. Should be avoided in an infected or poorly vascular recipient bed as allograft is essentially a piece of dead bone. Use of intercalary allograft with IM device has been described
- Bone substitute, e.g. use of hydroxyapatite chambers reported by Weiland

3.6.6   Method 5: Bone Transport
- Definition: a form of bone regeneration under tension stresses pioneered by Ilizarov
- Original idea: corticotomy to preserve endosteal circulation, minimise soft tissue trauma
- De Bastiani later showed that corticotomy is not always needed – more important is delay in distraction after the osteotomy of nor-

mally 7 days – possibly because needs time to re-establish the local blood supply and soft tissue repair, ± osteoblast do not respond to mechanical stimulation in the early post-osteotomy period

- Metaphysis as site of osteotomy usually since more osteoblasts
- Ilizarov recommended 1 mm/day in four increments, as he showed that many small increments results in better new bone formed than a small number of large increments
- Osteotomy, is followed by the distraction phase – here, formation of bone is by intramembranous ossification only if the construct has adequate stability
- This technique of callotasis/distraction osteogenesis allows simultaneous restoration of bone defect and correcting of LLD
- The final phase is docking – but there are many problems here, e.g. delayed union – which may require BG
- Other Cx during distraction: nearby joint subluxation and/or dislocations, neurovascular injuries, etc.

3.6.6.1 Main Types of Bone Transport

- Type 1: external method – bone segment transfixation with K wires, segment transported by movement of the rings. Advantage: simple construct, allows simultaneous limb length and deformity correction
- Type 2: internal method – the transfixing K wires introduced obliquely, transported to the desired position by distraction devices fixed to an immovable ring. Good for cases with no shortening and deformity. Disadvantage is the complex construct. Need to change the construct after transport is completed since compression forces generated by wires not enough
- Type 3: transport over an IM nail (Brunner 1990) reported
- Can transport at one (monofocal) or both sites at same time (bifocal)
- De Bastiani uses monolateral frame with success in more straightforward cases. Disadvantage: more pain (larger half pins), and more scarring. Also, the sliding component for dynamisation may not be effective due to eccentric positioning and binding of the frames

under axial loading (Paley 1990). Overall, monolateral frames are good for humerus and femur; while circular ones better if poor bone quality, in tibia/lower femur (use of hybrid frames has also been reported)

3.7   Appendix: Bone Graft Materials and Substitutes

3.7.1   Basic Terminology
- Osteogenicity/osteoprogenitor cells: substance containing living cells that are capable of differentiation into bone
- Osteoconduction: promotion of bone opposition to its surface, functioning in part as a receptive scaffold to facilitate enhanced bone formation
- Osteo-induction: provision of a biologic stimulus that induces local or transplanted cells to enter a pathway of differentiation leading to mature osteoblasts

3.7.2   What Is a Bone Graft Material?
- Definition: any implanted material that, alone or in combination with other materials, promotes a bone healing response by providing osteogenic, osteoconductive, or osteo-inductive activity to a local site

3.7.3   Main Classes of Bone Graft Materials
- Autograft
- Allograft
- Synthetic materials
    - Osteoconductive blocks or granules, cement
    - Osteo-inductive proteins, e.g. BMP
    - Composites

3.7.4   Historical Note
- Bone is one of the first types of tissue to be transplanted in the history of medicine
- First autograft – done in Germany in 1820

- First allograft – done in Scotland in 1881 by Macewen using the proximal humerus

3.7.5   Why Is There Increasing Demand for Bone Graft Materials?

- Reason for the recent high demand for allografts: more limb salvage surgery done, total joint especially revision total joint surgery, including periprosthetic fractures, management of massive bone defects, etc. But allografts have many disadvantages as we will discuss shortly
- Autografts are usually limited in availability, and massive harvest will cause significant donor morbidity and poor patient satisfaction
- So, is the booming market of synthetic graft materials the answer?

3.7.6   Why the Boom in Bone Graft Substitutes (Fig. 3.8)?

- This is because of:
  - Disadvantages of autografts
  - Disadvantages of allografts

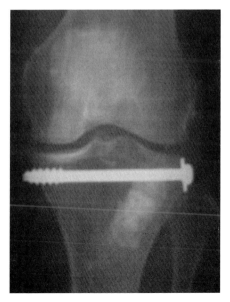

Fig. 3.8 This osteoporotic fracture of the tibial plateau was treated by bone graft substitute as well as screwing

3.7.7   Disadvantages of Allografts

- Rarely osteo-inductive except if we use demineralised bone matrix (DBM), since retains some BMP
- Fracture, especially easy during the process of creeping substitution. Also depends on the method of preservation. Need to avoid drilling and screwing of allografts to prevent fractures
- Non-union – hence sometimes we add autografts onto the junction between allograft and host bone
- Difficult to assess union
- Infection, e.g. bacterial and viral
- Size mismatch in cases in which we need to use massive allografts

3.7.8   Disadvantages of Autografts

- Limited availability
- Postoperative donor site morbidity
- Infection, haemorrhage, nerve damage, fracture, hernia, acute/chronic pain
- Increased operative time
- Operative blood loss

3.7.9   What Constitutes an Ideal Synthetic Graft Material?

- Biocompatible
- Minimal fibrotic reaction
- Can undergo remodelling
- Supports new bone formation
- Mechanical strength similar to cortical or cancellous bone
- Comparable modulus of elasticity to normal bone

3.7.10   Incorporation of Synthetics

- Depends on the type of agent we are using
- Most are osteoconductive, or have an osteoconductive carrier
- Most do not provoke clinically significant inflammatory response
- There are some concerns that wear debris may lead to bone resorption
- As well as extracellular mineral precipitation with crystal growth
- Bone usually forms by osteoblast-mediated bone formation

3.7.11 Remodelling of Synthetics

- Depends on whether there is successful incorporation or not
- Local mechanical loads may modulate the process
- Remodelling if present after incorporation may influence positively long-term graft integrity
- However, the mechanism and determining factors for incorporation of synthetics not completely understood

3.7.12 Common Types of Bone Graft Substitutes

- Allograft-based BG substitutes
- Cellular-based BG substitutes
- Factor-based BG substitutes
- Ceramic-based BG substitutes
- Polymer-based BG substitutes

3.7.12.1 Based on Allografts

- A prominent example is DBM
- Many models use bone chips contained herein as a mineral scaffold
- Available in the market in sheets, gel-like or putty like material; suiting the needs of individual patients

3.7.12.2 Based on Cells

- Most frequently used ones on the market employ the human mesenchymal stem cells

3.7.12.3 Based on Growth Factors

- Becoming popular include BMP-7 (OP 1 or Osteogenic Protein 1); BMP-2, etc.
- Other factors used include, e.g. TGF-beta, FGF, and the possibly promising osteogenic as well as regulatory effects of the Indian Hedgehog molecule

3.7.12.4 Based on Ceramics

- Ceramics sometimes used
- Some are calcium-ceramic based
- Bioglass-based

- Have osteoconductive action, and give mechanical support. Porosity similar to trabecular bone
- Bioglass acts by promotion of hydroxyapatite formation and cellular attachment
- Example: resorbable hydroxyapatite converted from corals; some brands mix this material with autogenous marrow

3.7.12.5 Based on Polymer
- Osteoconductive
- Example: injectable non-absorbable resins
- Can provide some mechanical support

3.7.12.6 Future
- We envisage the much awaited use of gene therapy in future clinical practice
- Gene therapy when applied to bone formation involves molecular control of bone formation by transfection of autologous cells in culture resulting in the secretion of substances like BMP to stimulate the osteoblast
- Local delivery methodology includes the ex vivo method as mentioned, can also be delivered in vivo by directly injecting transformed cells

General Bibliography

1. Bulkwalter J, Einhorn T, Simon S (2000) Orthopaedic basic science, 2nd edn. American Academy of Orthopaedic Surgeons

Selected Bibliography of Journal Articles

1. Boden SD (2000) Biology of lumbar spine fusion and use of bone graft substitutes: present, future, and next generation. Tissue Eng 6(4):383–399

2. Boden SD, Titus L, et al. (1998) The 1998 Volvo Award in Basic Science: lumbar spine fusion by local gene therapy with a cDNA encoding a novel osteoinductive protein. Spine 23(23):2486–2492

3. Keating JF, Robinson CM, et al. (2005) The management of fractures with bone loss. J Bone Joint Surg Br 87(2):142–150

4. Martin GJ Jr, Boden SD, et al. (1998) New formulations of demineralized bone matrix as a more effective graft alternative in experimental posterolateral lumbar spine arthrodesis. Spine 24:637–645

5. Mont MA, Jones LC, et al. (2001) Strut autografting with and without osteogenic protein. I. A preliminary study of a canine femoral head defect model. J Bone Joint Surg Am 83(7):1013–1022

6. Viggeswarapu M, Boden SD, et al. (2001) Adenoviral delivery of LIM mineralization protein-1 induces new bone formation in vivo and in vitro. J Bone Joint Surg Am 83:364–376

Contents

4.1   Fracture Fixation Principles: New and Old

4.1.1   Traditional AO Principles

- Anatomical reduction of the fracture fragments
- Preservation of blood supply
- Stable internal fixation
- Early active mobilisation

4.1.2   Determinants of Stability of Fixation in Fractures Fixed by the Traditional AO Method

- Local compressive preload
- Production of friction between the fragment ends
- Friction between fracture fragment ends will be improved by form fit between adjacent fracture surfaces

4.1.3   But Does Reduction Need to Be Anatomical?

- Yes, in the case of intra-articular fracture
- No, in many other situations, e.g. experience with locked nailing imprecise reduction of intermediate fracture fragments is well tolerated and compatible with healing by callus formation

4.1.4   Relevance of the Strain Theory in Fracture Healing

- To recapitulate, the strain theory as proposed by Perren – explains why impaired healing can occur in the presence of only an almost invisible gap; while fracture fragments subjected to relatively large displacements can result in good callus formation – this is because granulation tissue can tolerate 100% strain – it also explains why healing can occur in comminuted fractures, say, those treated by a neutralisation plate as the strain is now shared by the multiple fracture fragments

4.1.5   Indirect Reduction Principle
4.1.5.1   Introduction

- Mastery of the techniques and methods of indirect reduction is essential in treating many meta-diaphyseal fractures, especially by the popular minimally invasive technique, e.g. MIPO (minimal invasive plate osteosynthesis)

■ The book by Dr J. Mast published by Springer-Verlag is highly recommended in order to master techniques of indirect reduction

4.1.5.2 The Technique of Indirect Reduction

■ The indirect technique advocated by Mast uses long plates or the distractor as reduction tools, and minimises handling of soft tissues, hence fewer complications

■ The indirect technique emphasises a limited number of screws through the plate. Clinically, long plates with widely spaced screws have been shown to provide sufficient stability for fracture healing for meta-diaphyses. In addition, laboratory cantilever testing also reveals increasing strength for fixations with more widely spaced screws

4.1.5.3 Modalities That Can Be Used to Attain Indirect Reduction

■ Manual traction

■ Distraction device, such as the femoral distractor

■ Sometimes the implant itself can be used as a reduction aid, e.g. angled blade plate (discussed below)

■ The large fragment articulating tension device that can aid in distraction or compression of the fracture site

4.1.5.4 Traditionally Useful Implant: the Angled Blade Plate

■ The traditional use of the fixed angled blade technique is time-honoured (Fig. 4.1) and has proven efficacy, especially in good bone

■ The disadvantage is that it is not a very forgiving implant and there is frequent loss of fixation in osteoporotic bone

■ However, the traditional angled blade plate is still sometimes very useful in salvage surgery (e.g. salvage of failed DCS, Rn of nonunions)

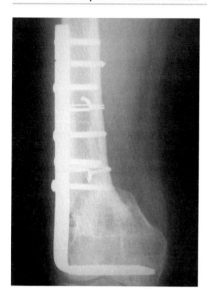

Fig. 4.1 The traditional blade plate is still useful in revisions and salvage surgery, especially for periarticular fractures

4.1.5.5 Use of Newer Implants (e.g. LISS)

■ The LISS (less invasive stabilisation system) plate, when you come to think of it, is based on similar reasoning to the angled blade plate (fixed angle device)

■ However, it is easier to use, especially in osteoporotic fractures, and in multi-fragmentary fractures

■ The LISS plate will be discussed in detail in the Sect. 4.3.2.5.4

4.2   General Stages of Development of Orthopaedic Implants

■ Awareness and definition of problems concerning standard treatment modalities

■ Idea, design and construction of a prototype, prototype testing, terminating in creation of a mature technical device

■ Continuous evaluation of the new technology

- Clinical evaluation
- Surveillance after the product is marketed
- Stage of maturity, which can be followed by further improvements and even more newly refined technology

4.3   Discussion of Traditional and New Implants

4.3.1   Screws

4.3.1.1 Definition of a Screw

- A screw is a device that converts a small applied torque into a large internal tension along the screw axis thereby enabling compression between two surfaces being held together (usually involving two fracture surfaces)

4.3.1.2 Components of a Screw

- Screw head
- Shaft
- Thread portion
- The screw tip

4.3.1.3 Design of the Different Components of a Screw

4.3.1.3.1 Screw Head

- Function: place where external torque is applied, acts to prevent the translational motion of the advancing screw, and effects compression of the fracture surfaces via the tension in the screw
- Most common design is the recessed hexagonal head, making it less likely for the screwdriver to slip. Other designs include Philips head and cruciate designs
- Most screw heads have a hemispherical under-surface that allows placement at different angles onto a plate, those with a conical under-surface need be aligned perpendicular to the screw hole in the plate
- A washer may be used just underneath the screw head to prevent subsidence of the screw head during compression in osteoporotic bones

4.3.1.3.2 Screw Shaft

- This is the region linking the screw head and the threads
- Its length is variable, e.g. it is longer in partially threaded cancellou screws
- The area between the shaft and the threads is a region of stress con centration and easier to break

4.3.1.3.3 Screw Threads

- Terminology regarding screw threads:
  - Pitch: means the distance between threads
  - Lead: means distance travelled by one full turn
  - Outer diameter: important factor determining pull-out strength represents the thread diameter
  - Core diameter: the diameter at the base of the threads; important factor determining the tensile and torsional strength of the screw

4.3.1.3.4 Screw Tip

- Commonly used screw tips and their uses:
  - Trocar tip – used in Schanz screws and in malleolar screws
  - Corkscrew tip – used in cancellous screws in which the tip helps clear the drilled pilot hole
  - Self-tapping tip – equipped with a flute that helps to cut threads and at the same time aid in removal of the bone chips. A screw that cuts its own thread helps ensure a tighter fit to the bone
  - Non-self-tapping tip – the tip here is round, and requires a special instrument (the tap) to cut the threads before insertion

4.3.1.4 Basic Types of Screw

- Cortical screws (Fig. 4.2)
- Cancellous screws (Fig. 4.3)

4.3.1.5 Summary of the Differences Between Cortical and Cancellous Screws

- Threads: cancellous > cortical

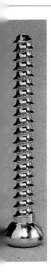

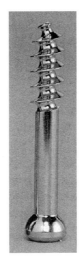

Fig. 4.2 The appearance of a cortical screw

Fig. 4.3 A partially threaded cancellous screw

- Pitch: cancellous > cortical
- Nature: cancellous is a modified wood-type screw, cortical is a machine-type screw
- Tap: no need for cancellous screws

4.3.1.6 What Is a Wood-type Screw

- A wood-type screw has large threads and when inserted into a small predrilled hole produces its own threads by compressing the softer material nearby (i.e., wood)
- The screw is much stiffer than the wood, and on insertion, it is the wood that deforms
- A cancellous screw is a wood-type screw since it cuts its threads in the soft cancellous bone

4.3.1.7 What Is a Machine-type Screw

- A machine-type screw has small threads packed closely together and needs tapping before insertion

- Unlike the wood-type screw, it is the machine-type screw that plastically deforms rather than the metal on insertion
- The design of the cortical screw takes after the machine-type screw Unlike the situation of the machine-type screw the cortical screw is stiffer than bone and deformation is at the bone and not the screw

4.3.1.8 Cannulated Screws

- This involves the insertion of a screw over a pre-positioned guide pin with over-drilling
- Clinical use: cannulated screws are used if very precise application is needed in regions where there is a small safety margin. A typical example is the use of cannulated screws in fixing fractures of the sacrum or fixing the sacroiliac joint
- Because of the larger root diameter, it has less holding power than non-cannulated screws of comparable calibre

4.3.1.9 Pull-out Strength of a Screw

- The pull-out strength of a given screw can be increased by the following factors:
  - Number of threads engaging the cortex (hence bicortical purchase has a stronger hold than unicortical purchase)
  - Thread type and profile: hence, the larger threads of the cancellous screw have a better hold
  - Bone quality: screws inserted into osteoporotic bones have a poorer hold
  - Bone–screw interface: this is the rationale of the use of hydroxyapatite-coated Schanz screws
  - Others: such as damage to the threads cut, poor technique, e.g. over-tightening of screws, measuring the screw track after tapping instead of before tapping

4.3.1.10 Clinical Applications of Screws

- As a lag screw: to effect inter-fragmentary compression, the cornerstone of the basic time-honoured AO principle
- As a positioning screw, e.g. fixing the plate to the bone

■ As a form of buttress: as in the "raft of screws" technique in tibial plateau fractures

4.3.1.11 The Screws in a Conventional Plate–Screw Construct

■ The conventional plate–screw construct functions by pressing the plate to the bone surface and creating friction at the bone–plate interface

■ In the screws of this plate–screw construct, the force along the long axis of the screw is several hundred kilograms and much higher than, say, that of the Schanz pins of the EF

4.3.2 Bone Plates

4.3.2.1 Function of Plates

■ Hold fracture ends and maintain proper fracture alignment
■ Transmit forces from one end of the bone to the other, protecting and bypassing the fracture area

4.3.2.2 Common Types of Plates

■ Neutralisation plating
■ Buttress plating
■ Compression plating
■ Tension band plating
■ Condylar plates

4.3.2.2.1 Neutralisation

Principle of Neutralisation

■ Systems of neutralisation are applied for purposes of stress shielding and minimisation of torsional bending, shearing and axial loading forces

Neutralisation Plate

■ Acts as bridge, as a mechanical link, bypassing the fracture
■ No compression
■ Can be used with lag screw(s), thus protecting from torsion, bending and shearing forces

Examples of Application of Neutralisation Principle
- Clinical application: segmental fracture, long bone with some comminution, short oblique fracture
- In the spine, examples include use of plates or rods inserted for protection of neural structures. Both anterior and posterior instrumentation are available

4.3.2.2.2 Buttress Plates
- Main aim is to prevent fracture from collapsing
- Designed to prevent axial deformity. Forces that cause axial deformity can be directly related to axial loading or may be secondary to bending or shear forces
- Buttress plates function to minimise compression and shear forces, and also act to minimise torque

Buttress Plating for Long Bone Fractures
- Main aim is to prevent the fracture from collapsing
- A correctly applied plate will apply a force that is perpendicular to the buttress plate
- Mostly for fractures at the metaphysis of the long bone, where the cancellous bone require support or buttress action besides prevention of collapse (or loss of length)
- In order to work, the plate should extend from the diaphysis to the metaphysis; and the large surface area of coverage is essential to enable a wide load distribution. It is essential that the plate be contoured to tightly fit the part of the bone to be buttressed in order to work
- Clinical application, e.g. tibial plateau fracture
- Careful contouring of the implant and preparation of the bony surfaces are essential in order to maximise contact surface area

Buttress Plating: Sequence of Screw Placement
- Screw insertion is begun closest to the area of potential motion (e.g. in the case of tibial plateau fractures, the area of potential motion is the fracture site)

- The remainder screws are placed in an orderly fashion towards the ends of the plate

Buttress Plating in the Axial Skeleton
- Example: anterior cervical locking plate system
- Example: anterior thoracolumbar locking plate system

4.3.2.2.3 Compression Plate

- Given the right fracture pattern, has an edge over the neutralisation plate by generating an axial compression force between fracture fragments
- Mechanism of compression depends on plate design, e.g. by means of "dynamic compression unit" in DCP (dynamic compression plates), or with the help of a tensioning device. Compression is effected at the fracture site, as a reaction to tension applied to the plate. A third mechanism used is the use of the method of eccentric screw placement

Dynamic Compression Unit
- In a self compression plate, the force applied as the turning torque of the screw head is transformed into a longitudinal force that will compress the bone ends
- Upon magnification of the unit, one sees that the screw hole resembles two half-cylinders placed at an angle. Upon screw insertion by twisting, the slope of the screw hole causes the plate to move at right angles to the direction of the descending screw

Static Versus Dynamic Compression
- A central time-honoured AO concept is absolute rigidity via interfragmentary compression
- Most of this basic principle is applied to static compression of the fracture (e.g. intra-articular fractures) that need anatomic reduction and absolute static rigidity
- However, there are situations, e.g. in eccentrically loaded bones like olecranon and patella fractures in which the AO teachings of tension

band principles is based on the use of dynamic compression of the fracture (see the Sect. 4.4 on tension band principles)

4.3.2.2.4 Use of Plates as Tension Bands

- Again, we refer to the application of plates to eccentrically loaded bones, e.g. the femur, the humerus, or the shaft of the radius and the ulna
- It is essential to apply the plate to the tension side when the forces are large as in the femur
- If the forces are not large, one does not always have to use the plate on the tension side and you may find in some areas that it is more convenient to use another approach only because the plate will lie there better or because of the nature of the fracture. Example: both volar and dorsal plating of the distal radius are well described

4.3.2.2.5 Condylar Plate

- Has both neutralisation and buttress function
- Typical clinical application is in fixing distal femoral fractures: where it is usually used in conjunction with lag screws that fix the intra-articular fracture fragments, and the plate helps to neutralise the deforming forces on the lag screws. As far as the buttressing function is concerned, it again helps fix the frequent metaphyseal comminution to the diaphysis

4.3.2.3 Pearls on the Use of Different Plates

4.3.2.3.1 Good Indications for Conventional Plating (e.g. DCP)

- Reconstruction of articular fractures
- Reconstruction of some long bone fractures like forearm fractures (since the radius–ulna articulation is nowadays regarded as a "joint" by most experts)
- Osteotomies – compression mode advisable
- Complex bone reconstruction procedures
- Pseudarthrosis

4.3.2.3.2 DCP

- Featured by having the DCU (Dynamic Compression Unit) geometry of the plate hole

4.3.2.3.3 Plate Mechanics

- With this standard plate and screw system, the tightening of the screws compresses the plate onto the bone. The actual stability results from the friction between the plate and the bone. Since the screw head is free to tilt within the plate hole, stability requires bicortical purchase of the screws
- Plate contouring is needed or there is the danger of loss of fracture reduction

4.3.2.3.4 Bone Healing

- Direct bone healing occurs under optimal conditions with direct osteonal bone healing that lead in one step to lamellar bridging of the fracture
- This type of healing is not as strong as indirect healing by callus (in fact resembles internal remodelling induced by necrosis). Hence, the usual recommendation is implant removal after 1–2 years to prevent re-fracture

4.3.2.3.5 Clinical Example

- In conventional forearm plating, it is generally accepted that four screws (eight cortices) should be anchored in each fragment except for simple transverse fractures where three screws may be enough

4.3.2.3.6 DCP Cx and the Use of LC-DCP

- Impaired blood supply of bone does not only affect healing, but also induces a cascade of deleterious reactions within the adjacent living bone
- In direct healing after conventional plating, the internal remodelling goes along with temporary porosity of the bone. When severe, and especially in the setting of infection, the bone may be rendered too

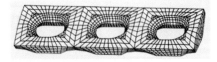
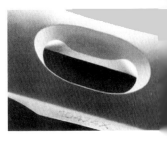

Fig. 4.4 The stress distribution of the LC-DCP

Fig. 4.5 Close up view
of the LC-DCP hole

weak to carry a load and the bone may sequestrate through conflu-
ent pores (sequester formation can prolong sepsis that is inaccessible
to antibiotics and needs debridement). To circumvent these short-
comings, the AO developed the LC-DCP or low-contact DCP that
helps preserve the periosteal blood supply by decreasing the surface
area of contact with the underlying bone. Other advantages of the
LC-DCP include: metallic finish is such that there are no unnecessary stress concentrations over the screw holes and so breakage is
less likely, even with contouring (Fig. 4.4), and more versatile direction of compression can be achieved by a re-design of the LC-DCP
screw hole (Fig. 4.5)

- Re-fracture: defined as fracture occurring after implant removal, either at the former fracture site or within the bone fragment affected
  by the plate ("secondary" fractures, in contrast, are those occurring
  with the implant in situ, with or without the presence of excessive
  loading)

4.3.2.4 Biological Plating
4.3.2.4.1 Principles of Biological Plating
- This involves:
  - Anatomical restoration of the articular surface in the traditional
    sense

- Maintenance of soft tissue attachments and vascularity to the cortical bone fragments
- Restoration of appropriate length, rotation, and alignment of the metaphyseal/diaphyseal region of the fracture, without preoccupation with exact anatomical restoration

4.3.2.4.2 Newer Plate

- Indirect healing after internal fixation is no longer regarded as a disturbance to healing, but is a goal in itself

4.3.2.4.3 Use of the Indirect Technique in the Setting of Plating

- The indirect technique advocated by Mast uses long plates or the distractor as reduction tools, and minimises handling of soft tissue
- The indirect technique emphasises a limited number of screws through the plate. Clinically, long plates with widely spaced screws have been shown to provide sufficient stability for fracture healing. In addition, lab cantilever testing also reveals increasing strength for fixations with more widely spaced screws

4.3.2.4.4 Resistance to Cantilever and Four-Point Bending

- Fewer but more widely spaced screws impart increased strength in cantilever and four-point bending in a lab model of plated fracture
- Another factor influencing the relative effects of screw number and placement on construct strength is the direction of cantilever bending, e.g. whether the plate is placed on the tension side or not
- Placing the plate on the non-tension side creates a much weaker construct, all being equal. If such a construct is pursued for whatever reason, it is more effective to increase resistance to cantilever bending by increasing the length of the plate rather than adding more screws to a shorter plate

4.3.2.4.5 Resistance to Torsion

- Torsional resistance depends on the number of screws securing a plate of a given width

- The length of the plate does not appear to have a significant effect on torsional resistance

4.3.2.4.6 Rationale of the Usual Practice of Placing Two Screws Near to Both Sides of the Fracture

- The clinical desirability of inter-fragmental control requires placement of a screw as close as practicable on each side of the fracture site
- Thus, in practice, most properly done plate-screw constructs included a screw in the plate hole nearest to the site of the fracture

4.3.2.4.7 Key to Success in Biological Plating

- Minimise the working length
- Maximise the plate length
- Length of the plate is more important than the number of screws placed in the plate with respect to bending strength
- A minimum of four screws may be adequate in more simple fracture patterns
- Occasionally, more screws are placed (>4) to prevent too much force concentration on the end screws, since the greatest concentration of applied force is usually located at the end screws

4.3.2.4.8 Advantages of Biological Plating

- The above-described minimal fixation constructs have increased inherent flexibility to allow enough micromotion for better callus formation
- Less soft tissue dissection and disruption confer biological advantages from less impairment of vascularity
- Perhaps the most important reason for respecting biology is that if biology is compromised, not only is healing slowed; but the potential Cx are severe – including non-union, infection, and sequestrum formation (whereas it is easier to salvage inadequate stability)

4.3.2.4.9 Mode of Failure of Biological Plating

- When longer plates fail, usually elastic deformation is seen to occur before distal screw pull-out
- (By contrast, in all short plate constructs, the bone usually fractures at the distal end of the plate – frequently with fracture lines extending through all three screw holes)

4.3.2.5 Newer Plating Systems

4.3.2.5.1 History

- The concept of preservation of blood supply by a design rationale rather similar to internal fixator technology is not new. Weber long ago described a plate with an elevated segment spanning the fracture site. The elevated part of the plate allows for better blood supply and can be used to hold cancellous bone graft

4.3.2.5.2 Introduction

- PC-Fix is a device for fixation of long bone fractures (e.g. forearm fractures) and is part of the by-product of scientific evolution towards the less invasive stabilisation system
- Designed by Perren and Tepic and made of titanium, its main goal is to optimise the preservation of biology, enhance fracture healing, and to improve resistance to infection
- Properly implanted devices (especially newer versions of PC-Fix) function as a completely implanted EF

4.3.2.5.3 PC-Fix

First Generation Design of PC-Fix

- Holes provide a precise fit to the conical head of the threaded bolts
- The surfaces in contact are constructed as steep cones. Such steep conical surfaces produce high friction upon application of an axial load. This minimises the torque transmittable to the thread, thus protecting the bone and the implant from overload. Thus, in the diaphysis, short monocortical screws provide sufficient strength against pull-out under a frictional bending load. The threaded bolts are self-cutting

- Looking from above, the "over-cuts" improve the flexural strength by displacing the edge of the holes towards the neutral axis of bending
- The under-surface is constructed with both longitudinal and transverse arches. The stiffness of the implant along its axis is evenly distributed
- The under-surface in contact with the bone is reduced to point contact
- Normally, the strength of the plates is weakest at the point of the weakest cross section at the screw holes. It should be noted that both PC-Fix and the LCP (which will be described in the Sect. 4.3.2.5.5) are designed to have similar stiffness along the plate without local stress concentration at the screw holes. Such a design will be more tolerant of a fracture gap of a given width

Second Generation Design of PC-Fix
- The design of PC-Fix 2 provides both angular stability of the screws as well as axial stability. Technically, this was made possible by machining a conical thread in both the screw head and the plate hole, whereby the plate–screw fixation does not even touch the bone

Advantages of PC-Fix
- Bone surface below PC-Fix is partly or fully vascularised
- Faster bone union – most fractures unite (90%) at the 4- to 6-month mark in one study (Injury 2001)
- Simplicity of application, less equipment, precise contouring of the plate is unnecessary
- Possibly less sepsis than DCP (improved vascularity)
- Less need for bone graft
- Shorter operative time (monocortical screws offered sufficient anchorage in diaphyseal bone)
- Less disturbance to intramedullary blood vessels with the use of monocortical screws
- Probably easier to monitor healing (than traditional plating)

Main Disadvantages of PC-Fix

- Not ideal for compression osteosynthesis since it is not possible to insert a lag screw at an angle through the holes in the device, nor can axial compression be effected by eccentric screw placement as in devices like LC-DCP and DCP (if compression is really needed, may have to bring the implant under tension and the bone under compression. Alternatively, compression by pre-bending and use of eccentric drill guide)
- Many experts do not recommend application of too short a PC-Fix, if only to increase the resistance to bending loads
- The bone cannot be aligned to the PC-Fix with screws

Other Disadvantages

- Implant removal is sometimes difficult because of jammed screws (6% in one series) or difficult to remove (jamming of the steep cone at the screw–fixator connection commonly due to the surgeon tightening the screw during implantation more than instructed or excessive torque)
- In one series (Injury 2001) there are occasional reports of non-union requiring secondary intervention, occasional malalignment and loss of anatomical reduction
- Caution to be exercised in using monocortical screws in metaphyseal bone
- Problems from extensive plate contouring: distortion of screw holes
- Putting monocortical screws with less "feel" and the surgeon may not feel accustomed to putting in monocortical screws first of all
- Stripping of the hexagonal head occasionally occurs
- Although monocortical screws are more biological, there is no grip in the near cortex, so that potentially more screws are necessary than in LC-DCP
- PC-Fix is now largely replaced by LCP

4.3.2.5.4 LISS Plating

Introduction

- Whereas the success of the use of PC-Fix in achieving the advantages of less infection, better healing and simplicity of application was proven in clinical multi-centre trials, the point fixator has become the "father" technology of the LISS (less invasive stabilisation system) and the LCP (locked compression plate)

▪ These modern devices work on the principle of "flexible elastic fixation"

The Flexible Elastic Fixation Concept

▪ The main aim of this fixation technique is to imitate spontaneous healing including its induction of callus formation, and allow early motion

▪ This technology supports MIPO

The Essence of Flexible Elastic Fixation

▪ The key is "elasticity"

▪ This implies that the displacement of the fracture ends under load must be reversible. The locked internal fixator technique takes advantage of the elastic properties of metals, especially that of pure titanium

▪ Since in fixing bones of limited strength (like osteoporotic bones) the deformability of the implant is key, LCP/LISS plate technology is also good for fixation of osteoporotic bone and enables the use of elastic flexible fixation

▪ Notice that one good point about elasticity in fixation is that the implant–bone construct/anchorage is less likely to fail in the event of a single high loading challenge to the construct, i.e. a more forgiving device

▪ The deformability of the implant is a key to fixation of bones of limited strength (especially osteoporotic bones). The locked internal fixator technique enables the use of elastic flexible fixation

The LISS Design (Fig. 4.6)

▪ Designed by Frigg and others (2001)

▪ The design was initially inspired by the favourable results of inter-locked intra-medullary nailing. In fact, the final construct resembles a pre-contoured condylar buttress plate equipped with insertion handle (to ease the MIPO technique), and with fixed angle locking screws

■ There are separate plate designs for the distal femur (Fig. 4.7) and proximal tibia to suit the different local anatomy in these regions

Screw Design of the LISS

■ The screws have a conically threaded profile, not only providing stable angular fixation, but also self-centring in the hole, and keeps the screw from backing out of the LISS plate (an obvious advantage if the MIPO technique is used)

■ The core diameter of the screws is enlarged to resist the increased bending moment and high shearing force

■ The above, plus the stable threaded screw–fixator interface, allows for unicortical screw placement

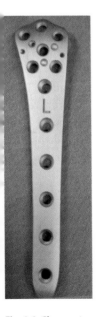

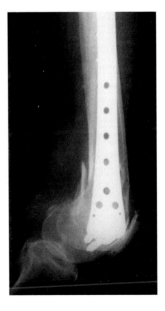

Fig. 4.6 Close up view of the LISS plate

Fig. 4.7 Lateral X-ray showing LISS plating for a fractured distal femur

- Unicortical screw usage permits the use of self-tapping and drilling screws and obviates screw length measurements as all the diaphyseal screws will then be of comparable length
- Percutaneous plate placement also necessitates the use of a water-cooled drill sleeve during percutaneous insertion of screws to minimise heat generation

Screw Orientation of the LISS
- The plate is so designed that the posterior screws do not penetrate the inter-condylar notch, and the anterior screws are parallel to the PFJ
- The screws are overall convergent to increase the surface area of contact with the (osteoporotic) bone
- The plate, equipped with the handle, is designed for percutaneous insertion

Other Features of the Screws of the LISS Plate
- It should be noted that just as self-drilling external fixation pins will push away the bone when inserted, the LISS screws also tend to push away the bone during screw insertion with a power drill
- One cannot expect the fixator to help achieve fracture fixation. Thus, the LISS can be expected to maintain, but not obtain, fracture reduction – this is in sharp distinction to the use of the 95° angled blade plate. Here, establishment of proper placement of the blade plate in the distal femoral region will ensure appropriate axial and sagittal plane alignment

Fine-Tuning During LISS Plating
- As the plate is not meant to be used as a reduction device, fine-tuning after LISS plate insertion is frequently needed to ensure fracture alignment
- Examples include the "Whirlybird" or pull screw, which allows for fine adjustment of frontal plane alignment

Indication
- Ideally to provide fixed angle support for metaphyseal fractures

- Especially in osteoporotic bones
- Also of use in periprosthetic fractures around TKR

Key to Success
- Ensure correct indication
- Use the correct plate: special LISS plates are available for tackling fractures of the distal femur and proximal tibia, also take care to use the correct side (i.e. right side vs left side)
- Ensure proper fracture reduction before plate insertion as the LISS plate is not meant to be used as a reduction aid
- Eccentric placement of the LISS plate should be avoided as this may lead to eccentric screw placement in the diaphysis
- FWB is only allowed when the callus is seen on serial postoperative radiographs

Modes of Failure of the LISS
- All screws literally slice through the cortex in a longitudinal manner
- All screws pull out of the bone

Complication of LISS
- Implant loosening – causes include premature FWB postoperatively, failure of the screws to lock in the implant, distance between the implant and the bone too great, plate too short
- Proximal screw pull-out of the LISS can be due to misplacing of the LISS on the shaft; this will lead to a tangential screw position with poor screw hold
- Implant breakage – in cases of delayed/non-union, lack of callus causes cyclic implant loading and subsequent implant failure
- Others: rotational malalignment, infection, etc.

4.3.2.5.5 *Locking Compression Plates*
Design
- Locking compression plates (LCP) designed by Frigg and Wagner
- Combine the features of internal fixator and compression plating – the surgeon is free to select the best treatment method to suit the fracture situation and make combinations as necessary

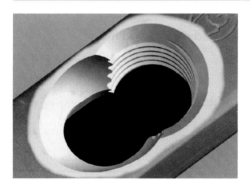

Fig. 4.8 Close-up of the combi-hole, a feature of the LCP

- The plate hole of the LCP is called the combi-hole (Fig. 4.8), which is a merger between DCU (dynamic compression unit) geometry of the LC-DCP with a conical threaded hole
- The shape of the conical thread is identical to that of the second generation PC-Fix and LISS
- The locking head screw is captured in the threaded part of the combi-hole through 200° – this new design was found in previous studies to provide sufficient angular *and* axial stability

Indications for Use of LCP
- Said to be good in fracture fixation of osteoporotic bone
- The new combi-hole allows the use of LCP in the management of more complex metaphyseal fractures with diaphyseal extension – in this situation, the locking head screws will be used to fix the fracture close to the joint; while standard screws will be used to apply axial compression between the metaphysis and diaphysis fracture fragments

Relation Between Distance of Separation from Bone and Plate Behaviour
- Previous lab studies on plastic tibiae indicate that if the separation is < 5 mm, implant behaviour is more like a plate, rather than like EF (J Trauma 1996)
- The larger the plate–bone separations, the more likely the non-contact plate behaves as an EF

Implications of LCP Behaviour Resembling an EF

- Previous biomechanical studies reviewed that fixation rigidity of EF can be improved by increasing the distance between pins in the same fragment, and an increase in the number of pins (J Orthop Res 1984)
- The implication is that in using LCP in load-bearing situation, we prefer to use longer plates; say, using a six- or eight-hole plate, instead of a four-hole plate

Complications of LCP

- In general, screws must all fail at the same time in order for the whole construct to fail, an obvious advantage in osteoporotic bone. Unicortical fixation has been shown to be weak in torsion, and is now falling out of favour with some experts, especially in osteopenic patients who have very thin cortical thickness
- Jamming of the locked screws – the steep conical fit requires the torque tightening to be minimal. Application of high torque to the screw head causes the screw head to lock and removal is difficult. A torque-limiting device should therefore be used
- Lack of feeling or feedback to the surgeon during screw insertion – the design of the LCP locks torque and tilting upon minimal axial pull within the screw, so that the screw cannot pull out during insertion. The disadvantage is that feedback to the surgeon regarding the engagement of the screw is minimal. The surgeon should ensure proper engagement of the screw within solid cortical bone
- Failure of monocortical screws – monocortical screws are prevented from tilting via a firm lock between the screw and the body of the fixator. However, even monocortical screws require anchorage within a proper cortex. It may theoretically fail if the thickness of the cortical shell is too low

Summarising the Comparison Between Conventional Versus Locked Plates

- Conventional plate: bicortical purchase is required to prevent screw toggle, and friction between the under-surface of the plate and the underlying bone provides stability to the construct. If the contact

between the plate and underlying bone is lost, all stability of the construct will be lost. Stable contact between the plate and the underlying bone can also compromise periosteal perfusion

- Locked plate: contact between the plate and the bone is not required
for stability since the corresponding threads of the plate and screw
prevent the screw from toggling; the plate essentially acts as a cortex.
Unlike conventional plating, the plate is frequently applied first, then
the screws are inserted. This assumes accurate closed reduction before locked screw placement, as was stressed before

Newer Locked Plate Designs and Their Advantages
- Newer polyaxial locked plates (POLYAX; DePuy, Warsaw, IN, USA)
offer some freedom of angulation of screws prior to final screw-plate
seating by virtue of a Bushing in the plate. Hoop stresses are generated as the conical screw engages the bushing, thereby locking the
screw at the chosen angle

Key Concept
- Locked plates and especially the screws that come with the system
are expensive and discretion is advised in implant selection. Not
each and every fracture benefits from the use of locked plates
- The best indication for locked plates is in periarticular fractures, especially in osteoporotic bones. Previous cadaver research highlight-
ing the role of locked plates in osteoporotic bones can be found in
the works of Zlowodski et al., who demonstrated the superior performance of locked constructs over conventional plating in osteopenic bone

4.4   Tension Band Principle

4.4.1   Definition
- It is a device that will exert a force equal in magnitude, but opposite
in direction to an applied bending force

.4.2 Introduction

- It is a classic engineering concept
- The tension band principle was introduced by Pauwels in the 1930s
- In orthopaedics, it is commonly applied to internal fixation of eccentrically loaded bone, in regions like the patella, olecranon, acromion, etc.

4.4.3 Illustration of the Principle

- The standard illustration (used in engineering drawings) is that of an I-beam connected by two springs and is found in all AO manuals
- If the I-beam is loaded right down the middle over the central axis, uniform compression of both springs is attained
- If there is an eccentric load (as happens with a lot of fractures in certain areas of the body), the spring on the same side compresses and the spring on the opposite side is placed in tension and stretches
- The crux of the matter is: if the tension band is applied before eccentric loading, there will then be uniform compression of both springs. That is the essence of the tension band principle

4.4.4 Application in Practice

- Only certain fractures are amenable to tension band wiring. The tension band material – plate, wire or suture – must counteract tensile forces
- The most common material used is stainless steel
- Example: in using tension band wiring (TBW) for the olecranon, the implant alone does not provide stability. It serves to guide the compression force
- In combination with antagonistic deforming muscles, TBW can help produce uniform compression at the fracture site
- The parallel wires or screws serve as rails along which the bone fragments slide

4.4.5 Use of Plates as a Tension Band

- Again, we refer to the application of plates to eccentrically loaded bones, e.g. the femur, the humerus, or the shaft of the radius and the ulna

- It is essential to apply the plate to the tension side when the force are large as in the femur
- If the forces are not large, one does not always have to plate on the tension side and you may find in some areas that it is more convenient to use another approach, only because the plate will lie there better or because of the nature of the fracture. Example: both volar and dorsal plating of the distal radius are well described

4.4.6   Contraindication to the Use of Tension Bands

- A common contraindication to the use of tension bands is comminution involving the opposite cortex
- Besides the above, attention to technical details is important or the tension-band principle will not work
- Example: TBW for a fractured patella. The patella fracture can end up with a juxta-articular gap if the wires are placed too far away from the joint. Try to place the wires closer to the joint. Also, the wires must be parallel to each other. The parallel wires serve as "rails" along which the bone fragments slide

4.5   Biomechanics and Function of Intramedullary Nails

4.5.1   IM Nail Biomechanics

- An IM nail by itself acts as an internal splint
- Only offers resistance to bending stress
- Subsequent introduction of locking allows resistance to: compression (prevents shortening) and rotation – these new nails thus extend the indication of the IM nail to other more unstable fracture patterns

4.5.2   Contraindication of IM Nailing

- Infection
- Fracture patterns outside the zone of indication (e.g. too proximal and too distal – example: a tibial nail is relatively contraindicated if the fracture is proximal to the bend in the tibial nail)

- Bone deformity
- Prosthesis in the way, e.g. THR prosthesis in situ

4.5.3 Advantage of the IM Nail

- If done well, healing is biological and even stronger than primary bone healing
- No need to open the fracture site and less chance of the fracture being infected
- Reaming actually may promote healing – by providing a source of autologous bone graft to the fracture site

4.5.4 Mechanical Features of the IM Nail

- Material strength: as defined by Young's modulus in the stress/strain curve
- Structural strength which depends on:
  - Stiffness = slope of load/deformation curve
  - Moment of Inertia (I) = needs to know the outer and inner diameter (Do vs Di respectively) $I = \pi(Do - Di)^4/64$. Hence depends much on the radius/diameter to the fourth power
  - Other geometric features:
    - Anterior bow (usually not exactly like the natural bow to create slight bone/nail mismatch to create some frictional stability)
    - Cross-section (most are clover-leaf-shaped, the clearance provided allows easier revascularisation after reaming – designs with flutes may jam better, but difficult to remove later)
    - Slot (allows radial compression during insertion and accommodates mismatch ± offers more frictional component of fixation gained through radial compression and a corresponding increase in hoop stresses in bone)
    - Size (some designs prevent abrupt loss of moments of inertia by increasing the thickness of its nails with a smaller diameter)

4.5.5 Causes of Implant Failure/Breakage

- Significant new trauma

- Weight-bearing too early, especially unreamed nails: Browner says weight bearing too early in locked nails increases stresses at the bolts and may fracture the bolts. This was found to be likely to occur in unreamed nails
- Delayed union of various causes – it all boils down to a race between bone healing and implant failure
- Fatigue failure of the nail – can occur even after apparent bone union, the nail continues some weight-bearing function, and cyclic loading can still cause fatigue failure
- Other reasons: not enough stability (e.g. too small nail in a large cavity), a defect/pre-existing micro-crack with eventual crack prolongation and propagation

4.5.6   Sites of Hardware Breakage
- Unlocked nails: most fracture at the slot-tip
- Locked nails: most fail through one of the interlocking holes: the more proximal of the two distal holes said to be more common
- Notice the site of breakage is sometimes at a pre-existing defect or a micro-crack

4.5.7   Advantages of Reaming
- Increases the contact area – hence, improves the fracture site stability by increasing the frictional component of fixation (does so mainly by enlarging the isthmus – the mid-shaft region of the bone with constant diameter), the effect abates after > 2 mm of reaming
- Stimulates fracture healing: by provision of a source of autogenous bone graft
- Allows a larger diameter, stronger nail to be inserted

4.5.8   Disadvantages of Reaming
- Risk of fat/marrow embolism – especially dangerous in the face of lung contusions in poly-trauma; design of new reamer head that may help decrease reaming pressure is needed (Fig. 4.9)
- Disruption of the endosteal blood flow – only temporary, and the periosteal blood supply has been shown to adequately compensate until the endosteal flow is reconstituted

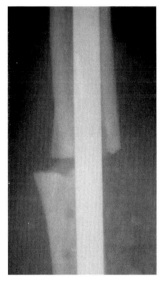

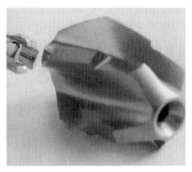

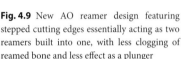

Fig. 4.9 New AO reamer design featuring stepped cutting edges essentially acting as two reamers built into one, with less clogging of reamed bone and less effect as a plunger

Fig. 4.10 Eccentric reaming needs to be avoided to prevent unnecessary bony damage

- Weakens the cortex – usually not problematic unless excessive thinning (by the equation of the moment of inertia I; luckily, we are removing only the innermost portion of bone – less effect) or by eccentric reaming (Fig. 4.10)

4.5.9   Finer Biomechanical Points

- Starting hole: the starting hole is the second important factor determining the degree of bone–nail mismatch (besides the built-in anterior bow). Too anterior placement with respect to the neutral axis of the medullary canal causes high hoop stresses at the fracture site and possible bursting of the anterior cortex. Medial/lateral deviation from the ideal starting hole should be avoided to prevent varus/valgus. Large but correctly placed holes cause less strength reduction than correctly sized but inappropriately placed holes

- Loads on the nail: these include bending, torsion and compression loads:
  - In bending: the lateral femoral cortex is subjected to tension and the medial cortex to compression
  - In compression: the force is due to the action of the muscles. Hence, if the nail is not locked, the fracture needs to be transverse and not comminuted or shortening will occur
  - In torsion: this form of loading occurs mostly in manoeuvres like rising from a chair

4.5.10   Effect of Fracture Configuration and Location

- The fracture location: determines how much isthmus contact the bone has with the IM nail on either side of the fracture. Midshaft fractures are therefore the optimal type for reaming
- Fractures that are proximal or distal to the isthmus are more difficult to treat with an IM nail since they only have cortical contact on one side of the fracture. Interlocking is therefore a must

4.5.11   About Interlocking

- Static interlock: a must for those oblique/comminuted fracture and for those rather proximal/distal fractures to control shortening and rotation. Weight-bearing too early in these cases risks screw breakage – better to wait until fracture consolidation has begun to occur; thus, the fracture site will begin to share some of the load
- Dynamic interlock: reserved for cases where one of the fracture fragments is felt to achieve adequate fixation with the isthmus. Has the advantage of early WB as there is no concern of screw breakage. Dynamic locking allows some gliding to occur (P.S. the initial fears of static locking creating a "non-union machine" have turned out to be unfounded, and routine dynamisation is no longer commonly administered)

4.5.12   Do We Still Perform Dynamisation?

- Routine dynamisation is no longer commonly administered, as explained

- If performed, it should be done early rather than late. Usually involves removal of the screw with the greatest distance from the fracture site
- However, it can be considered if the fracture is slow to heal in the following situations:
  - Stable fracture configuration
  - Sometimes for hypertrophic or oligotrophic non-unions or delayed unions

4.5.13 Advantages of IM Nail Compared with Plating
- Compared with plates:
  - Lower infection rate
  - Reduced soft tissue trauma
  - Decreased incidence of non-union
  - Improved biomechanical function

4.5.14 Dangers of Reamed Nailing
- Experimental studies revealed:
  - Inflammatory changes can occur (the inflammatory response induced by femoral nailing was comparable to that as a result of uncemented THR)
  - Impairment of immunity
  - Increased inflammatory capacity of PMN
  - High intramedullary pressure (from piston like effect) causing intravasated bone marrow
  - Animal model: reaming in the presence of lung contusions = marked increase in pulmonary vascular resistance

4.5.15 Theoretical Advantage of Unreamed Nailing
- Less release of inflammatory mediators
- Fewer abnormalities in pulmonary permeability
- Less ARDS in some clinical studies where one third of patients had concomitant severe chest injuries

4.5.16   In Practice

■ However, judging from the results of clinical studies, the effect of reamed and unreamed nailing on the incidence of post-traumatic complications is clinically not proven and seems to be difficult to evaluate

4.5.17   The Future

■ New reaming system: designed to minimise the local and systemic effects of reaming
■ Allows intraoperative irrigation and suction during reaming

4.6   External Fixation

4.6.1   Clinical Applications of External Fixators

■ As temporary stabilisation device: such as spanning a limb with open IIIB and C fractures, spanning a very unstable fracture dislocation, effect temporary skeletal fixation to buy time for urgent vascular repair, and as temporary fixation for very complex fractures, etc.
■ As definitive fracture fixation: such as in treating difficult periarticular fractures with too poor a soft tissue envelope for open reduction, e.g. use of hybrid EF in pilon fractures and tibial plateau fractures, etc.
■ As salvage: the ring fixators are especially good for salvaging for instance malunions and non-unions after failed fracture surgery, especially in the face of bone loss and a high-risk host such as a patient with a history of DM or vascular disease

4.6.2   Components of an External Fixator

■ Schanz screw
■ Clamps
■ Central body
■ Compression–distraction system

(The discussion that follows uses the Orthofix in fractured tibia as an illustrative example)

4.6.2.1 The Schanz Screw

- The Schanz screw, or half pin, is the mainstay of most EF constructs
- The Schanz screw has no head and a long shaft
- It can be inserted after pre-drilling since it cuts its own thread
- It is of two varieties: those with longer threads holding both cortices, and those with short threads holding only the far cortex. The latter type may provide the construct with greater stiffness

4.6.2.1.1 Comparing Schanz Screw Design with Screws Used in Conventional Plating

- The screws of the conventional plate are subject to only a minimal bending load, since conventional plate–screw constructs function by pressing the plate to the bone surface – thus creating friction at the interface of plate and bone
- The pins of the EF (and the screws of the newer implants like the internal fixators) transfer much more of a bending load than conventional screws; thus, their core is thicker than that of a conventional screw. Shallow threads suffice since the threads are only there to resist pull-out forces and do not need to produce or maintain compression between the implanted body and bone

4.6.2.1.2 Pearls Concerning Schanz Screws

- Pinholes < 30% of bone diameter
- 5-mm pin 1.5 times stronger than < 4-mm pin
- Separate pins greater than 45°

4.6.2.2 Clamps

- Act as a connection between the Schanz screw and the other fixator components

4.6.2.3 Central Body

- The main body can be just a connecting rod or a more elaborate system allowing, say, compression or distraction

4.6.2.4 Compression Distraction System
- Many Orthofix central bodies have a compression distraction mode
- Examples of clinical use are in bone transport or to effect fracture compression in, say, delayed unions

4.6.3   Main Types of External Fixators
- Pin and rod fixators
- Ring fixators
- Hybrids
- Ilizarov method

4.6.3.1 Pros and Cons of the Pin and Rod Fixators (Fig. 4.11)
- Advantages: simple and quick to construct
- Disadvantages: fracture needs to be reduced beforehand because once in place, little adjustability of the fracture alignment remains.

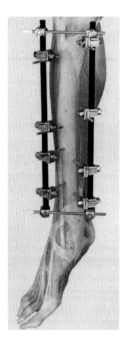

Fig. 4.11 Model showing the popular pin–rod construct

This cantilever system will not tolerate axial loading as in a ring fixator, and cannot allow weight-bearing; there is a theoretical danger of delayed union and non-union

4.6.3.2 The Circular EF
- More recent innovation
- Uses 1.8- to 2-mm wires
- An important feature: bending stiffness independent of loading direction

4.6.3.3 Pros and Cons of Ring Fixators
- Advantages: can correct complex multiple plane deformities, allows adjustability of alignment, even in the postoperative patient with the fixator in place, and allows early weight-bearing
- Disadvantages: bulky, many more pins and there is a higher chance of pin track problems, and possibly decreased compliance with long-term use

4.6.3.4 Pros and Cons of Hybrid Fixators
- Advantages: some special (especially periarticular) regions very useful and can avoid spanning the joint with the danger of joint stiffness; while at the same time, can control even complex comminuted fracture patterns. Examples include Pilon fractures, and fractured tibial plateau
- Disadvantages: rather bulky, pin track sepsis, etc.

4.6.4 Determining Factors of EF Stiffness
- Bone rod distance
- Number of Schanz screws/pins
- Separation between the Schanz screws
- Distance of the Schanz screw from the fracture site
- Number of rods
- Overall configuration of the EF construct
- Others: pin diameter, pin insertion angle, etc.

(The discussion that follows uses a unilateral, uniplanar, simple EF construct as an example)

4.6.5   The Final Mechanical Strength of EF

- Not based solely on the fixator, but on:
    - The composite structure as a whole
    - Strength of the host bone, etc.

4.6.5.1 Bone–Rod Distance

- Although decreasing the bone–rod distance of a unilateral fixator frame increases the stiffness, in practice space has to be left for dressing and in case there is increased soft tissue swelling

4.6.5.2 Number of Schanz Screws

- Increased stability with increased pin number
- But there are practical limitations, e.g. have to respect anatomical safe corridor, and there can be regions one needs to avoid, e.g. to make way for future flap surgery

4.6.5.3 Distance of the Schanz Screws from the Fracture Site

- Better fixator and fracture stability
- Hence avoid placing the Schanz pin too far from the fracture site

4.6.5.4 Separation Between the Schanz Screws

- In general, an increase in the pin–pin distance in a bone segment increases the bending stiffness

4.6.5.5 Number of Rods

- An increase in the number of parallel rods in a unilateral frame construct increases the bending stiffness

4.6.5.6 Configuration of the EF

- See the discussion that follows

4.6.6   Common Fixator Configurations

- Unilateral (uniplanar or biplanar)
- Bilateral (uniplanar or biplanar)
- Modular frame constructs

4.6.6.1 Unilateral Uniplanar

- This is a popular construct, because it is not bulky and the patient can sit more comfortably
- There are fewer scars or pin track sites
- It is the construct usually used in open tibial fractures

4.6.6.2 Unilateral Biplanar

- A more stable construct is used when a more prolonged EF application is expected
- Examples include cases where there is bone loss or significant soft tissue injury

4.6.6.3 Bilateral Uniplanar

- The main disadvantages include: it is weaker than a unilateral frame in the sagittal plane. Also, transfixing pins can cause neurovascular damage
- Advantages are few, but since it has transfixation pins in situ, application of the pre-load to the Steinmann pins can effect fracture compression

4.6.6.4 Bilateral Biplanar

- This is a stable construct as it can withstand bending moments in both the AP and sagittal planes
- Clinical uses: occasionally to temporarise in the presence of a segmental bone defect, say, in open tibial fractures, and occasionally in arthrodesis of some joints

4.6.6.5 Modular Frames

- Again with fractured tibia as an example, this construct usually involves two Schanz screws in each fracture fragment connected by a short tube. We then add a third tube to connect the two short tubes
- Advantage: this does permit some readjustment of fracture alignment as opposed to a standard unilateral, uniplanar construct

4.6.7   How Rigid Should an EF Be?

▪ See the following discussion on the concept of controlled micro-movement

4.6.8   Role of Micromotion in EF

▪ There is a trend using more flexible frames, or the adjustment of frames to allow dynamisation of the fracture, increasing the strain acting on the fracture site

▪ This is based on previous experimental and clinical studies that have shown that imposing small amounts of axial micro-movement for short periods each day may be beneficial for bone healing, especially if EF was used as the definitive device for fixation of fractures

4.6.9   Caution in the Administration of Micromotion

▪ However, recent papers suggest that although an element of micro-motion is beneficial for bone healing, the micromotion should be introduced relatively early. Late introduction may either be ineffective or even detrimental (e.g. it was shown in CORR 1998 that a high strain rate stimulus applied later in the healing period can significantly inhibit the process of bone healing). The beneficial effect, when applied early, on fracture healing may be related to the viscoelastic nature of the differentiating connective tissues in the early endochondral callus

4.6.10   Timing for Applying a Mechanical Stimulus to Encourage Bony Healing

▪ Most experts are of the opinion that if we were to use mechanical stimulation to promote healing, especially in fractures involving bones that heal more slowly (such as the tibia), then it is usually recommended that mechanical stimulation start upon seeing early signs of periosteal bridging callus

4.6.11   Dynamisation of EF

▪ The term "dynamisation" used in the context of the issue of bone healing in EF is rather imprecise. It often means adjustment of the frame to permit unconstrained axial loading of the fracture, with the hope of an increase in micromotion that is not easy to quantify, for there must be sufficient stability to maintain reduction

4.6.12 Timing of Dynamisation

- It is mostly given several weeks after fracture when early bridging has occurred
- Some brands of EF have sliding frames that allow axial stress to be applied through weight-bearing

4.6.12.1 Key Concept

- Previous studies revealed the extreme sensitivity of healing fractures to mechanical stimuli
- The secret of success may well be to adjust the prescribed regime according to the phase of healing. A given fracture may heal more rapidly in EF if the mechanical environment can be tailored according to the individual needs of the fracture and the patient
- Having said that, some experts feel that associated soft tissue injuries may be more important in the selection of EF configuration than its characteristics with regard to mechanical stability

4.6.12.2 Passive Dynamisation

- Due to pin bending
- Remove side bars and pins

4.6.12.3 Active Axial Dynamisation

- Weight-bearing – without pin-bending
- Relaxation of axial constraint

4.6.12.4 Controlled Axial Dynamisation

- Such as the use of the cam device

4.6.13 Complications of EF

- Pin track infection
- Premature pin loosening

- Possible increased chance of delayed union or non-union
- Neurovascular injuries
- Others: joint stiffness, etc.

4.6.14   How to Improve Pin–Bone Interface

- Apply half pins rather than wires
- Wash pins at the time of surgery
- Avoid thermal necrosis – hand drill
- Pre-loading

4.6.15   EF Disassembly

- Is controlled removal needed?
- Not much literature looking at this aspect
- Probably not necessary if there are signs of fracture consolidation, but controlled removal is frequently needed in difficult reconstructions, say, by the Ilizarov method. See the Sect. 4.7 on Ilizarov procedures

4.6.16   EF Summary

- External fixators are very versatile implants that can be used both in acute fracture fixations and in chronic reconstructions. It is relatively minimally invasive and, if properly applied, it burns no bridges; these are some of the major advantages of this type of implant
- The ideal construct for an external fixator is not known
- The modern trend is towards increased versatility, like making allowance for a change in compression/alignment
- Newer computer-aided frame constructs representing the state of the art such as the Taylor spatial frame were mentioned in Chap. 1

4.7   Principles of the Ilizarov Method (Fig. 4.12)

4.7.1   Introduction

- Ilizarov invented the technique of distraction osteogenesis in the 1950s, which, in his own words, works by "tension stress"

- In fact, the expression "distraction osteogenesis" that we often use does not wholly describe the procedure. This is because not only is there bone formation upon execution of the procedure, but soft tissue formation as well – such as muscle, vessel wall, tendon

4.7.2 Chief Use of the Ilizarov Method

- The main use is for bony lengthening (Fig. 4.13)
- This technique is particularly useful in complex situations where simultaneous bony lengthening and deformity correction need to be implemented

4.7.3 Other Uses

- Elective deformity correction of long bones
- Management of non-unions, by means of compression instead of distraction

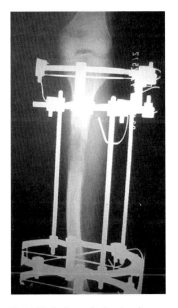

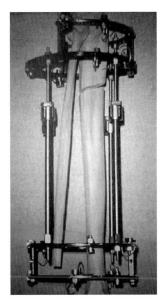

Fig. 4.12 Radiograph showing distraction osteosynthesis using the Ilizarov frame

Fig. 4.13 Model showing an Ilizarov frame construction

- Acute management of complicated fractures (an example will be pilon fractures with short distal fragments and a poor soft tissue envelope)

4.7.4   Mechanism of Action

- Given adequate rigidity and correct execution of the procedure, there is bone formation of the intramembranous type by distraction osteogenesis
- VEGF (vascular endothelial growth factor) appears to be involved
- In addition, the piezoelectric phenomenon in the new regenerate tissue and marrow is believed to be induced by the restricted elasticity of the tensioned wires used in the Ilizarov construct (Frankel and Golyakhovsky)

4.7.5   Histology

- Osteogenesis by intramembranous ossification is found on microscopy parallel to the applied distraction force

4.7.6   Why Choose a Circular Frame?

- The circular frame construct reproduces the shape of the cylindrical long bones such as the tibia
- This frame construct can resist deforming forces in different directions such as common bending and torsion stresses. In addition, it may confer an element of axial stability sometimes adequate enough for early weight-bearing – a feat that cannot be accomplished by a usual monolateral EF construct
- Word of caution: early weight-bearing is not always possible. Example: if the Ilizarov method was used in treating acute tibial pilon fractures with very distal ± small fragments, then early weight-bearing should be avoided

4.7.7   Why Choose Multiple Tensioned Wires?

- Believed to be able to induce a piezoelectric phenomenon via the restricted elasticity of the tensioned wires

- Small calibre wires reduce soft tissue trauma and avoid too many incisions
- Tensioning needed to confer adequate fragment stability

4.7.8   Determinants of Frame Stability

- Larger wire diameter
- Smaller ring size
- Olive wires
- More wires ± half pins
- Cross wires at 90°
- Increase wire tension
- Rings closer to the fracture (but has to allow for swelling)
- Closer adjacent rings

4.7.9   The Key Steps

- Period of latency: lasts 4–7 days after the corticotomy and fixator application
- Period of distraction (if distraction osteogenesis is planned)
- Period of consolidation
- Frame dynamisation lasting around 3 weeks
- Removal of frame ± brace application

4.7.10   Role of Corticotomy

- The aim of doing a corticotomy instead of the usual osteotomy is to:
  - Prevent disruption of the intramedullary blood supply
  - Prevent injury to the periosteum and preserve the periosteal blood supply
- The site of the osteotomy should avoid the position of the nutrient artery
- The corticotomy can be monofocal (done at one level) or bifocal (at two levels)
- Monofocal corticotomy can be used in most lengthening procedures within 5 cm, or bone transport up to 7 cm

4.7.11   The Three Main Methods of Distraction

- The external method – see section on bone defect management in Chap. 3
- The internal method – see section on bone defect management in Chap. 3
- Combined

4.7.12   Preparing for Removal

- An adequate period of consolidation is essential before removal is contemplated, or the regenerate may fracture
- Before removal, dynamisation, such as by loosening the nuts of the interconnecting rods, is advisable

4.7.13   Adaptations for Use in Deformity Correction

- Hinges are usually used, acting as pivotal point for correction of angulation and displacement
- Preoperative planning and long lower limb alignment films are needed to plan the location of the osteotomy. Also, the location, number and orientation of the hinges are important

4.7.14   Adaptations for Use in Non-unions

- Compression mode is usually used to effect compression of the non-union
- Please note that compression will not work for pseudarthrosis. Established pseudarthrosis needs to be resected

4.7.15   Complications

- Bony Cx
- Soft tissue Cx
- Pin track Cx
- Other complications, e.g. psychological, especially in children

4.7.15.1 Bony Cx

- Fracture of regenerate
- Very slow or inadequate consolidation of regenerate (Fig. 4.14)

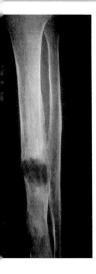

Fig. 4.14 This regenerate in a lengthened tibia
was slow to consolidate

- Lack of new bone formation (e.g. due to an unstable construct)
- If bone is transported, delayed union of the docking site

4.7.15.2 Soft Tissue Cx
- Nearby joint subluxation during lengthening
- Neural damage
- Vascular injury
- Soft tissue contractures or stiffness of nearby joints

4.7.15.3 Pin Track Cx
- Meticulous pin care needed
- Avoid skin tenting

4.8   Bioabsorbable Implants

4.8.1   Advantages
- Gradual transfer of the load to the healing skin tenting – less stress
  shielding

- No need to remove the implant
- The (local bony) anatomy may be better visualised on X-ray, since the view is not blocked, as with metallic implants

4.8.2   Disadvantages

- Synovitis and fibrous reactions – especially in those that degrade quickly (by hydrolysis)
- Possible mutagenicity
- No long-term studies for support
- Premature breaking loose occasionally – but this cannot be seen on X-ray since radiolucent
- Premature failure, e.g. micro-fracture, bending strength is seldom as strong as stainless steel and decreasing and tends to be more brittle

4.8.3   The Ideal Bioabsorbable Implant

- All advantages + no disadvantages

4.8.4   Common Types

- Polyglycolic acid – quick resorption looses strength quickly (PGA)
- Polylactic acid – slower resorption (PLA)
- Polydioxanone (PDS)
- Co-polymers (combined better properties of both)

4.8.5   Factors Influencing Rate of Degradation

- Local vascularity
- Porosity
- Crystallinity
- Molecular structure (such as L- and R-forms, e.g. of polylactic acid)

4.8.6   Examples of Clinical Application

- All-inside technique of meniscus repair
- Rotator cuff repairs (use of suture anchors)
- Bankart repairs/SLAB lesions (e.g. use of tags can sometimes obviate the complicated arthroscopic knot-tying)

Selected Bibliography of Journal Articles

1. ElMaraghy AW, Schemitsch EH, et al. (1998) Femoral and cruciate blood flow after retrograde femoral nailing. J Orthop Trauma 12:253–258
2. Fernandez AA, Galante RM, et al. (2001) Osteosynthesis of diaphyseal fractures of the radius using PC-Fix, a prospective study. Injury 32 [S-B]:44–50
3. Frigg R (2001) Locking compression plate (LCP). An osteosynthesis plate based on Dynamic Compression Plate and the Point Contact Fixator. Injury 32 [S-B]:63–66
4. Frigg R, Appenzeller A, et al. (2001) The development of the distal femur Less Invasive Stabilization System (LISS). Injury 32 [S-C]:24–31
5. Heim D, Schlegal U, et al. (1993) Intra-medullary pressure in reamed and unreamed nailing of the femur and tibia: an in vitro study in intact human bones. Injury 24 [Suppl 3]:S56–S63
6. Ip D, Wong SH, et al. (2001) Rare complications of segmental breakage of plastic medullary tube in closed intra-medullary nailing. Injury 32(9):730–731
7. Leung F, Kwok HY, et al. (2004) Limited open reduction and Ilizarov external fixation in the treatment of distal tibial fractures. Injury 35: 278–283
8. Peter RE, Selz T, et al. (1993) Influence of the reamer shape on intraosseous pressure during closed intra-medullary nailing of the unbroken femur. Injury 24 [Suppl 3]: S48–S55
9. Rhinelander FW (1968) The normal microcirculation of diaphyseal cortex and its response to fracture. J Bone Joint Surg Am 50:784–800
10. Schemitsch EH, Swiontowski MF, et al. (1994) Cortical blood flow in reamed and unreamed locked intra-medullary nailing. J Orthop Trauma 8:373–382

Special Types of Fractures

Contents

5.1   Stress Fractures

5.1.1   Introduction

- Commoner in athletes and military personnel
- Incidence: < 1% of general orthopaedic consultations, 20% in active runners, more in females overall
- Lower limbs > upper limbs, since lower limb bones are weight-bearing
- But specific types of stress fractures may be predisposed by special types of sports, e.g. fractured humerus in throwing sports

5.1.2   Normal Body Protective Mechanisms

- Muscle action – muscle fatigue therefore can lead to excess force exertion on bones
- Anatomy of Haversian canals – microscopic analysis of Haversian canal layout reveals that the anatomy helps prevent the propagation of microcracks should they occur

5.1.3   Aetiology

- Result of repeated excessive submaximal loading onto bones. This results in an imbalance between bone resorption and formation
- Role of intrinsic factors: e.g. hormonal factors may have a role in women (female athlete triad of amenorrhea, eating disorder and osteoporosis)
- Role of extrinsic factors: e.g. a sudden increase in the intensity, duration and frequency of physical exercise, especially in the absence of adequate periods of rest, has been found to cause an increase in osteoclast activity. The result may be bone formation lagging behind absorption

5.1.4   Histology

- Especially in high-risk stress fractures subjected to constant tensile forces, histology consists of only fibrous and granulation substances under the microscope
- Healing is more often expected to occur in non-high-risk locations

- Example: high-risk anterior cortex tibial stress fractures on microscopy usually consist of some local osteonecrosis and fibrous tissue with minimal or absent bone remodelling

5.1.5   Diagnosis
- Mainly clinical Dx
- Hx: typically, there is insidious onset of pain after a recent bout of intense exercise
- Physical examination: local tenderness/swelling if occurring in superficial bone, more differentials if presenting as pain in deep-seated bones, e.g. femoral neck
- Adjunctive investigations include: X-ray, bone scan, CT, MRI may help in confirming the Dx

5.1.6   Differential Diagnoses
- Stress reaction (bone still in continuity)
- Periostitis
- Exertional compartment syndrome (e.g. of the leg)
- Muscle sprain
- Avulsion injuries
- Sepsis
- Nerve entrapment
- Bursitis

5.1.7   Further Investigations
- X-ray: can be normal in the first 2–3 weeks. Periosteal reaction (Fig. 5.1) and cortical lucent lines may be seen in late cases
- Bone scan: much more sensitive and picks up Dx early. But non-specific as can be mimicked by stress reactions, etc. (differential diagnosis [DDx] of stress fractures from soft tissue injury as the former show increased activity in all three phases, the latter in the initial two phases)
- MRI: another option, higher specificity than bone scanning, but bone scanning is better in sites like the axial skeleton or pelvis

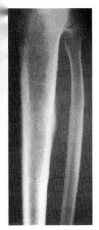

Fig. 5.1 Note the periosteal reaction at the proximal tibial shaft, subsequent bone scan confirms stress fracture in this athlete

5.1.8   Categories of Stress Fractures

- Low-risk group
- High-risk group: these are the ones that are prone to progress, and may displace or develop non-union. Owing to the high complication rate, high-risk categories of stress fracture should be treated in the same way as acute fractures

5.1.9   Common Sites of High-Risk Stress Fracture

- Tension side fracture of the femoral neck
- Anterior cortex tibia
- Medial malleolus
- Talus lateral process
- Fifth metatarsal diaphysis
- Navicular
- Patella
- Big toe sesamoid

5.1.10   Timeline for Healing of High-Risk Stress Fractures

- Healing of high-risk fractures can be slow

- Healing of displaced tension side femoral neck fractures, for instance, is slower than for acute fractures – may need as long as 3 months of protected weight-bearing

5.1.11 Treatment
- Low-risk stress fractures: most are treated conservatively, e.g. rest, activity modification, modify training programme, identify and treat predisposing factors such as nutritional and hormonal factors
- High-risk stress fracture: can still consider a period of protected weight-bearing in cast, except tension side fracture of the femoral neck. Otherwise operate

5.1.12 Surgical Indications
- Displaced stress fracture
- Stress fracture not responding to conservative treatment, especially high-demand athlete
- Chronic stress fracture with signs of chronicity on X-ray such as cystic changes, and intramedullary sclerosis

5.1.13 Prevention
- Proper coaching of athletes
- Proper exercise training protocol for professional and elite athletes
- Avoidance of sudden excessive repeated activities especially in non-athletes
- Proper nutritional and eating advice for female athletes

5.1.14 Stress Fractures in Different Body Regions
5.1.14.1 Femoral Neck
- An index of suspicion is needed since Dx not always straightforward since the hip is deep seated
- Most just present with weight-bearing hip pain, which increases with passive hip motion on exam
- Common predisposing factors include coxa vara, osteopaenia, and muscle fatigue

- Compression side stress fractures more common than tension side stress fractures
- If Dx not sure, consider MRI, or bone scan
- Some propose trying conservative Rn for compression-type fractures that mostly start at the inferior cortex of the femoral neck
- Tension side stress fractures are mostly treated operatively by urgent screw fixation and most fractures start at the superior cortex of the femoral neck since it may displace
- Non-weight-bearing should be initiated postoperatively since healing is slow

5.1.14.2 Patella

- Longitudinal or transverse stress fractures can occur in athletes although it is rare. One common DDx is bipartite patella
- Transverse fracture starts at the anterior patella surface since this is the area under high tensile stress from the pull of the patella tendon and quadriceps
- If left unrecognised, it may develop into complete fracture
- Early cases can only be picked up on bone scans
- May try conservative Rn, but fixation is needed if fracture is complete, especially in high-demand athletes

5.1.14.3 Tibia

- Common, reported in some series to account for half of all stress fractures
- Can occur on the compression side at the posteromedial cortex, or on the tension side at the anterior cortex. Tension side fractures more often associated with jumping or leaping sports
- Can either be longitudinal or transverse
- DDx: exertional compartment syndrome, medial tibial stress reaction, sepsis, tumours

5.1.14.3.1 Treatment

- Compression side fractures mostly respond to activity limitation and weight-relieving braces

- Tension side fractures, if early, can only be seen on bone scans or MRI. Only later can the typical v-shape defect be seen on X-ray
- Tension side fractures, if Dx early, can try conservative Rn. If no response, or if chronic changes already present on presentation like gap widening and local bone hypertrophy; fixation by IM device should be considered

5.1.14.4   Medial Malleolus

- Most occur at the junction between the medial malleolus and tibial plafond
- Most are vertical or nearly vertical, and most are in jumping athletes
- High risk of healing problem since under high shear
- Can be Dx by bone scan or MRI if not yet seen on X-ray
- Rn includes operative fixation ± BG if element of chronicity

5.1.14.5   Talus

- Rare. If occurring, usually at the lateral process
- Present with lateral ankle pain near sinus tarsi
- May be difficult to see on X-ray, CT may be required
- Most require a period of non-weight-bearing cast immobilisation

5.1.14.6   Navicular

- Mostly present as medial arch pain of the foot in sprinters
- More commonly located in the relatively less vascular mid third of the tarsal navicular
- Not easy to see on X-ray, may need CT
- If Dx early, NWB (non weight bearing) casting can be considered. Late presentation or fracture displacement needs fixation ± BG

5.1.14.7   Fifth Metatarsal

- Stress fractures can occur at proximal diaphysis
- Mostly present with pain at the lateral part of the foot
- May try a course of NWB casting, but have a low threshold for operative intervention since prone to non-union and re-fracture
- Delayed presentation cases may also need BG

5.1.14.8 *Big Toe Sesamoid*

- Stress fractures not common, but can occur with repetitive dorsiflexion of the great toe during running, with exacerbation of pain on foot push-off
- Increased tensile forces can cause transverse fracture
- Fracture of both sesamoids is rare, medial side more common
- For Dx use standard X-ray, a sesamoid view may be helpful ± bone scan
- DDx bipartite sesamoid
- If refractory to NWB casting, may need excision

5.2   Open Fractures

5.2.1   Introduction

- Incidence around 3%
- Incidence of higher Gustilo's grades of open fracture in countries with well-developed highways with more high-energy road traffic accidents, and in areas with more farm accidents since soil contamination automatically changes the open fracture to grade III
- Areas affected: most common are the tibia and phalanges of the hand

5.2.2   Gustilo's Classification

- Type I: wound clean, <1 cm
- Type II: wound >1 cm, no extensive soft tissue damage or avulsions
- Type III: includes cases of soil contamination, open segmental fractures, extensive soft tissue damage, traumatic amputation and gunshot injuries
  - IIIA: adequate periosteal cover
  - IIIB: periosteal stripping, contamination usual
  - IIIC: presence of arterial injury that needs repair

5.2.3   Goal of Treatment

- Prevention of infection at all costs – since infected non-union is very difficult to treat
- Restore function to the limb
- Healing of fracture in acceptable alignment
- Prevent clostridia myonecrosis especially in the presence of (soil) contamination

5.2.4   Principles of Treatment

- Adequate debridement
- Pulsatile lavage
- Antibiotic treatment
- Skeletal stabilisation
- Dead space management
- Management of bone defect
- Issues of soft tissue coverage

5.2.4.1 *Adequate Debridement*

- Our goal is to obtain a clean wound free of non-viable tissues and reduce the chance of infection
- Most require some wound extension to assess the maximum extent of the injury (the Gustilo's classification assigned may change on careful exploration)
- All necrotic and avascular tissues are debrided, but large articular fragments are retained usually
- Newer methods of vacuum-assisted debridement by the use of Venturi principle may be helpful
- A second-look operation is the norm within 48–72 h, especially in type III open fractures

5.2.4.2 *Pulsatile Lavage*

- Adequate irrigation is important since the solution to pollution is dilution
- To be effective, copious volumes of lavage needed, say between 8–12 l

■ But the merits and demerits of pulsatile lavage under pressure are:
  — Pros: helps decrease the rate of infection
  — Cons: added soft tissue injury, driving contaminated material to other tissue planes, effect on bone healing, topical antibiotics in fluid can be toxic to local tissues

5.2.4.3 Antibiotic Treatment

■ Study on infection rates published in 1974 by Patzakis:
  — 13.9% infection in patients who received no antibiotics
  — 9.7% in patients who received penicillin
  — 2.3% in patients who received cephalothin (Keflin)
■ Recommended antibiotic regime:
  — Cephalosporin (with an aminoglycoside in 3B open fractures)
  — Synthetic penicillin (with an aminoglycoside)
  — Penicillin should be added to above combinations in farm injuries

5.2.4.3.1 Role of Wound Cultures

■ Usefulness of initial wound cultures has been controversial
■ Previous retrospective studies have often failed to identify the causative organism

5.2.4.3.2 Timing for Giving Antibiotics

■ Antibiotics should be commenced immediately
■ There is evidence to suggest an increased infection rate if started > 3 h (Clin Orthop Relat Res 1989)
■ The successful use of local antibiotic impregnated beads has been reported and this difference reached statistical significance in the difficult type III fracture (J Bone Joint Surg Br 1995). An added advantage of polymethyl methacrylate (PMMA) beads is that they can aid in closing any dead space

5.2.4.4 Skeletal Stabilisation

■ Early skeletal stabilisation is part of our strategy for prevention of infection

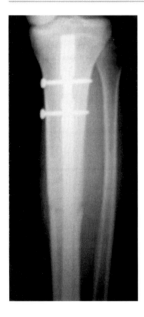

Fig. 5.2 Unreamed tibial nails as shown have few advantages over reamed nails, except arguably in some type III open fractures

- Even in the setting of low-grade sepsis, maintenance of fracture stability is essential as has been shown in experiments in the past
- IM nailing has been shown to be effective by Court-Brown for open fractured tibia up to Type IIIA, whether unreamed nails have an advantage in type III open fractures is subject to debate (Fig. 5.2). If used, a period of protected weight-bearing is needed to avoid premature failure of locking bolts
- Type IIIB and C cases mostly need EF (although some of these patients may even need amputation)
- Use of plating can be considered for open forearm fractures if the bed is not heavily contaminated

5.2.4.5 Dead Space Management
- One should prevent the formation and fill up deep spaces in our management of open fractures (especially those showing early signs of infection) to prevent the collection of sero-purulent material

- In infected beds, use of topical antibiotic beads and bead pouch is advisable and has been shown to be of help in the management of infected open fractures

5.2.4.6 Management of Bone Defects
- Management of bone defects was discussed in Chap. 3

5.2.4.6.1 Secondary Procedures to Stimulate Healing
- Early bone grafting can be considered in the presence of bone defects or delayed healing
- Timing of bone grafting in the presence of bone defects is 4–6 weeks, and usually after proper soft tissue coverage. Grafting for delayed union is usually done around 8–12 weeks
- A wait of a few weeks for BG after soft tissue reconstruction is a prudent way to ensure no active on-going sepsis, which, if present, will make BG procedures futile

5.2.4.7 Timing of Wound Closure in Open Fractures
- There are merits and demerits of early closure
- Pros: no need for second delayed operation
- Cons: possible retained necrotic tissue, borderline vascularity tissues may turn necrotic given time, chance of infection higher in presence of necrotic tissue

5.2.4.7.1 Conclusion on Time for Wound Closure
- The optimal time remains controversial
- Early closure is contraindicated in the face of heavy contamination and soft tissue degloving
- Even in more stable wounds, many require a second look for further debridement
- The results of an on-going prospective randomised trial on timing of wound closure is eagerly awaited

5.2.4.8 Issues of Soft Tissue Coverage
- Discussed in Chap. 2

5.2.4.8.1 Average Healing Time with Rn (After Court-Brown)

- Type I: 14 weeks
- Type II: 24 weeks
- Type IIIA: 27 weeks
- Type IIIB: 38 weeks
- Type IIIC: 74 weeks

5.3   Periprosthetic Fractures Around Total Joint Replacements

5.3.1   Risk Factors

- Rheumatoid arthritis
- Osteopaenia
- Osteolysis (Fig. 5.3)
- Anatomic: e.g. anterior notching of the femur
- Mechanical: e.g. presence of stress risers
- Others: advanced age, steroids, etc.

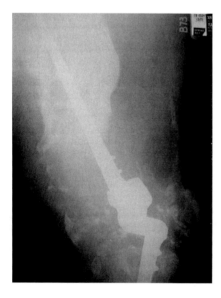

Fig. 5.3 Marked osteolysis will definitely predispose the bone to fractures

.3.2 Key Principle

- Key: prevention is most important

.3.2.1 Prevention of Periprosthetic Fractures in Primary THR (Acetabular Side)

- Avoid under ream > 2 mm, even in strong bone, by using the cementless cup
- Advise line to line reaming in osteoporotic bones if fixation with cementless cup planned, may add on screws for better hold
- Avoid force in hammering the cementless cup

.3.2.2 Prevention of Periprosthetic Fractures in Primary THR (Femoral Side)

- If previous plates/screws present, avoid their removal before hip dislocation
- Avoid excess force during hip dislocation
- Bypass stress risers with long stems extending at least two times diameter of femoral shaft beyond the stress riser (if not long enough, add cerclage)

.3.2.3 Prevention of Periprosthetic Fractures in Revision THR

- Avoid excess reaming in the weakened bone
- Have preoperative plan to tackle bone defects
- Avoid force in inserting the cementless cup
- Opening a window may help removal of a cemented component
- Well-fixed cementless stems may need to split femur before it can be removed
- X-ray guidance sometimes needed to guide against eccentric reaming of medullary cavity
- All stress risers need autograft, but structural grafts may be required if large

5.3.2.4 Prevention of Periprosthetic Fractures in Primary TKR

- Avoid anterior notching by using anterior referencing instrumentation

- Avoid forceful drawing of the tibia, can consider cutting the poster ior femoral condyle first
- Remove old implants (like blade plates) a few months before, to al low healing of defect, or if removed intraoperatively, then conside long stem
- In posterior-stabilised TKR, avoid eccentric cut of the inter-condyla box
- Avoid forceful patella eversion, in difficult cases consider rectus snip tibial tubercle osteotomy, or quads turn-down
- Avoid eccentric reaming of femoral canal during IM guide insertion

5.3.2.5 Prevention of Periprosthetic Fractures in Revision TKR

- Use long femoral stem to bypass not only stress risers, but areas o bone weakened by osteolysis
- X-ray can be considered as a guide to prevent eccentric reaming o medullary canal
- Avoid everting the patella by force

5.3.3   Periprosthetic Acetabular Fractures Around THR

- Incidence said to be low, but in fact many undisplaced fractures ma go unnoticed especially in the setting of cementless THR
- Incidence rising with the increased popularity of cementless acet abular components in THR

5.3.3.1 Aetiology

- Technical causes: e.g. over-reaming of the medial acetabular wall over-zealous hammering of press-fit acetabular components
- Implant-related causes: more in cementless THR
- Related to local bone anatomy/biomechanics: presence of stress ris ers or bone defects predispose to fractures and may affect the type o fracture that occurs
- Related to local bone quality: RA, osteoporosis, osteolysis, etc.

5.3.3.2 Classification

- Type 1: stable acetabular component

- Type 2: unstable acetabular component

(May look very simple, but reported in respectable papers, e.g. from Mayo by Lewallen et al.)

(In general, need to consider type of fracture – whether the wall or column involved, concomitant bone defects and bone stock in decision-making)

5.3.3.3 Treatment of Different Scenarios

- Intraoperatively, stable component, wall involved: screw/buttress wall, augments for cup
- Intraoperatively, stable component, column affected: buttress plating for column, augment cup
- Postoperatively, stable implant, minimally displaced fracture: mostly conservative, touch-down weight-bearing (TDW)
- Postoperatively, stable implant, displaced fracture: likely to need ORIF ± BG
- Intraoperatively, unstable component, wall involved: buttress plating
- Intraoperatively, unstable component, fracture column: buttress plating for column ± lag screw p.r.n. if other column lag screw
- Postoperatively, unstable implant, undisplaced fracture: revise component, BG + internal fixation (IF)
- Postoperatively, unstable implant, displaced fracture: revise component + may need acetabular roof reinforcement/BG/IF

5.3.4 Periprosthetic Femoral Fractures Around THR

- Incidence 0.5–1%, 3–5-fold in revision THR
- Rising trend

5.3.4.1 Aetiology

- Technical causes: e.g. excessive hammering of press-fit stems, eccentric reaming
- Implant-related causes: more in cementless THR
- Related to local anatomy/biomechanics: local femoral deformity, local stress risers

■ Related to bone quality: RA, osteoporosis, osteolysis, neuromuscular weakness

5.3.4.2 Vancouver Classification

■ Type A: at inter-trochanteric region (Figs. 5.4, 5.5): AG – involves greater trochanter; AL – involves less trochanter
■ Type B: at/distal to the stem
  – B1 – implant not loose
  – B2 – implant loose (Fig. 5.6)
  – B3 – B2 + poor bone stock
■ Type C: below the stem

5.3.4.3 Treatment

■ Type A:
  – Most are not displaced and are treated conservatively
  – Fix displaced, sizeably greater trochanter fracture
■ Type B treatment:
  – B1: options include cable/wiring, screw–plate construct ± onlay struts ± autograft

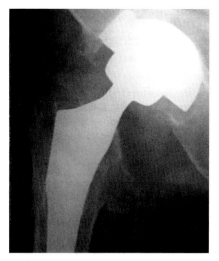

Fig. 5.4 Note periprosthetic fracture in the inter-trochanteric region of this well-fixed THR

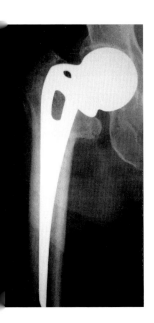

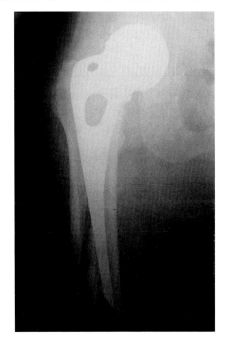

Fig. 5.5 Fracture in the inter-tro-chanteric region occurred in this subsided (and probably unstable) Moore's prosthesis

Fig. 5.6 This periprosthetic fracture occurs in a lower region just stopping short of the stem tip

- B2: long-stem revision THR ± IF (cementless long stem more common than cemented stems)
- B3: allograft/prosthesis composite, proximal femoral replacement prosthesis, etc.

■ Type C treatment: plate–screw construct ± cables (Fig. 5.7) ± strut grafting

5.3.5   Supracondylar Periprosthetic Fractures Around TKR

■ Incidence: 0.5%, but 5-fold in revision TKR
■ A rising trend

5.3.5.1 Aetiology

- Technical causes: anterior notching, hammering in press-fit stems
- Implant-related causes or predisposition: posterior stabilised implants with need to cut a large inter-condylar box
- Related to local anatomy/biomechanics: bony deformity of the femur, local stress risers
- Related to bone quality: RA, osteoporosis, osteolysis, poor knee/hip ROM

5.3.5.2 Classification: Rorabeck (1999)

- Type A: fracture undisplaced, implant not loose
- Type B: fracture displaced, implant not loose
- Type C: fracture undisplaced, implant loose
- Type D: fracture displaced, implant loose

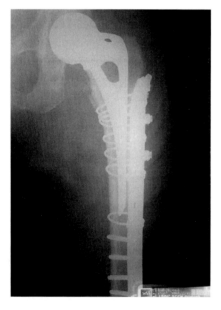

Fig. 5.7 Cables are very useful adjuncts to plates in revision fixation of periprosthetic fractures of the proximal femur

.3.5.3 Treatment

- Type A: common, treat with screws
- Type B: IM rod (Fig. 5.8) preferred unless the femoral component not spacious enough or fracture too distal. If very distal and/or osteoporotic consider LISS
- Type C: revision TKR (e.g. long-stem ± BG ± IF)
- Type D: revision TKR (e.g. long-stem ± BG ± IF)

(Goal: fracture healing with > 90° ROM, < 2 cm shortening, < 5° varus/valgus, < 10° sagittal malalignment and no pain)

5.3.5.4 Advantage of LISS in Supracondylar Fractures Around TKR

- Fixed angle screws give optimal fixation around the femoral fixation
- Less soft tissue dissection
- Lowered sepsis – minimal fracture exposure
- Less use of BG

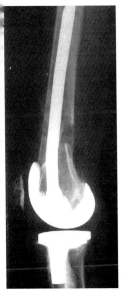

Fig. 5.8 The DFN is useful in fixing common supracondylar-type periprosthetic distal femur fractures

5.3.5.5 Disadvantages of LISS for Supracondylar Fractures Around TKR

- Reduction difficulties of the metaphyseal diaphyseal component of the fracture and difficulty in optimal plate placement
- Loss of distal fixation and/or toggling of distal screws can lead to varus angulation and fracture fixation failure

5.3.5.6 Comparison of Distal Femur Nail Versus LISS

- Not all TKR femoral components can accommodate distal femur nail (DFN)
- LISS is possibly better in patients with marked osteoporosis since it provides a larger contact surface area between the implant and the cancellous bone than does DFN (even with spiral blade insertion). Essentially, the multiple fixed angle screws are like multiple fixed angle devices

5.3.5.7 Pearls

- Many cases need elaborate preoperative planning. Need also to assess position of cement mantle, evidence of implant loosening, bone stock
- Suggest at least four screws to be placed proximally and distally to the fracture if significant osteoporosis

5.3.6 Fractured Proximal Tibia Around TKR

- Incidence: rare, only 0.5%
- May see a rise in future as the number of revision TKR increases

5.3.6.1 Aetiology

- Technical causes: hammering too heavily, eccentric reaming, etc.
- Implant-related causes: more with cementless implants, hinges, long-stem components
- Related to local biomechanics: malalignment, presence of stress risers
- Related to quality of bone: RA, osteoporosis, osteolysis, neuromuscular weakness

5.3.6.2 Classification: Felix (1997)

- Type 1: fractured tibial plateau – 1A (not loose), 1B (loose), 1C (intra-operatively)
- Type 2: fractured meta-diaphyses – 2A (not loose), 2B (loose), 2C (intraoperative)
- Type 3: fracture shaft below tibial component – 3A (not loose), 3B (loose), 3C (intraoperative)
- Type 4: disrupted extensor mechanics

5.3.6.3 Treatment of Type 1

- Type 1A: mostly conservative
- Type 1B: revision with long-stem tibial component and manage bone defects (wedges, grafted, or use cement)
- Type 1C: change intraoperative to long stem and fix the fracture anatomically

5.3.6.4 Treatment of Type 2

- Type 2A: displaced fractures need ORIF, for undisplaced may try casting, but elderly tolerate this poorly
- Type 2B: revise with a long stem and bone grafting in most cases
- Type 2C: most require ORIF

5.3.6.5 Treatment of Type 3

- Type 3A: most require ORIF
- Type 3B: rare, consider revision
- Type 3C: rare, may need options like long stem, and/or internal fixation
- Type 4: tension band wiring needed for fixing the tibial tubercle

5.3.7 Patella Fractures and TKR

- Incidence: 0.3% in resurfaced patella
- Can be higher than this figure with certain types of patella implant, e.g. related to the implant peg design

5.3.7.1 Aetiology
- Technical causes, e.g. excessive lateral release devascularising the patella, patella too thin
- Implant related (just mentioned)
- Related to bone quality, e.g. RA, osteoporosis

5.3.7.2 Classification: Goldberg (1988)
- Type 1: fracture not extended to implant interface, intact extensor mechanism
- Type 2: either fracture extension to implant interface, or disrupted extensor mechanism
- Type 3: fractured inferior pole: either with (3A) or without (3B) rupture of patella tendon
- Type 4: patella dislocated

5.3.7.3 Treatment
- Mostly conservative Rn
- Consider surgery if loosening or loss of extensor mechanism

5.4   Pathologic Fractures (Fig. 5.9)

5.4.1   Introduction
- In this section, we are mainly describing pathological fractures due to tumour deposits in bones
- Although in the strict sense, osteoporotic fractures are a form of pathological fracture (in fact they come under the heading of metabolic bone disease), the management of this large category of fracture will be discussed separately

5.4.2   Goal of Surgery for Pathological Fractures
- Relieve pain
- Improve function – usually ADL or ambulation
- Painless fractures in terminal patients especially of the upper extremities do not always need surgery

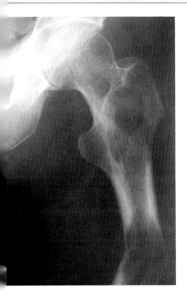

Fig. 5.9 Many pathological fractures such as this one occur in the highly stressed subtrochanteric region

5.4.3 Who Should Receive Prophylactic Surgery to Prevent Pathological Fracture? (Fig. 5.10)

- Traditional guidelines:
  - ≥ 2.5-cm bony lesion
  - ≥ 50% bony cortex involved
  - Especially if tumour is radio-resistant
- Newer popular guideline: Mirel's Score

5.4.4 Mirel's Score

- Based on calculation of scores. Scores are assigned to four parameters as follows:
  - Site of lesion: UL (1 point); LL (2 points); pertrochanteric (3 points)
  - Pain level: mild (1 point); moderate (2 points); persistent, affecting function (3 points)
  - Nature of lesion: blastic/scelerotic (1 point); mixed (2 points); lytic type (3 points)

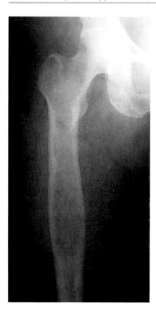

Fig. 5.10 Mirel's scoring aids our decision-making regarding whether to fix, for instance, long bones at risk of fracture

- Lesion size: <one-third circumference (1 point); between one-third–two-thirds (2 points); >two-thirds diameter (3 points)
- Total score: ≥ 9 points, consideration of prophylactic surgery

5.4.5   Before Proceeding Ask Yourself
- How sure are we it is a metastatic lesion?
- Is it an unknown primary?
- Better characterise the pathologic fracture by noting – whether the Dx is clinical vs radiological (any displacement, symptoms, ± infected)

5.4.6   General Work-up
- Before operation: if possible, better define the local patho-anatomy – skin, neurovascular status, joint, bone stock, fracture personality
- Define our goal, whether curative (e.g. amputation vs limb salvage in, say, pathologic fractures that are Cx of primary osteogenic sarcoma)

or palliative (e.g. pathological fractures in patients who already have multiple metastases)

- If major reconstruction planned, approach must be extensile; pre-operatively cooperate with oncologist on tackling of residual microscopic disease (e.g. adjuvant chemo- or radiotherapy) and plan ahead for skin and soft tissue coverage. Assess need for frozen section documentation

5.4.7 What Are the Surgical Principles?

- We must assume:
  - The fracture being involved by abnormal cells may not have the potential to heal
  - We need to assume the occurrence of abnormal deposits in the rest of the affected bone either currently or at a given time
- In view of above:
  - A surgical option should be selected that has low risk of failure – usually implies prosthetic replacement in peri-articular region, or a strong intramedullary device (such as a long cephalomedullary IM nail, say, in the case of a typical subtrochanteric fracture)
  - In the case of LL fractures especially, early mobilisation and ambulation should be allowed

5.4.8 What Are the Determining Factors if Multiple Options Exist?

- Disease factor, e.g. prognosis according to the opinion of the oncologist, the expected response of the disease to radiotherapy (RT) and chemotherapy (CT)
- Facility factors, e.g. availability of implants
- Surgeon factors, e.g. personal experience with the different surgical options
- Patient factors, e.g. whether medical co-morbidities contraindicate surgery, and his or her own personality

5.4.9 Approach to Pathological Fractures by Regions

- Fractured proximal humerus: options include prosthetic replacement with long stems, or long plates ± cementation if voids exist

- Fractured shaft of humerus: options include IM nailing spanning the whole humerus, avoid retrograde nail if deposits near elbow. If peri-articular regions affected by tumour hindering locking, consider plates ± cementation of voids
- Fractured distal humerus: options include plate fixation ± cementation for voids, even arthroplasty if bone stock poor
- Fractured femoral neck: prosthetic replacement is the mainstay, cannulated screws not recommended since assume fracture will not heal. If acetabular side eroded, may need THR
- Inter-trochanteric hip fractures: either a long IM device (e.g. Russell Taylor, long Gamma); or in difficult cases proximal femoral replacement. The usual DHS ± cementation may not hold out for a long time, but still an option since limited life expectancy
- Subtrochanteric hip fractures: most need a strong IM device like a Russell Taylor or long Gamma nail (Fig. 5.11). Proximal femoral replacement as a last resort

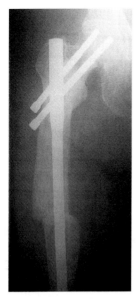

Fig. 5.11 Cephalomedullary nailing is useful in fixing pathological femur fractures

- Femoral shaft fractures: locked cephalomedullary nail is commonly used. Avoid retrograde nails. Rarely, inter-calary prosthesis if defect is large
- Distal femur fractures: either select plating with ± cementation or retrograde nailing reaching the region of the lesser trochanter and making sure there are no hip deposits. Another option is prosthetic replacement. (As a last resort, either total femoral replacement or amputation have been reported in patients with deposits spanning the whole femur especially if radio-resistant and chemo-resistant with intractable symptoms)

5.4.10 Main Determinants of Outcome

- Bone biology = biology and mechanics of diseased bone
- Pathology = natural history of disease progression and the effects of treatment on the tumour
- Function = assess whether the fracture altered the patient's activity level and lifestyle and can surgery improve it

5.4.11 Principal Reasons for Failure of Operation

- Prolonged immobilisation with non-operative treatment and fracture not healing – healing likelihood depends on histology, response to adjuncts like RT, etc.
- Hardware fails since construct relies on fracture healing – choose construct not relying on fracture healing, and stable enough for full weight-bearing, or endoprosthesis
- Early failed fixation from poor bone stock – inspect bone stock on either side of lesion (if it was a periprosthetic fracture) prior to surgery
- Early failure due to tumour recurrence – especially if RT/CT-resistant. – sometimes a primary resection (such as amputation) may even be less morbid > a failed fixation in a radiated field
- Protect the whole bone – weary of any additional metastases
- Use the most rigid implant available

(P.S. Those with UL fractures only, since not weight-bearing, more options will be available)

5.5   Osteoporotic Fractures (Fig. 5.12)

5.5.1   Introduction

- Osteoporotic bone has no impairment of its capacity for fracture healing
- The main problem in the past in operating on patients with osteoporotic fractures centred on the fixation of the implant to the bone

5.5.2   Epidemiology

- In one recent survey, the annual incidence of fragility fractures in USA:
  - Vertebral fractures 700,000
  - Hip fractures 300,000
  - Wrist fractures 250,000
  - Others 250,000

5.5.3   Key Principle

- It is increasingly being realised that any fragility fracture represents a risk factor for the development of other fragility fractures. In other words, the occurrence of a fragility fracture, be it at the wrist, hip, etc., warrants active measures of treatment for osteoporosis and prevention of further fracture

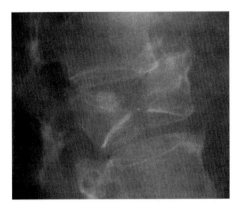

Fig. 5.12 Osteoporotic fractures are on the rise, of which vertebra fractures are very commonly seen

5.5.4   Role of Prevention

- Prevention is always better than cure
- To prevent fragility fractures, strategies include:
  - Fall prevention programme (see Chap. 15)
  - Education of the general public
  - Prevention and treatment of osteoporosis (discussed in detail in the companion volume of this book)
  - Adequate nutrition and exercises like Tai Chi are essential components of primary prevention
  - Other measures, e.g. use of hip protectors

5.5.5   Key Determinants of Future Fragility Fractures

- Age
- History of fragility fractures
- Bone mineral density

(There are of course other factors that may come into play, e.g. question of bone geometry and femoral neck length in the case of hip fractures; but the above are the three major factors)

5.5.6   Main Strategies to Tackle Osteoporotic Fractures

- Measures to improve the hold of the implant–bone interface interactions
- Increase surface area of the interface
- Use of implants with better mechanical advantage such as intramedullary nails
- Decrease the porosity of the fragile bone by introduction of foreign material
- By replacing the (frequently comminuted fracture) with a prosthesis
- Improvement in implant design

5.5.6.1   *Improving the Bone–Implant Interface Interactions*

- We take the bone–screw interface as an example in this discussion
- Hydroxyapatite coating, for instance, has been in use to decrease the chance of early screw loosening in osteoporotic bones. Examples of its use include coating of Schanz screws in EF, and hydroxyapatite coating of pedicle screws in fixation of the axial skeleton

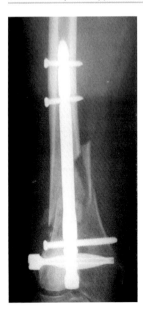

Fig. 5.13 The invention of the spiral blade not only has the advantages as mentioned in the text, but it is easier to revise should implant failure occur since it is bone-preserving

5.5.6.2 Increase the Surface Area of the Interface

- This is best exemplified by the development of the novel locking systems such as the spiral blades (Fig. 5.13) to replace standard locking bolts to increase the surface area of contact and hold of the implant–bone interface

5.5.6.3 Use of Implants with Better Mechanical Advantage

- This is best exemplified by the increased use of intra-medullary devices in the proximal femur fracture, especially those with unstable fracture patterns (e.g. use of Gamma nails, proximal femoral nail (PFN), intramedullary hip screw [IMHS])
- This move is because the IM nails have a better mechanical advantage and is ideal if the fracture is under high bending stresses such as the subtrochanteric region, etc.

5.5.6.4 Decrease the Porosity of the Fragile Bone by the Introduction of Foreign Material

- This is best exemplified by the currently very popular procedures of vertebroplasty and kyphoplasty for fragility wedge compression fractures of the axial skeleton
- This method has found application elsewhere, e.g. injection of Norian skeletal repair system (SRS) in the case of distal radius fractures, injection of cement in fixation of peri-trochanteric hip fractures

5.5.6.5 By Replacing the (Frequently Comminuted) Fracture with a Prosthesis

- Joint replacement in the form of hemi-arthroplasty or total joint replacement has found a place in comminuted peri-articular fractures both in the hip (e.g. THR in fractured acetabulum), around the knee (e.g. tibial plateau fractures), as well as the shoulder (e.g. three- or four-part fragility fractures) and elbow (e.g. comminuted low distal humerus fragility fractures)

5.5.6.6 Improvement in Implant Design

- This is best exemplified by the new locking compression plate systems (LCP), which are especially good in tackling peri-articular fragility fractures by dint of its angular stability and its increased pull-out strength
- A detailed discussion of LCP was presented in Chap. 4

5.5.7 Causes of Fracture Fixation Failure

- Loss of bone mass
- Significant mismatch between the modulus of elasticity of the implant and the osteoporotic bone
- Inability of the elderly to tolerate protected weight-bearing
- General tendency to fall

5.5.8 Relevant Biomechanics

- Bone is like a stiff spring. It deforms under load and regains the original form when unloaded

- The implant for fracture fixation and the bone differ in their moduli of elasticity, thus the presence of an implant distorts this phenomenon to a certain extent
- Thus, in theory at least, a pedicle screw made of titanium may have less tendency to loosen because of less mismatch or discrepancy between the moduli of elasticity with respect to bone
- Implants that rely on the holding power of screws in bone are dependent on the material properties of the bone, in a different manner from implants that achieve their structural stability by locking bolts, such as reamed nails. This holding power of screws is correlated in linear fashion to loss of bone mass
- In plate osteosynthesis of long bones, the stability of the fracture depends on friction between the cortical bone surface and the plate, generated by the hold of the screws. The stress in the implant–bone construct in fragile bones is high, and the holding power of the screws is low and cut-out with subsequent implant loosening is likely. Also, progressive instability can affect fracture healing
- In the case of IM nailing, when the implant–bone construct is stressed, it may temporarily be slightly deformed without jeopardising the function of the inter-locking bolts and the integrity of the construct
- The cortical hold of the bolts is not primarily responsible for stability of the osteosynthesis. The negative effect of the instability also has less effect on bone healing
- In the case of the EF, the EF acts as a bridging function. The fixator pins no longer function as screws, and thus the pull-out strength of the pins is not the primary problem
- The framework that the EF creates with the bone becomes an intrinsically stable system. Here again, a certain degree of instability no longer endangers the fixation, and may favour bone healing
- The downside, however, includes pin track infection, bulkiness of the EF, etc.

5.5.9 Strategies to Improve Fixation

- The intrinsic stability of the bone–implant construct may be increased by angular-stable devices such as the traditional AO angle blade plate and the newer LCP and LISS plates from the AO group
- Unlike the LCP and other new locked internal fixators, the traditional AO angle blade can still fail, but screws loosen and cut out from the osteoporotic bone
- In fact, the strategy of locking the screws to the plate is not entirely new. The old problem of loss of fixation of the screws in anterior cervical spinal plating was solved by locking the screws to the plate
- Subsequent reports of introduction of similar device known as "Schulis" also works on the principle of angular stability

5.5.10 Summary

- The newer devices are not quite dependent on the holding power of screws alone, but on the mechanical stability of the bone–implant construct
- Also, changing the characteristics of the cortical screw by increasing the core diameter and changing the pitch of the threads added to decreased reliance on the holding power of the screws on the (osteoporotic) bone

5.5.11 Prevention

- Prophylaxis and treatment of osteoporosis (covered in detail in the companion volume published by the author: *Orthopaedic Principles – A Resident's Guide*)
- Fall Prevention Programme – for secondary and primary prevention. Discussed in detail in Chap. 15 of this book

General Bibliography

1. Callaghan J, Rosenberg A, Rubash H (1998) The adult hip, vols 1 and 2. Lippincott Williams & Wilkins, Philadelphia
2. Insall J, Scott N (2001) Surgery of the knee, vols 1 and 2, 3rd edn. Churchill Livingstone, New York

Selected Bibliography of Journal Articles

1. Gliatis J, Panagiotopoulos E, et al. (2005) Midterm results of treatment with a retrograde nail for supracondylar periprosthetic fractures of the femur following total knee arthroplasty. J Orthop Trauma 19(3):164–170

2. Gosselin RA, Gillespie WJ, et al. (2004) Antibiotics for preventing infection in open limb fractures. Cochrane Database Syst Rev CD003764

3. Kruzic JJ, Scott JA, et al. (2005) Propagation of surface fatigue cracks in human cortical bone. J Biomech http://dx.doi.org/10.1016/j.jbiomech.2005.01.025

4. Parivizi J, Hozack WJ (2004) Treatment protocol for proximal femoral periprosthetic fractures. J Bone Joint Surg Am 86 [Suppl 2]:8–16

5. Templeman DC, Gustilo RB, et al. (1998) Update on the management of open fractures of the tibial shaft. Clin Orthop Relat Res 350:18–25

6. Tharani R, Vince KG, et al. (2005) Periprosthetic fracture after total knee arthroplasty. J Arthroplasty 20 (4)[Suppl 2]:27–32

7. Tornetta P III, Bergman M, et al. (1994) Treatment of grade IIIB open tibial fractures: a prospective randomized comparison of external fixation and non-reamed locked nailing. J Bone Joint Surg Br 76:13–19

8. Wolf RE, Enneking WF (1996) The staging and surgery of musculoskeletal neoplasms. Orthop Clin North Am 27:473–481

Contents

5.1   Definition of Osteoporosis

- Osteoporosis is a systemic skeletal disease characterised by low bone mass and micro-architectural deterioration of bone tissue, leading to enhanced bone fragility and a consequent increase in fracture risk (WHO Definition 1994)
- It is well known that the traditional definition of osteoporosis by the WHO involves a T-score of < -2.5

6.2   Explanation of the T-Score

- T-score:
  - Named after a researcher working in the field of densitometry
  - T-score calculation: {(patient BMD) – (mean young adult BMD)/ 1 SD of young adult BMD}

6.3   Further T-Score Elaboration

- It is clear from examining the formula for calculating T-scores that the result is dependent on the mean and standard deviation (SD) of the reference population, and that changes in these values can change the T-score, even when the patient's BMD is the same. T-scores are used for diagnostic classification in postmenopausal women and men aged 50 or more

6.4   Viewing the WHO Definition in the Correct Perspective

- To ease understanding, the definition can be re-phrased as follows: osteoporosis represents a disease affecting the bony skeleton and is characterised by increased ease of fracture even with low-energy trauma, caused either by low bone density, or deterioration of micro architecture or both

- This elaboration is important because low BMD according to traditional WHO criteria (T-score –2.5) is not always present in patients with fragility fractures; in some cases it is the bony quality that is mainly at fault. In the past, there has been excessive emphasis on the BMD, which is essentially a number, and the WHO is now correcting this old concept by re-emphasising the importance of risk (especially absolute risk) calculation (Iki 2007)
- Remember we just highlighted the fact that osteoporosis can result from alteration in bone quality or bone mass or both; not every patient with a fragility fracture has a T-score < –2.5
- This has led some experts to propose: in the presence of a fragility fracture, a clinical diagnosis of osteoporosis may be made independently of BMD, provided that other causes of fracture have been ruled out

6.5   Normal Versus Abnormal Bone Turnover and Maintenance of the Skeleton

- Bone resorption and formation are linked to preserving the skeleton: the molecular mechanism of the coupling of resorption and formation is under the control of three proteins involved in the TNF (tumour necrosis factor) signalling pathway
- These include two membrane-bound cytokine-like molecules called RANK (receptor activation of nuclear factor – KB), which is found on the pre-osteoclast cell membrane, and the RANK ligand, produced by osteoblasts, together with a secreted glycoprotein called osteoprotegerin (OPG), also produced by osteoblasts
- RANK and the RANK ligand bind with high affinity: this interaction with M-CSF (macrophage-colony stimulating factor) is sufficient for osteoclastogenesis. Osteoprotegerin (OPG) is a potent inhibitor of osteoclastogenesis that is also produced by osteoblasts and binds to the RANK ligand as a decoy, blocking RANK/RANK ligand interaction. Under-expression causes severe osteoporosis in mice

- One tenth of the human skeleton is remodelled every year; thus, in 10 years the entire skeleton can be replaced. Bone remodelling occurs in discreet foci in bone. Remodelling occurs in a stereotyped sequence at each site with activation and resorption preceding formation, the entire sequence taking about 4 months in adult humans

6.5.1 Scenario 1: Normal Bone Turnover

- If bone formation equals bone resorption, at an instantaneous point in time, there is transient increased porosity in bone. This is potentially reversible bone loss, since over time these cavities can be eventually filled back up with bone leading to no net bone loss

6.5.2 Scenario 2: High Bone Turnover

- High turnover state can be caused by increased resorption, decreased formation or both. Examples of increased absorption include calcium and vitamin D insufficiency with occult secondary hyperparathyroidism, or caused by secondary causes of osteoporosis like hyperthyroidism, steroids, etc. Post-menopausal state can cause a decrease in formation due to dwindling female sex hormones

6.5.3 Scenario 3: Low Bone Turnover

- It is well known that bisphosphonates work by suppression of bone resorption (anti-resorptive) and markers of bone turnover like NTX decrease with its use. One disadvantage of prolonged bisphosphonate use is over-suppression of bone remodelling, causing the bone to be more brittle ± slow accumulation of micro-damage
- An example of a disease state with greatly decreased bone turnover is osteopetrosis

6.6 Latest WHO Fracture Risk Assessment Tool (WHO-FRAT) to Help Compute 10-Year Fracture Risk

- Age
- Gender

- Prior fragility fracture (> age 50)
- Low BMD
- Parental Hx of fracture
- Low BMI
- Smoking and alcohol intake
- Past steroid use
- Secondary causes

6.7   Risk Factors Seen from the Correct Perspective

- Most experts agree that of all the risk factors listed by the WHO, three emerge as the most important:
  - Prior fragility fracture
  - Advanced Age
  - Low BMD
- However, to make the picture complete, risk of (particularly hip) fracture also depends very much on the risk of falls, especially in the elderly presenting with fractures around the eighth decade of life

6.7.1   Important Role of Previous Fragility Fractures

- The concept that fragility fractures predict further fragility fractures should be borne in mind
- Research in the past showed that in general, an index fragility fracture at least increases the future chance of fragility fractures at least 2-fold, e.g. index hip fracture increases future hip fracture 2.3-fold, future spine fracture 2.5-fold and future forearm fracture 1.4-fold (Klotzbuecher et al. 2000)
- Whereas an index spine fracture increases future spine fracture up to 4.4-fold, future hip fracture 2.3-fold and future forearm fracture 1.4-fold (Klotzbuecher et al. 2000)
- Similar meta-analysis of previous fractures and subsequent fracture risk was reported by Kanis et al. (2004)

7.2 Important Role of Age

- Ten-year probabilities of hip fracture were computed in men and women at 10-year intervals from the age of 50 years and lifetime risks at the age of 50 years from the hazard functions of hip fracture and death (Kanis 2001)

- A recent study from the Royal Infirmary of Edinburgh revealed that the incidence of re-fracture rises very sharply after around the eighth decade in a follow-up study of patients admitted from 1988 to 1999 (Robinson et al. 2002)

7.3 Important Role of BMD

- For every 1.0 SD decrease in T-score the fracture risk in postmenopausal women approximately doubles. Other clinical risk factors, especially age and history of fragility fracture, also contribute to the risk of future fractures

6.8 Concepts of Relative Versus Absolute Risk

- It is important to differentiate between relative and absolute risk in risk calculation

- This is easier to understand if we look at standard published tables containing the 10-year probability of fragility fracture with relative and absolute fracture risk, together with corresponding T-score and age such as by Kanis in J Bone Min Res 2001. Thus, given the same age, the relative risk of future fracture increases as the T-score decreases from 0 to –2.0. However, the absolute risk of future fracture increases markedly given the same T-score of, say, –2.0 for a 70-year-old lady relative to a much younger 50-year-old lady (absolute risk 5.3% vs. 1.1% only for the younger lady)

6.8.1 Examples of Relative Risk for Hip Fracture in White Women

BMD T-score < –4.5	15.0 (RR value)
BMD T-score < –2.5	4.5

Maternal hip fracture < 80 years	2.7
Previous wrist fracture	1.9
Previous spine fracture	1.9
Current smoker	2.1
Inability to arise from chair	2.1
Use of anticonvulsants	2.1

6.8.2   Key Concept

■ It is important to realise that the absolute benefit of our treatment to patients with fragility fractures depends mainly on the reduction of the *absolute* risk of fragility fracture
■ Relative risk reduction is independent of absolute fracture risk

6.9   Osteoporosis Management

6.9.1   Summarising Management Options

■ Non-pharmacological, e.g. weight-bearing exercise, attention to diet and life style
■ Important role of calcium and vitamin D
■ Drugs used in prevention and treatment of osteoporosis
   – Prevention only: hormonal therapy
   – Prevention and treatment: bisphosphonates, SERM, etc.
   – Treatment only: calcitonin, pulsatile PTH therapy (especially for severe osteoporosis)

6.9.2   Role of Calcium and Vitamin D

6.9.2.1 Introduction

■ The great importance of ensuring replete calcium and vitamin D among our patient population with fragility fractures in particular has not been stressed enough in many standard orthopaedic textbooks in the past

- The importance lies in the fact that calcium and vitamin D intake modulate age-related increases in the PTH levels of bone resorption and occult PTH increases do in fact contribute to the pathogenesis of osteoporosis and lessen the effects of whatever expensive anti-osteoporosis medications our patients may be taking
- It is common knowledge that the serum calcium level of humans has to be maintained within narrow limits for neuromuscular tissues in particular and a multitude of other cellular functions including enzymes to work. Our body's store of calcium is found mainly in our skeleton as hydroxyapatite crystals. Its in-built homeostasis system is such that the above-mentioned calcium level in the circulation must be properly maintained, even at the expense of resorption of the skeleton if and whenever the need arises
- Vitamin D plays an important role in the regulation of calcium levels as well as bone mineralisation, among many other functions, and in fact vitamin D is now regarded as a hormone. Its deficiency causes osteomalacia, or rickets, while a lack of vitamin D can exacerbate osteoporosis. Other important roles include gait balance strength, particularly in the elderly, and its effect on the immune system. In addition, the Framingham Study revealed that low intake and low serum level of vitamin D are in fact associated with increased risk of OA progression
- Sub-clinical vitamin D deficiency and secondary hyperparathyroidism is very common in patients with osteoporosis, but this fact is very often underestimated (Utiger 1998)

6.9.2.2 WHO Guidelines

- Current WHO guidelines on the "Consultation on Mineral Requirements in Human Nutrition" highlighted the international recommendation nowadays of calcium intake of at least 1,200 mg per day. For the elderly, especially those living alone and in institutions like nursing homes, calcium supplementation is highly recommended. At the same time as avoiding excess animal protein (which may outweigh the effect of calcium intake), other foods rich in calcium can be considered for the elderly, such as fresh green vegetables, tofu cheese, etc., although these choices are of course suitable for the general population as well

■ Studies in the US indicate that only about 50% of the adult population is meeting its calcium and vitamin D needs, and an estimated 80% or more vitamin D deficiency has been reported in a hospitalised fracture population. Minimal healthy vitamin D serum level is at least 30 ng/ml. If <30 ng/ml, parameters of secondary hyperparathyroidism are usually present and contribute to the development of osteoporosis. More recent recommendations by workers like Holic and others advise a level between 35 and 55 ng/ml, instead of the traditional figure of 30 ng/ml

6.9.2.3 Calcium/Vitamin D and Fracture Risk Reduction

■ Calcium supplementation and vitamin D slow the loss of BMD, decrease bone turnover over 4 years and reduce fracture incidence in elderly adults. It is a cost-effective, weak anti-resorptive and can decrease hip fractures by 7–25% in 3 years (McClung 1999). In fact, recent evidence showed that the addition of supplemental calcium to alendronate treatment resulted in a statistically significant additional reduction in NTx, which is a commonly used bone resorption marker (Curr Med Res Opin 2007). However, as expected, we find that speakers in international symposia representing different drug companies producing expensive anti-osteoporosis agents seldom highlight the importance of calcium and vitamin D

■ In both prevention and treatment of osteoporosis, adequate dietary calcium and vitamin D are necessary to maintain the skeleton, other expensive anti-osteoporosis drug therapy assumes a calcium- and vitamin D-replete patient (NIH 2000)

■ The importance of ensuring a calcium- and vitamin D-replete patient is that calcium and vitamin D intake modulate age-related increases in the PTH levels of bone resorption, and occult PTH increases contribute to the pathogenesis of osteoporosis and lessen the effects of anti-osteoporosis medications, and this cannot be over-emphasised

- It is important to note that in the most recent meta-analysis on this issue just published in the Lancet 2007, the authors found that the fracture risk reduction was significantly greater (24%) in trials in which the compliance rate was high ($p < 0.0001$). The treatment effect was better with calcium doses of 1,200 mg or more than with doses less than 1,200 mg ($p = 0.006$), and with vitamin D doses of 800 IU or more than with doses less than 800 IU ($p = 0.03$)

6.9.2.4 Therapeutic Guidelines from the Royal College of Physicians (2000)

- If one refers to guidelines from well-respected institutions like the Royal College, those therapeutic agents with grade A evidence of the prevention of future hip fractures include only alendronate, risedronate, calcium + vitamin D (besides the use of hip protectors)

6.9.3   Strontium Ranelate

6.9.3.1 Introduction

- Mechanism of action: despite the fact that an occasional expert in osteoporosis has commented that the mechanism of action of strontium ranelate is largely unknown, studies from France have suggested that strontium has the dual action of simultaneously increasing bone formation and decreasing bone resorption (Marie et al. 2001). This comes about via a simultaneous increase in the replication of pre-osteoblasts, resulting in an increase in osteoblasts, as well as a decrease in the differentiation of pre-osteoclasts into osteoclasts and a decrease in the bone-resorbing action of osteoclasts. Despite the above-mentioned, many researchers feel that in humans as opposed to animal models, the bone formation stimulation effect may actually be less than in animals
- Role in vertebral fracture prevention: vertebral fracture risk reduction was demonstrated in both the TROPOS trial as well as an earlier SOTI (Spinal Osteoporosis Therapeutic Intervention) study. The latter involved 1,649 post-menopausal ladies, in whom a dose of strontium ranelate at 2 g/day orally reduced the relative risk of new vertebral fractures by 49% at 1 year and 41% over 3 years (Meunier et al. 2004)

- Role in non-vertebral fracture prevention: in a recent multi-centre TROPOS trial (Treatment of Peripheral Osteoporosis Study) involving most European countries and some Scandinavian countries, the authors found that the relative risk of experiencing a hip fracture in the ITT (intention-to-treat) population was reduced by 15%, but that this figure did not reach statistical significance, as this study was neither designed nor powered for this parameter. However, it was found in a post-hoc analysis that in the high-risk fracture subgroup, i.e. ladies >74 years of age with a femoral neck BMD T-score of ≤ −3.0 treatment was associated with a 36% reduction in risk of hip fracture (Reginster et al. 2005)

6.9.3.2 Cochrane Review for Strontium Ranelate

- There is evidence to support the efficacy of strontium ranelate for the reduction of fractures (vertebral and to a lesser extent non-vertebral in postmenopausal osteoporotic women and an increase in BMD in postmenopausal women with/without osteoporosis. Diarrhoea may occur however, adverse events leading to study withdrawal were no significantly increased with taking 2 g of strontium ranelate daily. Potential vascular and neurological side-effects need to be further explored (O'Donnell et al. 2006)

6.9.3.3 Key Concept

- At this juncture, strontium ranelate have reasonably good safety record up to the 5-year mark, and the latest literature has it that the drug is best used in the "oldest old" say around the eighth decade up elderly with fragility fractures. It can also be considered for those who developed side effects after bisphosphonate therapy or despite attempted re-challenge. The sachet can be conveniently taken at night before retirement to bed. *There are some recent reports of allergic reactions in the form of Steven-Johnson like syndrome and the patients should be cautioned about this potential side effect as well.*
- There is no current literature to support the combined use of strontium and bisphosphonates

6.9.4 Pulsatile Teriparatide Therapy (Fig 6.1)

6.9.4.1 Introduction

- Mechanism of action: it was previously found that continuous high-dose PTH infusion causes a catabolic effect on bones, while a low-dose once daily administration will have anabolic effects instead
- The catabolic effect of continuous PTH infusion is mediated by ↑RANKL, ↓OPG, with stimulated osteoclastic-mediated bone resorption activity with concomitant rise in serum calcium
- The anabolic effects of PTH once-daily dose comes about by means of the stimulation of bone-lining cells, ↓RANKL ↑OPG, ↓osteoblast apoptosis, and possibly also stimulates BMP, IGF, cbfa1 and Wnt signalling. The overall effect results in enhanced osteoblast function and population, thus bone formation. The anabolic action outweighs the stimulation of osteoclasts, which was believed to be mediated via interleukin-6 gene expression in a previous animal experiments in rats (Chiba et al., J Vet Med Sci 2002)
- Clinical effect of decreased bone resorption markers (e.g. NTx) and increased formation markers (e.g. PINP) achieved by teriparatide but not alendronate was demonstrated in the FACT study (McClung et al. 2005)

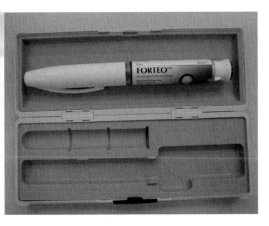

Fig. 6.1 Illustration showing the drug teriparatide commercially marketed as Forteo

- PINP stands for amino-terminal propeptide of type I procollagen and is an indicator of osteoblastic activity, currently used to monitor therapy after teriparatide treatment. Development of an algorithm for using PINP to monitor treatment of patients with teriparatide (Eastell et al. 2006)
- In fact, studies have shown that teriparatide injection once daily also improves bone micro-architecture (Jiang et al. 2003) in the form of better trabecular volume, cortical thickness, and better connectivity on checking serial transiliac crest bone biopsies, and improved mineralisation pattern (Misof et al. 2003)
- In peripheral long bones like the distal radius, 18 months of teriparatide increases cortical thickness, improves overall geometrical diameter, thus indirectly improving the polar moment of inertia (Zanchetta et al. 2003)

6.9.4.2 Bioavailability and Side Effects

- The current drug is not the same as the endogenous 1-84 PTH, but a shorter peptide so that the calculated bioavailability and action are such that 20 μg of teriparatide will cause a pulsatile surge of PTH action lasting for about 3–4 h in the body; thereafter, before the due time for another subcutaneous injection the following day, there is usually complete suppression of endogenous PTH
- The recommended duration of therapy is 18 months
- Side effects include hypercalcaemia; thus, monitoring of the calcium level is important. Other drawbacks include high cost, and a black box warning that there are some initial reports of associations with osteosarcoma in animals, but this is now thought to be dose- and species-related; thus, clinical trials proceeded and the drug has now been FDA-approved

6.9.4.3 Comparison of Action of Teriparatide Versus Bisphosphonates

- Anti-resorptive therapies increase bone strength by decreasing bone turnover. This lower bone turnover results in a higher mean mineralisation and decreases the number of active resorption pits within bone at any given time. These resorption pits are speculated to be areas of focal weakness and a higher number of them would, if all other things were equal, result in greater fragility. Parathyroid hormone therapy increases the rate of bone remodelling, which introduces many resorption pits, but this source of strength loss is thought to be compensated for by rapid increases in bone mass (Davidson et al. 2006)

6.9.4.4 Combined Use with Bisphosphonates Contraindicated

- In another recent clinical study, teriparatide significantly increased markers of bone turnover that peaked at 6 months (serum procollagen type I N-terminal propeptide, 218%, and urinary N-telopeptide corrected for creatinine, 58%; $p < 0.001$), while alendronate significantly decreased the markers at 6 months (−67% and −72% respectively; $p < 0.001$; McClung et al. 2005)

6.9.4.5 Key Concept

- Never prescribe teriparatide therapy with bisphosphonates for they have opposite mechanism of action
- Upon completion of Teriperatide therapy at 18 months, patients should afterwards be given anti-resorptive therapy.

6.9.4.6 Clinical Trials on Teriparatide: Fracture Prevention Trial

- This clinical trial showed that treatment of postmenopausal osteoporosis with parathyroid hormone (1–34 PTH) decreases the risk of vertebral and non-vertebral fractures; increases vertebral, femoral and total-body bone mineral density; and is well tolerated. Although the 40-μg dose increased bone mineral density more than the 20-μg dose, it had a similar effect on the risk of fracture and was more likely to cause side effects (Neer et al. 2001)

6.9.5   Bisphosphonates
6.9.5.1 Introduction

- Mechanism of action: these are pyrophosphate analogs that bind to exposed mineral surfaces of bone and are incorporated into newly formed matrix. Then, ingested by osteoclasts, they interfere with the activation and function of osteoclasts

- Bisphosphonates also interrupt the mevalonate pathway for cholesterol biosynthesis, preventing formation of the ruffled border of osteoclasts (Wimalawansa 2000)
- Bone remodelling effects: decreases bone turnover by decreasing the depth of resorption cavities, and decreases the activation rate of the new remodelling units
- Newer bisphosphonates inhibit osteoclast bone resorption at doses that do not impair mineralisation, unlike first generation bisphosphonates
- Bisphosphonates improve osteoblast and osteocyte preservation by decreasing apoptosis
- BMD gained during bisphosphonate therapy is frequently sustained after withdrawal, especially with those with long half-lives in bone, more so in older patients (Ravn 2000)

6.9.5.2 Side Effects

- Oral bisphosphonates should be swallowed whole with 6–8 oz of plain water while in an upright position, in order to be certain that the tablets enter the stomach. If the tablets stick in the oesophagus they can irritate it – in fact, besides oesophagitis, it has recently been reported that it can cause significant oesophageal ulcers (Endoscopy 2006). One should not lie down for 60 min after taking ibandronate for similar reasons
- *Patients should avoid taking bisphosphonate medication together with calcium tablets at the same time. Calcium tablets should thus be taken separately*

6.9.5.3 Pregnancy

- Pregnancy: bisphosphonates have been shown to cause foetal damage in animals, but there are no data on the risk to the foetus in humans. Bisphosphonates should be used during pregnancy only if the physician feels that its potential benefit justifies the potential risk. It is therefore usually contraindicated to give bisphosphonates to premenopausal ladies who desire to become pregnant

.9.5.4 Contraindications

- Not FDA-approved for premenopausal women, pregnant women, or children
- Patients with oesophageal problems, especially with stricture or motility. Could try with simple reflux, if reflux is well controlled by proton pump inhibitors
- Patients with the inability to stand or sit upright for 30 min
- Hypersensitivity to the drug
- Hypocalcaemia
- Renal insufficiency (creatinine clearance of less than 35)

.9.5.5 Special Side Effects

- The really long-term safety of bisphosphonates like alendronate has been documented in reports of follow-ups of up to 10 years, while raloxifene and strontium ranelate have similar reports with follow-ups of up to 8 and 5 years respectively
- There have been recent worries among orthopods, however, that in those patients being put on chronic bisphosphonates for around 10 years sometimes there may be too much suppression of bone turnover, affecting fracture healing, and there may also be an increased risk of increased brittleness of long bones ± accumulation of micro-damage
- Whether the newer generation of much more potent bisphosphonates that are currently very popular will cause even more hypermineralisation or potential for micro-damage accumulation is unknown

.9.5.6 Bisphosphonates Versus Fracture Healing

- Fracture healing: at doses used to treat osteoporosis, bisphosphonates do not appear to inhibit fracture healing, but may mildly delay remodelling of the callus (Morris 2005)

.9.5.7 Duration of Therapy: the FLEX Study

- The FLEX Study (Fracture Intervention Trial Long-term Extension) revealed that women who discontinued alendronate after 5 years revealed a moderate decline in BMD, with a gradual rise in biochem-

ical bone markers, although there is no suggestion of heightene
fracture risk (except for clinical vertebral fractures), compared with
those who continued the drug. Many experts propose that the drug
should be continued to around the 10-year mark. The author feel
this advice is particularly sound if the patient has multiple associated
risk factors

6.9.5.8 Is There a Case for Lifelong Use?

- The reader should note in passing that there are insufficient data to
  tell whether bisphosphonates need to be given past the 10-year mark
  not to mention whether or not routine lifetime use is indicated

6.9.5.9 Newer Bisphosphonates: Ibandronate

- Both ibandronate and zoledronate are third generation bisphosphonates with cyclic side chains. Being more potent, they can be given in
  smaller doses and with longer dose intervals
- Ibandronate may be taken daily, but it is the *only* oral bisphosphonate that has been approved for monthly oral administration. Thus
  the dose is either 2.5 mg daily or 150 mg once a month. The tablet
  should be taken on the same day of each month if monthly dosing is
  prescribed to patients

6.9.5.10 Efficacy of Intermittent Dosing: the DIVA Study

- The DIVA study showed that oral daily (2.5 mg) and intermittent
  ibandronate (dose interval of >2 months), delivering a similar cu-
  mulative exposure, were evaluated in 2,946 osteoporotic women
  with prevalent vertebral fractures. Significant reduction in incident
  vertebral fracture risk by 62% and 50% respectively was shown after
  3 years. This is the first study to prospectively show anti-fracture efficacy for the intermittent administration of a bisphosphonate
- However, the incidence of non-vertebral fractures was similar in the
  ibandronate and placebo groups after 3 years (9.1%, 8.9% and 8.2%
  in the daily, intermittent and placebo groups respectively; difference
  between arms not significant)

- Although subsequent findings from a "post-hoc" analysis showed that the daily regimen reduces the risk of non-vertebral fractures (69%; $p = 0.012$) in a higher-risk subgroup (femoral neck BMD T-score <−3.0), it seems premature to conclude without an element of doubt at this juncture of the efficacy of ibandronate in reducing significant non-vertebral fractures like hip fractures; however, monthly ibandronate did seem in this trial to be at least as effective and well tolerated as the currently approved daily ibandronate regimen in postmenopausal osteoporosis

6.9.5.11 Newer Bisphosphonates: Zoledronic Acid

- Zoledronate represents another one of the injectable bisphosphonates just like etidronate (Didronel) and pamidronate (Aredia)
- A once-yearly infusion of zoledronic acid over a 3-year period was found to significantly reduce the risk of vertebral, hip and other fractures (Black et al. 2007)
- Adverse events, including changes in renal function, were similar in the two study groups. However, serious atrial fibrillation occurred more frequently in the zoledronic acid group (in 50 vs. 20 patients, $p < 0.001$)

6.9.5.12 Tackling "Breakthrough" Fractures Despite Patient Being on Bisphosphonates

- Recheck drug compliance all along
- That is why sometimes we do a DXA 1 year after the start of bisphosphonates
- Doing a biochemical screen in these cases is advisable, such as assay of Ca PO4 1,25di(OH) vitamin D, 24-h urinary calcium, bone formation markers like ALP and resorption markers like NTX
- Consideration should also be given to other treatment choices like strontium, or pulsatile PTH therapy
- If it is felt safe to continue bisphosphonates, and the compliance has been marginal, the long-acting bisphosphonates like ibandronate can be considered, or other yearly injection derivatives, although they have more side effects

6.9.6   Selective Estrogen Receptor Modulators

■ As the name implies, selective estrogen receptor modulators (SERM) are not compounds like the pure anti-estrogens (e.g. ICI 182,780) which antagonises the effect of estrogens in all tissues including bone, uterus, breast and cardiovascular system

■ Different classes of SERMs exhibit both agonist *and* antagonist effects on the above tissue, depending on the tissue in question and the hormonal milieu. The estrogen receptor changes its shape when there is binding by SERM. The resultant shape will then determine which gene will be activated, hence the type of proteins produced (Yang et al. 1996)

■ The only type of SERM licensed to manage osteoporosis are the benzothiophene derivatives (e.g. raloxifene), rather than the other major group of triphenylethylene derivatives (e.g. tamoxifen)

■ We will not discuss this group of drugs in detail, for its efficacy was mainly demonstrated for vertebral, but not non-vertebral fractures. The interested reader is referred to details of the MORE study, and the newer EVA study comparing raloxifene with alendronate

6.9.7   New Drug Under Clinical Trial: Denosumab (also Called AMG 162)

6.9.7.1 Introduction

■ The drug denosumab was developed by the world's biggest bio-technology company, Amgen. It is engineered to be given as a twice-yearly subcutaneous injection of 60 mg. Denosumab is designed to target RANK ligand, a protein that acts as the primary signal to promote bone removal. In many bone loss conditions, RANK ligand overwhelms the body's natural defence against bone destruction. Preclinical models have demonstrated that inhibiting RANK ligand leads to significant improvements in cortical and trabecular bone density, volume and strength

6.9.7.2 Potential Uses of Denosumab Besides Osteoporosis Management

- Denosumab is currently being studied for its potential in a broad range of bone loss conditions including osteoporosis, treatment-induced bone loss, bone metastases, multiple myeloma and rheumatoid arthritis

6.9.7.3 Denosumab: Early Results

- The ongoing, multi-centre, phase 2 dose-ranging trial includes results from 337 healthy post-menopausal women with low BMD who completed 2 years of the study. Researchers reported denosumab (60 mg) increased BMD of the lumbar spine by 7.4% in women administered the therapy twice yearly and 6.2% for Fosamax (70 mg weekly). Across all doses and dosing intervals, denosumab increased the BMD of the lumbar spine by 4.3 to 9.0% over baseline
- Researchers also reported that twice-yearly injections of denosumab (60 mg) increased total hip BMD by 5.1% after 24 months. Fosamax (70 mg weekly) produced a 3.4% increase during the same time period. Denosumab, at all doses and dosing intervals studied, increased total hip BMD by 2.8 to 5.1%. Across all doses and dosing intervals, distal one-third radius BMD increased by 0.6 to 2.5%, and total body BMD increased by 0.9 to 4.5%

6.10   Secondary Prevention of Fragility Fractures

6.10.1   Introduction

- One of the main challenges facing the orthopaedic surgeon in managing osteoporotic fractures is how to bring what we know about osteoporosis and fragility fractures from evidence-based medicine and our current understanding of the topic as afore-mentioned, into clinical practice. This is of pressing importance as the projected incidence of for instance fragility hip fractures will rise to staggering levels, especially in Asia (Cooper et al. 1992)

6.10.2   The Need for a Proper Systematic Referral Mechanism or Program for Secondary Fragility Fracture Reduction

▪ There are many studies that point to the low to very low incidence of patients suffering from fragility fractures that require hospital admission who are eventually in receipt of osteoporosis treatment at the 1-year mark. The author recently reported an incidence of only 30% (Ip et al. 2006), and only 15% was reported by Panneman et al. 2004. Also, as far as osteoporosis management is concerned, it is worthwhile noting the recent AAOS (American Academy of Orthopaedic Surgeon) Position Statement stressing the need not only to enhance the care of patients with hip and fragility fractures, but the importance of prevention as well, which is very much an obligation of orthopaedic surgeons. There is also a move towards possibly making the important topic of osteoporosis evaluation and treatment a potential medico-legal requirement in the future (http://www.aaos.org/wordhtml/papers/position/1159.htm)

6.10.3   New Approach to Fracture Risk Reduction: Fracture Liaison Service

▪ In Glasgow, UK, different medical centres have come up with a more cost-effective way of effecting secondary prevention of fragility fractures by mainly targeting patients at high absolute risk of future fracture. The aim of the Fracture Liaison Service (FLS) currently set up in the UK and in an increasing number of countries worldwide is to offer all women and men aged >50 who present with a new fracture (excluding traffic accidents, falls from above head height) a standardised structured referral mechanism for the assessment and treatment of osteoporosis and secondary fracture prevention (McLellan et al. 2003)

6.10.3.1   Initial Success of the FLS

▪ Some of the elements contributing to the success of the FLS include:
  − FLS links secondary and primary health care providers
  − FLS links orthopods, osteoporosis clinicians, radiologists, nurses, primary care clinicians, physiotherapists and nurses to form a

multi-disciplinary service. The two key persons in the FLS include a fracture liaison nurse who help to co-ordinate matters, as well as a lead clinician with the necessary enthusiasm and clear, achievable objectives

— Assess to the DXA service and channel the DXA service to give priority to patients with high calculated absolute fragility fracture risks

▪ Other areas: keeping of a database, software templates, standardised protocols, written forms to ease data entry by the fracture liaison nurse as well as the GPs, lobby for support from health administrators, publications and incorporation into national guidelines or standards of care. Last, but not the least important, introduce the success story to other nations by holding international conferences. The author has also had the honour of attending one such conference and learned a lot from world experts in this area like Dr. Alastair McLellan and Dr. Stephen Gallacher from Glasgow, UK

6.10.3.2 Implementation of a FLS Pilot Programme in the Author's Regional Hospital

▪ The author has implemented a pilot program based on the teachings of the FLS and modified to suit the local resources and health care environment; this will be discussed in Chap. 14 on hip fracture rehabilitation protocol

General Bibliography

1. Vitamin and mineral requirements in human nutrition. Report of the Joint FAO/WHO Expert Consultation. Geneva, World Health Organization

Selected Bibliography of Journal Articles

1. Bonnick S, Broy S, et al. (2007) Treatment with alendronate plus calcium, alendronate alone, or calcium alone for postmenopausal low bone mineral density. Curr Med Res Opin 23(6):1341–1349

2. Davidson KS, Siminoski K, et al. (2006) The effects of antifracture therapies on the components of bone strength: assessment of fracture risk today and in the future Semin Arthritis Rheum 36(1):10–21

3. Eastell R, Krege JH, Chen P, Glass EV, Reginster J-Y (2006) Development of an algorithm for using PINP to monitor treatment of patients with teriparatide. Curr Med Res Opin 22:61–66

4. Iki M (2007) Absolute risk for fracture and WHO guideline: WHO model for assessing absolute risk of fracture. Clin Calcium 17(7):1015–1021

5. Ip D, et al. (2006) Elderly patients with two episodes of fragility hip fractures from a special subgroup. J Orthop Surg 14(3):245–248

6. Klotzbuecher CM, et al. (2000) Patients with prior fracture have an increased risk of future fractures: a summary of the literature and statistical synthesis. J Bone Miner Res 15(4):721–739

7. McClung MR, San Martin J, et al. (2005) Opposite bone remodeling effects of teriparatide and alendronate in increasing bone mass. Arch Intern Med 165(15):1762–1768

8. McLellan AR, et al. (2003) The fracture liaison service: success of a program for the evaluation and management of patients with osteoporotic fracture. Osteoporos Int 14:1028–1034

9. Marie PJ, Ammann P, Boivin G, Rey C (2001) Mechanisms of action and therapeutic potential of strontium in bone. Calcif Tissue Int 69:121–129

10. Meunier PJ, Roux C, et al. (2004) The effects of strontium ranelate on the risk of vertebral fracture in women with postmenopausal osteoporosis. N Eng J Med 350(5):459–468

11. Miller PD, McClung MR, et al. (2005) Monthly oral ibandronate therapy in postmenopausal osteoporosis: 1-year results from the MOBILE study. J Bone Miner Res 20(8):1315–1322

12. Neer RM, Arnaud CD, et al. (2001) Effect of parathyroid hormone (1–34) on fractures and bone mineral density in postmenopausal women with osteoporosis. N Eng J Med 344(19):1434–1441

13. O'Donnell S, et al. (2006) Strontium ranelate for preventing and treating postmenopausal osteoporosis. Cochrane Database Syst Rev (4):CD005326

14. Panneman MJ, et al. (2004) Under treatment of anti-osteoporosis drugs after hospitalization for fracture. Osteoporos Int 15(2):120–124

15. Reginster JY, Seeman E, De Vernejoul MC, et al. (2005) Strontium ranelate reduces the risk of nonvertebral fractures in postmenopausal women with osteoporosis: treatment of peripheral osteoporosis (TROPOS) study. J Clin Endocrinol Metab 90:2816–2822

16. Robinson CM, et al. (2002) Refractures in patients at least forty-five years old: a prospective analysis of twenty-two thousand and sixty patients. J Bone Joint Surg Am 84-A(9):1528–1533

17. Tang BM, Eslick GD, et al. (2007) Use of calcium or calcium in combination with vitamin D supplementation to prevent fractures and bone loss in people aged 50 years or older: a meta-analysis. Lancet 370:657–666

18. Utiger RD (1998) The need for more vitamin D. N Engl J Med 338(12):828–829

19. Yang NN, Venugopalan M, et al. (1996) Identification of an estrogen response element activated by metabolites of 17beta-estradiol and raloxifene. Science 273(5279):1222–1225

Minimally Invasive and Computer-Aided Surgery

7.1   General Introduction

7.1.1   Introduction: Technique of Indirect Reduction

- It is essential to note that one has to master the indirect reduction techniques of fractures
- This is because many of the minimally invasive plate osteosynthesis (MIPO) techniques described are based on indirect reduction

7.1.2   Definition

- Indirect reduction refers to a technique that avoids direct fracture exposure and further muscle stripping of the various small bone fragments in the fractured zone

7.1.3   Rationale

- It relies upon the technique of ligamentotaxis in which we restore the overall position of the fracture fragments, thereby avoiding periosteal stripping and devascularisation
- By protecting the viability of the fracture fragments, it may obviate the need for a subsequent bone graft and may result in a lower infection rate
- We do need, however, to restore mechanical alignment, but not absolute anatomical alignment for these meta-diaphyseal fractures

7.1.4   Fracture Healing Associated with Indirect Reduction

- Unlike the traditional AO concept of absolute stability, which now still holds for intra-articular fractures, with indirect reduction, the result is relative stability as evidenced by callus formation

7.1.5   Preoperative Work-up

- Evaluate the fracture configuration
- Utilise implant templates
- Plan the method of fixation construct
- Step-wise approach of surgical tactics
- The details can be found in the book written by Dr J. Mast published by Springer-Verlag

7.1.6   Commonly Used Instruments to Effect Indirect Fixation

- Universal distractor
- Articulated tensioner
- Laminar spreader
- Dental pick
- Clamps
- Weber's clamp

7.2   Minimally Invasive Plate Osteosynthesis

7.2.1   Background Terminology (Krettek)

- MIPO: minimally invasive plate osteosynthesis
- MIPPO: minimally invasive percutaneous plate osteosynthesis (for extra-articular fractures)
- TARPO: trans-articular approach with percutaneous plating for intra-articular fractures

7.2.2   What is MIPO?

- MIPO by definition avoids direct exposure of the fracture site. If used with a conventional plate, the plate is used as an extra-medullary splint, and thus does not depend on compression or lag screw application
- Since the conventional plates may not be ideally suited to MIPO, new, recently developed plates are now used to complement this technology, e.g. LISS plating

7.2.3   Traditional Concepts

- Traditional AO concept of open reduction and rigid IF resulting in direct bone healing
- Over-emphasis on mechanics at the expense of biology, although Allgower did advocate "care in soft tissue handling"

7.2.4   Newer Developments

- Mast came up with the concept of "indirect reduction"

- The principle is to take advantage of the soft tissue connection of the bone fragments, which align spontaneously when traction is applied to the main fragments
- Advantage: reduces surgical dissection, less compromise of vascularity, thus possibly better healing and less sepsis

7.2.5 Latest Developments

- New insight: observation that IF based purely on reduction of fragment mobility without the bone fragments touching may also result in solid bone healing
- Result = principle of absolute stability by interfragmentary compression replaced (at least in the situation of many meta-diaphyseal fractures) by the principle of "pure internal splinting"
- Ganz coined the term "biological fixation"

7.2.6 Indication for MIPO

- Best indicated for situations in which biology is the most important concern (e.g. in the face of significant soft tissue trauma)
- Although it is still possible to perform minimally invasive plating with the use of conventional plates, the newer point contact fixators and the latest LCP that do not require pre-contouring (together with self-drilling and self-tapping screws) are the best adjunct to go with the MIPO technique

7.2.7 How Does MIPO Compare with IM Nailing and EF?

- Although IM nailing permits a minimally open approach, the advantages are offset by the extensive damage to the intramedullary circulation, and local + general intravascular thrombosis
- Although the EF preserves the biology of the fracture fragments, healing is slow and sometimes delayed at the expense of patient comfort

7.2.8 New Innovations in Plate Design and Technology to Complement the MIPO Technique

- Special design help in the tunnelling of the new plate systems such as LISS and LCP

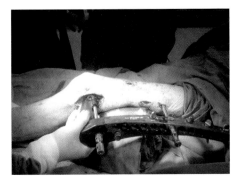

Fig. 7.1 The less invasive stabilisation system (LISS) plate was designed for the minimally invasive plate osteosynthesis (MIPO) technique

- Examples:
  - The end of the LISS plate is pointed
  - The LISS (Fig. 7.1), which is mostly used to fix metaphyseal or meta-diaphyseal fractures, is pre-contoured to fit into the anatomy of most femurs and tibiae
  - The aiming handle helps insertion and screw insertion since the locked unicortical screws require alignment of the implant and the bone axis within comparably narrow limits
  - Screws are self-drilling and self-tapping to minimise the difficulty in finding the initial drill hole, and the added steps of measuring and tapping of conventional plating

7.2.9   What About the Argument by Some That "Blind Tunnelling Itself Causes Significant Soft Tissue Trauma"?

- Previous studies done by Krettek and others regarding the effect of the ligation of the perforating arteries, for example, during the open surgical approach to femoral fractures, have disproved the argument

7.2.10   Virtual Fluoroscopy Versus MIPO: Are They Complementary?

- This is affirmative

- Example is shown in the setting of the LISS: in LISS plating, the distal fragment of the fracture comes under direct vision of the operating surgeon. However, one intraoperative challenge for the surgeon is that the proximal fragment must be accurately reduced and fixed properly to the LISS as eccentric plate placement causes early pullout of the monocortical screws

- This requires the surgeon to control six degrees of freedom at the same time. But a single fluoroscopic image provides information only on three degrees of freedom. It is difficult for the surgeon to maintain length, fracture alignment, and fracture rotation using imaging in only one plane at a time

- Virtual fluoroscopy allows the plate and proximal fragment to be tracked independently in ≥ two planes, during reduction of the fracture

- In future, implant-specific software may come of age to aid the trauma surgeon in obtaining adequate images to allow accurate restoration of length, alignment and rotation, especially during minimally invasive plate osteosynthesis

7.3 MIPO in Different Body Regions

7.3.1 MIPO in the Proximal Tibia

7.3.1.1 Introduction

- One common problem with the fixation of proximal tibial fractures arises from soft tissue complications, say, after ORIF with traditional plating. The MIPO technique can help in this respect

7.3.1.2 Cases of Tibial Fracture in Which to Consider MIPO

- Metaphyseal or combined metaphyseal-articular fractures of the proximal tibia

7.3.1.3 Problems of Fracture Around the Proximal Tibia

- Difficult to reduce

- Difficult to align
- Difficult to stabilise
- Easy to develop soft tissue and wound Cx
- Infections

7.3.1.4 Common Surgical Approaches

- Medial
- Lateral
- Combined
- Main advantage of the medial approach as opposed to the lateral approach is that the plate can be subcutaneous instead of submuscular – and has been used by Krettek successfully – especially if the main pathology is on the medial side (P.S. to visualise any articular component of the fracture, we may need to extend the incision to allow for a submeniscal arthrotomy. We perform MIPO only after articular reconstruction)

7.3.1.5 Advantage of MIPO in Proximal Tibial Fractures

- Allows for stabilisation of both the medial and the lateral column using a single approach, if used with the newer locking plates that provide angular stability
- Many of the locking plates for the proximal tibia are designed for the lateral proximal tibia (e.g. LISS-PT) to be used in conjunction with a lateral approach for submuscular tunnelling beneath the tibialis anterior
- Krettek emphasised that certain injuries are best treated with subcutaneous medial plating if the main pathology is on the medial side, or occasionally if the soft tissues on the lateral side are greatly traumatised

7.3.1.6 The Case for Adjunctive Fibula Fixation

- To obtain a lateral weight-bearing strut
- Offers a fulcrum when fine tuning the tibial alignment prior to fixation of the main distal tibial fragment
- Correction of length

7.3.1.7 The Spanning of the Plate

- The plate should bridge the metaphyseal-diaphyseal fracture fragment, extending distally from the level of the joint, so that at least three bicortical diaphyseal screws can be used for distal fixation

7.3.1.8 Disadvantages of a Lateral LISS Plate

- Do need to elevate the muscle with some unavoidable devitalisation of the fracture
- Risk of peroneal nerve injury, especially when a 13-hole LISS is used
- Risk of compartment syndrome

7.3.1.9 Advantages of the Medial Approach

- Allows fixation of the bicondylar fracture through a single incision
- No muscle stripping
- Especially effective if there is mostly medial comminution or in the presence of traumatised lateral soft tissue and/or if the compartment pressure is increased

7.3.2 Distal Femur MIPO

7.3.2.1 Disadvantages of the Traditional AO Technique

- Decreases bone perfusion beneath the plate
- Decreases rate of fracture vascularisation
- Increases susceptibility to infection

7.3.2.2 Development of the MIPO Technique for the Distal Femur

- The idea is mainly to decrease surgical dissection, again working on the principles of ligament axis
- The feasibility of performing MIPO techniques for the distal femur was reinforced thanks to previous cadaveric studies performed by Krettek
- The AO LISS plating system was well suited for the performance of the MIPO technique in the region of the distal femur, the details of which have already been discussed in Chap. 4 and also in the section on fractures of the distal femur in Chap. 10 and will not be repeated here

7.3.3   Minimally Invasive Reduction of Fractures of the Proximal Humerus

7.3.3.1 Indications

- Can usually only be considered in the presence of soft tissue bridging the fracture fragments in order to gain benefit from ligamentaxis
- Recent works of Hertel et al. show that the vascularity of the humeral head is more likely to be maintained if:
  - There is an intact medial hinge of soft tissues
  - A lengthy metaphyseal head extension is noted on analysing the fracture pattern
- Common indications:
  - Valgus impacted fracture of the proximal humerus
  - Three-part fractures

7.3.3.2 Advantages of the Minimally Invasive Technique

- In the absence of fracture exposure, adhesion within the surrounding gliding surfaces is reduced and the rehabilitation period is possibly shorter than open surgery. More detailed discussion can be found in Chap. 9
- Less chance of sepsis
- Less bleeding
- Probably less pain and quicker rehabilitation

7.3.4   Minimally Invasive Technique for Articular Fracture of the Distal Radius

7.3.4.1 Work-up of Complex Intra-articular Fractures

- CT scanning is of help for the surgical planning of fixation of displaced intra-articular fractures
- The wrist joint has a low tolerance for articular incongruity, and careful preoperative planning is essential

7.3.4.2 Indication of Minimally Invasive Techniques

- Minimally invasive techniques should be considered if close reduction fails

■ For those cases in which CR is successful, a combination of EF + multiple K-wires can be used to maintain reduction (although large fragments are best held by plates and screws)

7.3.4.3 *Methods of Reduction of Articular Fracture*

■ It was shown by Jupiter that a 2-mm articular step-off is predictive of post-traumatic arthrosis and poor functional result. AVN is rare in intra-articular distal radius fractures because of the good blood supply, but can occur in high energy injuries
■ The methods of reduction include:
  − Open reduction using standard incisions (involves more soft tissue dissection)
  − Smaller incisions are now possible thanks to the development of new low profile, fracture-specific implants for intra-articular fractures of the distal radius
  − Mini-open reduction (sometimes mini-incisions for the purpose of BG)
  − Arthroscopic-assisted reduction – gaining popularity

7.3.4.4 *Columnar Classification and Development of Fracture-Specific Implants*

■ The Columnar Classification is an increasingly popular classification for intra-articular fractures of the distal radius. The distal radius in this classification is divided into the lateral or radial column, the intermediate column, and the medial or ulna column. New low-profile plating systems have now been developed to tackle each of the columns. For example, if only the dorsal ulna corner is fractured, we only need to use the corresponding plate to tackle the fracture and minimise soft tissue dissection and surgical trauma. Further discussion on this topic will be found in Chap. 9

7.4   CAOS and Surgical Navigation

7.4.1   Surgical Navigation – How It Works

- Uses a camera to locate the position and alignment of a surgical instrument
- Positional feedback is then provided in real time on a monitor
- Feedback is either given with respect to medical images of the patient or an intraoperatively defined, patient-specific referencing system

7.4.2   Componentry/Requirements

- Non-deformable rigid object, e.g. bony skeleton of the spine or lower extremities – thus it is difficult if not impossible to navigate soft tissue
- A modern set of navigation systems and special instruments
- Virtual object as representation of the real rigid object – obtained either by 3D imaging using CT, 2D virtual fluoroscopy, or landmark-based reference system

7.4.3   Basic Principles and Workflow

- Optical localiser system with camera
- Process of registration – can be "image-based" or "image-less":
  - Image based – involves a process of correlating the patient's anatomy and the images
  - Image-less – involves a process of defining a patient-specific, landmark-based referencing system intraoperatively, as in "image-less" system used in some TKR systems
- Patient tracking/dynamic referencing – involves a process of tracking the position and to compensate for relative movements of the object during surgery

2.2.2.1 Main Component 1: Optical Localiser System
7.4.3.1.1 Function

- It detects the said special navigation instruments intraoperatively, but does not detect the patient

7.4.3.1.2 Mechanism

■ There are two common mechanisms:
  - Passive optical localisers – passive systems involve instruments fitted with passive reflective marker spheres. Here, the infrared light required for instrument localisation comes initially from the camera and is only reflected by the above-mentioned reflective marker spheres, just like the ones used in many gait analysis laboratories
  - Active optical localisers – more popular nowadays, used by popular navigation systems like Stryker
■ Optical localiser systems use cameras that can detect infrared light
■ The cameras are calibrated, most feature a 3D co-ordinate system
■ Capability to calculate the exact location of an infra-red light source with respect to the camera
■ The above-mentioned active systems require the use of active LED (light-emitting diodes). The infrared light in the active system comes in fact from the LED on the instrument

7.4.3.1.3 Advantages of Active over Passive Systems

■ The more popular active systems often come in a wireless format, and are more accurate than the passive systems. Also, fluids such as blood intraoperatively will affect the reflective marker spheres of the passive systems. One example of an active system is that developed by Stryker, where there is the added advantage that instruments allow fully remote software control from the sterile field

7.4.3.1.4 Pitfalls/Cautions

■ If an active system is employed, ensure the LED faces towards the camera or the camera will not see anything
■ If a passive system is used, avoid blood or other liquid contaminating the reflective marker spheres

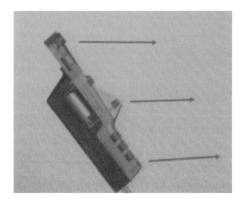

Fig. 7.2 Picture showing an "active" optical tracker system in the form of light-emitting diodes (LED), here marketed by stryker.com

7.4.3.2 Main Component 2: Localising Navigated Instruments
7.4.3.2.1 Mechanism/Functionality

- In the active systems described above, the instruments with built-in LED must be designed in such a way that there must be at least three light-emitting/reflecting sources, arranged in a non-collinear manner (Fig. 7.2). This arrangement is needed to define a non-ambiguous instrument co-ordinate system, and calibrate the said instrument

7.4.3.2.2 Calibration

- Calibration of the instrument is needed for the system to detect the dimension and geometry of the light-emitting/reflecting sources, and the location of the tip of the instrument relative to the light-emitting sources
- If the geometry of at least three light-emitting sources of an instrument is known, the optical localiser system can then calculate how close the instrument is to the camera; orientation of the instrument with respect to the camera (e.g. whether facing the camera or tilted), and location of the tip

7.4.3.2.3 Pitfall

- Never accept any instrument with a bent tip – even most active systems cannot compensate for a bent tip

- With the tip bent, the initial calibration data and the real tip position will no longer correspond and accurate surgical navigation can no longer proceed
- This has led some fool-proof advanced active systems like the Stryker system to require a validation step of the geometry of the tip. Manual override is possible, but is not recommended. If the surgeon detects any bending of the tip after the validation process, the surgeon should stop and reject the bent instrument

7.4.3.3 Main Component 3: Dynamic Referencing

7.4.3.3.1 Workflow

- Involves attaching a tracker to the patient – usually a stable bony landmark, in order to determine the position of the patient, and compensate for movements between the camera and the relevant anatomy after registration

7.4.3.3.2 Pitfall

- The patient tracker must be fixed rigidly, and must not move relative to the relevant anatomy
- Movement of the patient tracker intraoperatively will lead to inaccuracy in surgical navigation

7.4.4 The Process of Registration

7.4.4.1 What is Registration?

- Registration is the calculation of a mathematical transformation that relates corresponding data referenced in different co-ordinate systems
- It is rather like the process of figuring out how to correlate different representations of the same thing (e.g. a tourist trying to find his way in an unfamiliar city that he visits by holding a road map on his hand – the city map is a simple representation of the city streets)
- We alluded to the process of registration for 2D virtual fluoroscopy (with a 2D C-arm, the image is registered automatically by the system – needs a C-arm tracker with a phantom attached to the C-arm. The phantom allows the position of the X-ray source and the focal

length to be calculated, and compensates for image distortions, the C-arm can be moved away and the position of the calibrated tools is projected onto the saved images). What about 3D registration techniques?

7.4.4.1.1 Point-to-Point Registration

■ Requires a set of common points to be identified that can be easily selected on both the patient and the image

■ This allows the system to relate each point of the image space to the corresponding point in the surgical space

■ With correct registration, the software can now show exactly how the position of the instruments corresponds to the medical images used for planning and registration

■ Reference points must be spaced adequately far apart and the points must not be collinear to avoid ambiguity and inaccuracy, spreading out in all three dimensions

7.4.4.1.2 Surface Matching

■ Acts as a refinement of the initial point-to-point registration process

■ Involves correlation of the surface of the 3D image model with multiple points digitised on the patient's surface anatomy

■ Pitfalls include: ensure the surface rendered represents truly the relevant anatomy, one needs to spread out the points in three dimensions in a non-collinear fashion

7.4.4.2 A Word About "Image-less" Registration

■ Image-less registration is the process of defining a patient-specific reference system, based on the digitisation of anatomical landmarks

■ Image-less registration requires a patient tracker on the relevant anatomy. The patient tracker acts as a reference point, defining the co-ordinates of the surgical space

■ The positions of the landmarks are digitised with respect to or within the 3D coordinate system defined by the tracker and recorded. Options for landmark digitisation include methods like motion analysis, vector digitisation, surface mapping, etc.

■ Always ensure the tracker does not move relative to the bone, or the accuracy of the surgical navigation will be compromised. The system does not "see" the patient and thus cannot compensate for inaccurate landmarks

.4.5   Details of CT-Based Navigation

■ This method involves:
  - The need for preoperative CT
  - A registration step: whereby to relate a 3D virtual model to an actual object in the theatre

.4.5.1 Advantages

■ Decreases operative time
■ Decreases radiation exposure

7.4.5.2 Disadvantages

■ Requires preoperative CT – thus not suitable for fracture cases where reduction will be performed *after* CT has been obtained
■ Need for a registration step
■ Cost

7.4.6   Details of Virtual Fluoroscopy: Computer-Aided Fluoroscopic Navigation

7.4.6.1 Introduction

■ Involves:
  - Tracking the position of the patient and fluoroscopic unit by opto-electronic and electromagnetic markers
  - Storage and harvest of 2D C-arm X-ray images in the OR
  - Use of the stored images for surgical navigation by displaying the position of the optically-tracked instruments with respect to the images
  - The images can be readily updated (e.g. post-reduction mano-euvres)
  - Virtual fluoroscopy displays the predicted position of surgical instruments and implants relative to stored images. These systems have an inherent error of < 2 mm or < 2°. It is good for, say, screw

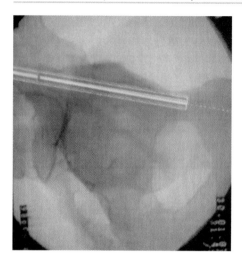

Fig. 7.3 Virtual fluoroscopic aided insertion of the screw at the anterior column of the acetabulum

insertion in areas with a low margin of error such as when fixing acetabular fractures (Fig. 7.3)

■ After, say, the fitting of the optical tracking arrays (e.g. via use of light-emitting diodes) to both the C-arm and the patient to allow tracking of the fracture, the calibration target and a software package are used to warp each X-ray image to render them optically correct

■ Requires interface with a CAOS workstation and computer

■ After storing the images, the real-time position of the surgical instruments can be overlaid upon stored images

■ Real-time feedback is possible as the instruments are moved

7.4.6.2 Advantages of Virtual Fluoroscopy

■ A preoperative 3D model is not necessary

■ Involves storage and harvesting of 2D C-arm fluoroscopic images in the operating room

■ Electromagnetic or optoelectronic markers are used to mark the position of the patients and the fluoroscopic unit

■ Stored images are employed to provide surgical guidance and can be readily updated after, say, fracture reduction has been performed

7.4.6.3 Disadvantages

- Cost
- Has an inherent error as reported by the system manufacturer
- The system does not have the capability to track an implant once it is inserted into bone; thus, error in screw positioning may occur, for example, in the event of guide wire deflection

7.4.6.4 Summary of Comparison Between CT-Guided Navigation and Virtual Fluoroscopy

- 3D CT-based CAOS systems are not suitable for aiding the three critical steps of, say, the femoral nailing procedure. The technique also requires preoperative CT and is not suitable for fracture cases in which a reduction will need to be performed after obtaining the CT. However, with the advent of virtual fluoroscopic techniques, surgical navigation of these three critical steps can be performed. Virtual fluoroscopy means simultaneous navigation on a multitude of fluoroscopic images taken at different angles, thus increasing control and reducing the total number of images needed for surgery
- This new technique decreases the amount of ionising radiation to which the orthopod is exposed. The disadvantage is the expense incurred by procuring specialised equipment and instruments

7.4.6.5 Clinical Example: Virtual Fluoroscopy in Long Bone Nailing

- Use of surgical navigation (virtual fluoroscopy) in nailing long bone fractures
- In search of a proper insertion site for the IM nail: the starting point (for nail insertion) can be identified by virtual fluoroscopy. The trajectory "look-ahead" feature can be used to align the drill guide with the femoral canal in two planes; the guide wire is then inserted into the piriform fossa. Overdrilling and reaming follow
- Fracture reduction: a special reduction rod with an array of light-emitting diodes can be inserted into the proximal fragment and negotiated to the fracture via virtual fluoroscopy. Fracture manipulation follows until the virtual axis of the proximal fragment aligns with the distal fracture fragment (a new femoral fracture reduction

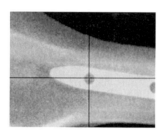

Fig. 7.4 Virtual fluoroscopy in action

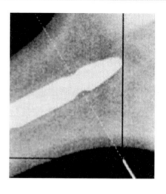

Fig. 7.5 Use of virtual fluoroscopy as an aid to locking bolt insertion in intramedullary nailing

software package that is said to be able to obtain accurate reduction in sagittal and coronal planes and restoration of anteversion will soon become available. With this technology, both fracture fragments are instrumented and tracked. Docking points will match up when the fracture is reduced)

- Placement of locking screws (Figs. 7.4, 7.5):
    - The technique can aid in controlled insertion of the proximal screws in cephalomedullary nailing as well as confirming the version and depth of nail insertion
    - Virtual depth gauge for selection of proper screw length of distal interlocking screws is possible thanks to the trajectory length feature of this new technology

General Bibliography

1. International Commission on Radiological Protection, Publication 60. Recommendations of the International Commission on Radiological Protection

Selected Bibliography of Journal Articles

1. Foley KT, Simon DA, et al. (2000) Virtual fluoroscopy. Oper Tech Orthop 10:77–81
2. Helfet DL, Shonnard PY, et al. (1997) Minimally invasive plate osteosynthesis of distal fractures of the tibia. Injury 28 [S-A]:42–48
3. Rampersaud YR, Foley KT, et al. (2000) Radiation exposures to the spine surgeon during fluoroscopically-assisted pedicle screw insertion. Spine 25:2637–2645
4. Simon DA, O'Toole RV, et al. (1995) Accuracy validation in image-guided orthopedic surgery. Proceedings of the 2nd International Symposium on Medical Robotics and Computer-Aided Surgery

Contents

8.1   Compartment Syndrome

8.1.1   Definition of Compartment Syndrome

- A condition in which an increased pressure within an enclosed osteo-fascial space that reduces the capillary blood perfusion below a level necessary for tissue viability

8.1.2   Classification

- Acute: severe and usually following trauma
- Chronic: mild, recurrent, resolve with rest, bilateral involvement

8.1.3   Common Causes of Acute Compartment Syndrome

- Fracture (closed or open), especially those resulting from high energy trauma
- Crushed injury
- Reperfusion injury
- Tight plaster and/or dressing

8.1.4   Pathophysiology (After Matsen)

- Increase in volume (content): haemorrhage, post-ischaemic swelling, reperfusion, arterial venous fistula
- Decrease in compartment size: plaster too tight, constrictive dressings, pneumatic anti-shock garments, closure of fascial defects
- Increase in compartment pressure → decrease in capillary blood flow: causing ischaemia, increased microvascular permeability, increased tissue fluid (intra-cellular and extra-cellular oedema) and pressure rises, thus further decreasing capillary blood flow. Results in a vicious cycle
- Arterial spasm

8.1.5   Other Theories of Pathophysiology

- Muscle ischaemia: (after Whitesides)
    - Electrically responsive up to 3 h and surviving for as long as 4 h
    - Irreversible damage after 8 h

- Variable results after 6 h
- Nerve ischaemia:
  - Survive 4 h with only neuroplexic damage
  - Axonotmesis after 8 h
- Net muscle perfusion:
  - Mean arterial blood pressure minus the compartment pressure
  - 20 mmHg → irreversible muscle damage
  - 40 mmHg → surgical decompression by fasciotomy
  - Resistance to ischaemia is decreased in tissue damaged by injury
  - Elevated tissue pressure acts synergistically with ischaemia to produce more cellular deterioration than ischaemia alone
  - Muscle subjected to 6 h of antecedent ischaemia demonstrated a lower tolerance to increased tissue pressure than normal muscle

8.1.6 Diagnosis

- Clinical mainly:
  - Pain out of proportion, not relieved by analgesics
  - Pain caused by passive stretching of the muscles in the compartment concerned
  - Tense or swollen compartment
  - Paraesthesia
  - Weakness
  - Presence of pulse alone does not exclude compartment syndrome and its absence is a late sign
  - Capillary refill not reliable

8.1.7 Compartment Pressure Measurement

- Especially important in head injury patients, unconscious patients, in cases of drug overdose, equivocal S/S, multiple trauma, concomitant nerve injury
- Adjunct to clinical assessment
- Differential pressure (diastolic minus compartment pressure) of 30 mmHg (McQueen and Court-Brown 1996)
- Direct compartment pressure of 45 mmHg (Matsen)

— Lowering or raising the systemic blood pressure may affect the level of direct compartment pressure that results in ischaemic compromise

8.1.8   Compartment Pressure Measurement Method

- Whitesides infusion technique
- Stryker STIC system
- The wick catheter
- The slit catheter
- Highest tissue pressure is usually recorded at the level of the fracture or within 5 cm of the fracture

8.1.9   Management

- Remove all (tight) plaster and bandage (if any)
- Emergency fasciotomy once diagnosis made
- Do not elevate the involved limb

8.1.10   Indication for Decompression – Fasciotomy

- High index of suspicion
- Clinical evaluation
- Supplemented by compartment pressure measurement and monitoring

8.1.11   Relevant Anatomy of Regional Compartments of the Body

8.1.11.1 Arm Compartments

- Anterior
- Posterior
- Deltoid

8.1.11.2 Forearm Compartments

- Volar
- Dorsal
- Mobile wad
- Pronator quadratus

8.1.11.3 Hand Compartments
- Central palmar compartment
- Adductor compartment
- Thenar compartment
- Hypothenar compartment
- Interosseous compartment (four dorsal, three palmar)
- Carpal tunnel

8.1.11.4 Digit Compartments
- Neurovascular bundle bounded by Cleland's and Grayson's ligament

8.1.11.5 Foot Compartments
- See section on foot injuries in Chap. 10

8.1.12 Principles of Fasciotomy
- Full skin incision to avoid skin necrosis
- Fasciotomy – skin alone produces only a slight reduction in compartment pressure (Gelberman)
- Epimysiotomy – no pressure drop after epimysiotomy (Mubarak 1976), indicated when muscle appears pale, tense and avascular (Eaton and Green)
- Forearm compartments are interrelated – volar fasciotomy alone lowered pressure in the dorsal compartment significantly (Gelberman)
- Muscle compartments in the hand are isolated and require individual release
- Adequate decompression of the median nerve – at lacertus fibrosus, edge of pronator teres, proximal edge of flexor superficialis and carpal tunnel
- Carpal tunnel – raised pressure in the forearm/hand; compartment syndrome, release of the carpal tunnel, also indirectly releasing Guyon's canal

8.1.13 Location of Fasciotomy Incisions
- Arm

- Anterior and deltoid compartment – incision from elbow just medial to the lateral bicipital sulcus to the acromion
- Posterior compartment – posterior incision from the olecranon along the lateral side of the triceps
- Anterior and posterior compartment – single medial incision over medial intermuscular septum from shoulder to elbow (Green)
- Volar forearm compartment
  - Henry's approach
  - Ulnar approach
  - Minimise damage to the cutaneous nerves and longitudinal veins
  - Create skin flaps to cover the median nerve at the wrist and the ulnar nerve at the elbow
- Dorsal forearm compartment
  - Straight linear incision from 2 cm lateral and 2 cm distal to the lateral epicondyle towards the midline of the wrist
- Dorsal surface of the hand
  - Interosseous compartments and adductor compartment
  - Two longitudinal incisions over the I/F and R/F
- Palmar surface of the hand
  - Extended carpal tunnel release
  - Thenar compartment – longitudinal incision over the radial side of the first metacarpal
  - Hypothenar compartment – longitudinal incision over the ulnar side of the fifth metacarpal
- Fingers and thumb
  - Mid-lateral incision along the non-dominant side of the digits
- Leg fasciotomy
  - Double incision (Mubarak 1976)
  - Perifibular (Matsen)
  - Fibulectomy– contraindicated in trauma patients
- Foot fasciotomy
  - Two dorsal incisions
  - One medial incision (Henry)

8.1.14   Complications of Compartment Syndrome

8.1.14.1 Volkmann's Ischaemic Contracture

- Irreversible tissue ischaemia because of delayed or incomplete fasci otomy → muscle necrosis and scar down → contracture
- Forearm: elbow flexion, forearm pronation, wrist flexion, thumb ad duction, MCPJ extension, IPJ flexion

8.1.14.2 Volkmann's Ischaemic Contracture: Treatment

- Splinting
- Physiotherapy
- Surgery – muscle excision, muscle sliding, tendon transfer, free mus cle transplantation (gracilis muscle)

8.1.15   Delayed/Late treatment of Compartment Syndrome

- ≥ 24 h
  - Increased rate of infection and amputation after fasciotomy
  - Observe and reconstruct later

8.1.16   Fasciotomy Wound Management

- Dressing
- Primary suture
- Secondary intention
- Skin grafting

8.1.17   Chronic Compartment Syndrome

8.1.17.1 Clinical Features

- Most associated with exercise
- Frequently bilateral
- Pressure and cramping in the involved compartment, associated numbness and weakness
- Resolved with rest
- May evolve into acute compartment syndrome
- Most common anterior and lateral compartments of the leg
- Muscle hernia (occurs in 60% in Reneman's series, more obvious after exercise), lower third of the leg between the anterior and lateral

compartments where there are branches of the superficial peroneal nerve

8.1.17.2 Dx of Chronic Compartment Syndrome
- Compartment pressure measurement (before and after exercise)
- Resting pressure ≥ 15 mmHg
- One minute post-exercise pressure ≥ 30 mmHg
- Five minutes post-exercise pressure ≥ 20 mmHg
- Recent near-infrared spectroscopy (non-invasive)

8.1.17.3 DDx of Chronic Compartment Syndrome
- Stress fracture, periostitis, tendinitis, nerve entrapment, vascular claudication, venous stasis, neurogenic claudication

8.1.17.4 Treatment of Chronic Compartment Syndrome
- Activity modification
- Fasciotomy – smaller incision

8.2 Deep Vein Thrombosis and Pulmonary Embolism

8.2.1 Nature and Pathophysiology of DVT
- Thrombus formation in the venous system of the lower limbs
- Can occur anywhere from the pelvic veins down to the calf veins
- Proximal DVT carries a higher risk of developing PE
- Often silent and asymptomatic
- Usually resolves, seldom leading to long-term venous insufficiency
- Thrombus dislodgement can lead to PE
- Pathophysiology:
  - Venous stasis
  - Endothelial injury
  - Hypercoagulability

8.2.2 Risk Factors
- Old age

- Obesity
- Varicose veins
- Immobility
- Pregnancy
- High-dose oestrogen therapy
- Thrombophilia
- Malignancy
- Heart failure
- Nephrotic syndrome
- Trauma
- Surgery of long duration
- Pelvic and lower limb surgery

8.2.3   Operations with Highest Risk in the Field of Orthopaedics

- Total hip replacement
- Total knee replacement
- Multiple trauma, especially pelvic-acetabular fractures
- Spinal cord injury

8.2.4   Incidence (Without Prophylaxis)

Total DVT	40–80%
Proximal DVT	15–50%
Fatal PE	0.3–0.5%

8.2.5   Diagnosis of DVT

- Clinical – calf pain, swelling, Homan's sign, fever, tenderness
- USG – sensitive, operator-dependent
- Venogram – sensitive, gold-standard
- I^{125}-fibrinogen scan – limited accuracy

8.2.6   Diagnosis of Pulmonary Embolism

- Clinical – chest pain, shortness of breath, tachycardia
- Ventilation/perfusion scan – screening
- Pulmonary angiogram

- Spiral CT
- MR angiogram

8.2.7 Prophylaxis of Thromboembolism

- Mechanical
  - Compression stockings
  - Pneumatic compression boots
  - Continuous passive motion
- Pharmacological
  - Warfarin
  - Heparin
  - LMW heparin
  - Aspirin
  - Dextran
- Type of anaesthesia

8.2.7.1 Mechanical Methods of Prophylaxis

- Compression stockings
  - No proven value when used alone
  - Have to be combined with other modalities
- Pneumatic compression boots
  - Increases venous blood flow
  - Reduces the rate of DVT
  - May be less effective against proximal DVT
- Foot pump
  - Intermittent plantar compression
  - Mimics walking
  - Early studies are promising
  - DVT rate of 13% in THR patients
- Continuous passive motion
  - No proven value

8.2.7.2 Pharmacological Prophylaxis

- Warfarin
  - The most commonly used agent in the past 20 years

- ↓ DVT by 60%
- ↓ Proximal DVT by 70%
- DVT rate: 20% after THR, 35–50% after TKR
- 10% of DVT cases are proximal (without prophylaxis 40% of DVT after THR are proximal DVT)
- Rate of significant bleeding 1–2%
- Maintain INR between 1.8 and 2.5
- Advantages: oral administration
- Low cost
- Disadvantages: delayed onset of action
- Bleeding
- Monitoring of INR
- Drug interactions

■ Heparin
- Standard fixed low dose is not effective in the prevention of proximal DVT
- Adjusted-dose heparin is more effective
- Slight effect on coagulability
- Prolongs the APTT by 1–5 s
- No increase in bleeding complications

■ Low molecular weight heparin (LMWH)
- Derived from enzymatic or chemical depolymerisation of standard heparin
- Similarly as effective as heparin
- Inhibits platelet function less; therefore, produces less bleeding
- 90% bioavailability
- Less binding to plasma proteins
- Four times longer half-life than heparin
- Allows once or twice daily dose
- Laboratory monitoring not required
- Reduces rate of proximal and distal DVT by 70%
- 6% after THR; 25% after TKR
- Comparison with warfarin:
    - Lower rate of DVT

- No significant difference in proximal DVT and symptomatic
- For PE: rate of bleeding 2–4 times higher
  - Disadvantages: parenteral; high cost
- Aspirin
  - Anti-platelet action
  - Inhibition of cyclo-oxygenase
  - Lower symptomatic PE rates in some non-randomised studies
  - No reduction in DVT rate in randomised studies
- Dextran
  - Moderately effective in preventing DVT after total joint replacement
  - 57% reduction in risk of DVT
  - If not popularly used, can cause:
    - Volume overload
    - Hypersensitivity reactions
    - Bleeding
    - High cost

8.2.8   Influence of Anaesthesia

- Use of epidural/spinal anaesthesia in THR leads to a ↓ rate of DVT (compared with GA): sympathetic blockade, vasodilatation, increased blood flow
- Hypotensive epidural anaesthesia further reduces blood loss
- Preserves blood volume and ↑ blood flow to the lower extremity
- Minimises activation of the clotting cascade
- Reduction of DVT only observed in patients not receiving prophylaxis

8.2.9   Prophylaxis: Current Status and Unresolved Issues

- Routine prophylaxis has been the standard of care since 1986
- Unresolved issues:
  - Role of routine surveillance
  - The type of prophylaxis
  - Duration of prophylaxis

8.2.10   Treatment of DVT
8.2.10.1   Aim of Treatment
- To prevent fatal PE
- To reduce the morbidity of DVT

8.2.10.2   Definitive Treatment
- Heparin
    - To prevent extension of the clot
    - Full heparinisation within 5 days of major bleeding due to joint replacement
    - LMWH is an effective alternative
    - Switch to warfarin for 3–6 months
- Inferior vena cava filter
    - When heparinisation is contraindicated
    - When there is recurrent PE

8.2.10.3   Management of Isolated Calf DVT
- Controversial
- Precursor of proximal clot propagation in 20% of patients
- Either anticoagulation or serial surveillance
- Risk of late postoperative DVT continues for 3 months
- LMWH reduces new symptomatic DVT identified 3 weeks later (from 19% to 7%)
- Current opinion supports continued prophylaxis beyond acute hospitalisation

8.3   Fat Embolism

8.3.1   Introduction
- Represents a contributing cause of death in patients of multiple trauma
- Fat can be found in the lungs of almost all patients with major trauma
- Clinical syndrome of fat embolism is found in about 5% of these patients

- Macroglobules of fat in both the pulmonary and systematic circulation, causing the fat embolisation syndrome, consisting of respiratory insufficiency, cerebral dysfunction, petechial haemorrhages

8.3.2   Aetiology of the Fat Embolism

- Pelvic or long bones fracture:
    - When fracture occurs, there is damage to the medullary venous sinuses, with fat globules from marrow
    - Enters the blood via the sinuses, then the pulmonary and systemic circulation
    - Also during manipulation and stabilisation of the fracture
- Massive trauma may disrupt adipose tissue especially high velocity gun shots, explosions and extensive burns
- Total joint replacement: during the intramedullary procedure in hip and knee replacement
- During reaming of an intramedullary nail

8.3.3   Pathological Mechanism of the Fat Embolism

- There are two main theories for the causative mechanism of fat embolism

8.3.3.1 Mechanical Theory

- Many fat globules are trapped by the pulmonary capillaries, some through the pulmonary capillaries or pulmonary AV anastomoses, and enter the systemic circulation, embolising the organs with high blood flow such as the brain, kidney or heart

8.3.3.2 Metabolic Theory

- Lipoprotein lipase on the capillary endothelial walls breaks down the large fat globules to release free fatty acid
- Pulmonary lipase also breaks down neutral triglycerides into toxic unsaturated FFA, causing endothelial damage with an inflammatory response and increasing capillary permeability
- Results in extravasation of proteinaceous fluid, even intra-alveolar haemorrhage

8.3.4   Associated Abnormal Physiology

- Mechanisms cause hypoxia due to ventilation/perfusion mismatch, shunting, diffusion impairment, congestive atelectasis, decreased compliance and increased dead space/tidal volume ratio
- Coagulation abnormalities may occur (DIC)
- Cerebral effects persist despite correction of hypoxaemia and in the absence of direct cranial trauma
- Hypovolaemic shock exacerbates right heart failure

8.3.5   Signs and Symptoms

- Usually a history of fracture of the long bone of the lower limb, patient transport with insufficient fracture immobilisation, occasional arthroplasty
- Onset 1–2 days after injury. Earliest symptoms are dyspnoea and tachypnoea, with cyanosis, cough and production of frothy, blood-stained sputum
- In about 25–50% of patients, there is a petechial rash involving the upper thorax, axillae, neck, soft palate and conjunctiva, which may be due to occlusion of the capillaries by fat globules or as a result of thrombocytopenia (by DIC)
- Mental changes include confusion, drowsiness, decerebrate signs, convulsion and coma
- 60% of patients have mild to moderate pyrexia associated with tachycardia
- Fat globules and petechiae are seen on retinal examination

8.3.6   Laboratory Test

- Arterial blood gas – low PaO2 and low $PaCO_2$, respiratory alkalosis (hyperventilation)
- Hypoxaemia is the hallmark of FES
- Urine and sputum – fat globules
- Haemoglobin – mild anaemia, haemolytic features with falling serum haptoglobin
- Coagulation – increased fibrin degradation products, thrombocytopenia, and coagulation abnormalities

- Ca level – fall in serum calcium combined with the free fatty acids to form soaps
- Fat macroglobulinaemia > 8 μm, by cryostat test (clotted blood is frozen, sectioned and stained for fat)
- CXR – diffuse opacification of both lung fields, features of ARDS
- ECG – evidence of right ventricular strain, T wave inversion, RBBB
- (Note: The tests are often too insensitive and non-specific. The diagnosis essentially remains a clinical one)

8.3.7 Management
8.3.7.1 Introduction
- It is a self-limiting disease, the treatment is mainly supportive, and there is emphasis on the maintenance of oxygen delivery to the peripheral tissues

8.3.7.2 Prevention
- Rapid immobilisation of the fracture site prior to transport of the patient
- Early operative fixation of fractures of long bones
- Evidence shows that the use of sharp reamers, with deep flutes and small reamer shafts, and slowly advancing the reamer generates less fat embolism
- No evidence can confirm that an unreamed nail has an advantage over a reamed nail in terms of reducing fat embolism
- Evidence shows that pulsatile lavage before cementation in arthroplasty decreases the fat embolism
- Over-reaming of the femoral canal can decrease incidence in TKA

8.3.7.3 Managing More Severe Scenarios
8.3.7.3.1 Pulmonary Ventilatory Support
- Oxygen by face mask and continuous positive airway pressure (CPAP)
- Mechanical ventilatory support with positive end expiratory pressure (PEEP) if PaO_2 cannot be maintained above 8 kPa
- Intensive care monitoring is essential

- Repeated ABG analysis over the first 48 h is the most valuable guide to diagnosis and therapy

8.3.7.3.2 Adequate Circulating Volume
- Normal circulating volume must be ensured. Untreated shock is associated with poor prognosis in FES

8.3.7.3.3 Role of Steroids
- Use of steroids remains controversial
- Methylprednisolone with a dosage of 10mg/kg is shown to play a prophylactic role only
- Some other studies show that large doses of steroids diminish hypoxaemia, when given early

8.3.7.3.4 Other Agents: Aspirin, Dextran, Heparin
- Some evidence shows that they may be of limited benefit in decreasing platelet adhesiveness and formation of fibrin-fat emboli aggregates
- They are not used routinely
- They may exacerbate bleeding from sites of recent trauma

Selected Bibliography of Journal Articles

1. Anand S, Buch K (2007) Post-discharge symptomatic thromboembolic events in hip fracture patients. Ann R Coll Surg Eng 89(5):517–520
2. Glover P, Worthley LI (1999) Fat embolism. Crit Care Resusc 1(3):276–284
3. Jeong GK, Gruson KI, et al. (2007) Thromboprophylaxis after hip fracture: evaluation of 3 pharmacologic agents. Am J Orthop 36(3):135–140
4. McQueen MM, Court-Brown CM (1996) Acute compartment syndrome in tibial diaphyseal fractures. J Bone Joint Surg Br 78(1):95–98

Trauma to the Upper Extremities

Contents

9.1 Sternoclavicular Joint

- Stability determined by strong soft tissue structures, i.e. capsular ligament, inter-clavicular ligament, costo-clavicular ligament and intra-articular disc
- Other anatomic features: similarity with distal clavicle in having intra-articular disc and costoclavicular ligament, which is rather like coracoclavicular (CC) ligament

9.1.1 Sternoclavicular Joint Dislocation

- Anterior >> posterior dislocation, but posterior much more dangerous – look for altered breathing, circulation, BP, etc.
- One of the least dislocated body joints, physeal injury < 20 s is in fact more common
- Dx – clinical (not always accurate in assessing direction of dislocation); X-ray (Rockwood favours caudocephalic tilt X-ray and comparing both clavicle positions by an imaginary horizontal line, called serendipity because this X-ray view was discovered by chance), ± tomograms. CT is the best investigation, can also see physeal injury cases better in younger patients

9.1.2 Clinical Signs to Suggest Dangerous Posterior Dislocation

- Shortness of breath
- Upper limb venous congestion
- Palpable sternal corner on ipsilateral side
- Compromised arm circulation
- Swallowing difficulties

9.1.3 Reduction Manoeuvre

- Anterior – closed reduction (CR) manoeuvre: direct pressure or try figure-of-eight strapping
- Posterior – support in between shoulders or seated with knee of surgeon, then pull shoulders back/in some cases try the use of towel clip. Try to have early reduction, not later than 4 days

- Posterior dislocation cases = always have the thoracic surgeon ready in case massive bleeding from torn vessels occurs
- Post-reduction stability: posterior dislocation cases more stable than anterior

9.1.4   Main Pitfall
- In young patients labelled with this Dx, need to carefully differentiate from physeal injuries using CT scanning

9.1.5   Complications (Posterior Injuries)
- Superior vena cava (SVC) laceration
- Pneumothorax
- Thoracic outlet syndrome
- Oesophagus rupture ± tracheo-oesophageal (TE) fistula
- Death from haemorrhage

9.2   Acromioclavicular Joint Dislocation

- Usually result of a fall at the tip of the shoulder
- Clinically sometimes indistinguishable from a very distal fractured clavicle with displacement
- Check integrity of the other components of the suspensory ligament complex of the shoulder girdle region (will be discussed below)
- Only the treatment of type 3 is controversial

9.2.1   Rockwood Classification
- Type 1 – sprained acromio-clavicular ligament
- Type 2 – acromio-clavicular joint (ACJ) subluxates
- Type 3 – no more contact (CC ligament ruptured)
- Type 4 – clavicle driven posteriorly into trapezius
- Type 5 – very marked displacement (torn delto-trapezial fascia)
- Type 6 – clavicle under acromion, very rarely seen

9.2.2   Management

- Treatment by types:
  - Type 1: conservative
  - Type 2: conservative, chronic symptomatic cases as type 3
  - Type 3: controversial. Proposers of operative Rn still have to demonstrate that result of operation brings near normal function
  - Type 4: most operate
  - Type 5: operative, since skin impingement and associated soft tissue tears significant
  - Type 6: operative, may need distal clavicle excision ± Weaver-Dunn (modified) by substitute coraco-acromial (CA) ligament to replace the torn CC ligament
- Operative options for types 3 and 5
  - Historic – transfer coracoid (with muscles attached) to under-surface clavicle. Little used since musculocutaneous palsy and pain common
  - Transfix ACJ – danger of damaging the intra-articular (IA) disc and degenerative changes later; pin migration lethal
  - CC screw (Fig. 9.1) more popular than implants like the hooked plate (Fig. 9.2), which can cause impingement
  - Resect distal clavicle ± with modified Weaver-Dunn

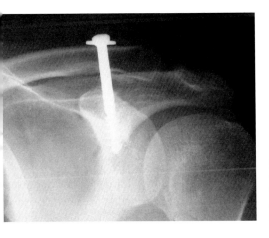

Fig. 9.1 Radiograph of patient illustrating the use of the coraco-clavicular screw in operative treatment of ACJ dislocation

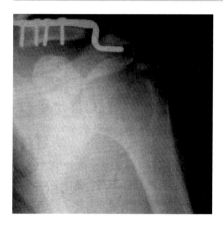

Fig. 9.2 The hooked plate illustrated here is not as popular as it frequently causes shoulder impingement

9.3   Shoulder Dislocation and Instability

9.3.1   General Concepts

- Matsen proposes two ends of the spectrum:
  - TUBS: traumatic unidirectional instability from Bankart lesion that may require surgery: (repair, capsular shift, etc.); vs.
  - AMBRI(I): atraumatic multidirectional instability, that tends to be bilateral, needs rehabilitation, and only if fails inferior capsular shift needed ± closing the rotator interval
- Qualify any dislocation by the following:
  - Acute vs. chronic/locked, or recurrent
  - Position of the humeral head
  - Direction of dislocation
  - Voluntary vs. involuntary
  - Dislocation or subluxation

9.3.2   Facts and Myths of Anterior Dislocation

- Myths:
  - Bankart lesions are the only essential lesions (although present in 90% of cases, capsular plastic deformation frequently coexists, lab tests seem to show that Bankart *alone* does not in fact frequently lead to dislocation)

- Recurrence in young patients: first time dislocators quoted as 90% by Rowe in JBJS in the 1950s (Bigliani feels that true figure more likely to be around 50–60%, quoted by Simonet and Cofield 1984). There are still no long-term results to support whether these shoulders routinely need to be fixed
- Period of immobilisation varies among centres; most use Bigliani's protocol of 3 weeks in young patients and less, say, 1–2 weeks, in older patients in whom stiffness is more of a concern
- Avoid sports in younger patients for 6 weeks at least

.3.3   Investigations

- X-rays: in two planes (axillary and AP) are most useful
- Special X-ray views to pick up Hill Sachs lesions (Stryker Notch) and for viewing the glenoid (West Point). Hill Sachs lesions can sometimes be seen on axillary view (Fig. 9.3)
- MR arthrogram: helps pick up not only Bankart lesions (Fig. 9.4), but also other associated lesions such as cuff injuries, humeral avulsion of glenohumeral ligaments (HAGL) or superior labral anterior posterior (SLAP) lesions

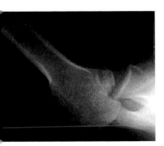

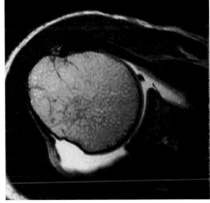

Fig. 9.3 This axillary view is a good illustration of the Hill Sachs lesion

Fig. 9.4 The anterior Bankart lesion is seen here on this MRI arthrogram

9.3.4   Anterior Dislocation: Treatment Principles

- Check for any generalised ligament laxity or any signs of multidirectional instability. Ask for all details of initial trauma events, its severity, position of arm, and treatment received
- Acute dislocations CR manoeuvres: most use the Hippocrates method, ruling out neurovascular injury and especially cuff tears in old folks, look out for any associated fractures (Fig. 9.5)
- Mostly immobilised for 3 weeks, followed by shoulder rehabilitation
- Role of arthroscopy mainly:
  - To tackle pain from debridement loose flaps
  - To tackle strategic lesions like Bankart repair (Fig. 9.6) and capsular side. Contraindication if inexperienced, pear-shaped glenoid, engaging Hill Sachs lesions ± need to assess any deficient glenoid bone stock in recurrent cases
- Open repair
  - Obsolete procedures include, e.g. PuttiPlate, where too much undesirable stiffness results, or bony procedures, like proximal

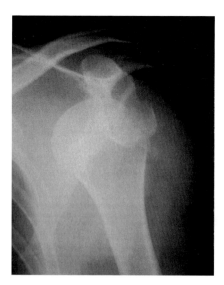

Fig. 9.5 This patient suffers from anterior fracture dislocation of the shoulder

humeral osteotomy, since in most cases of acute dislocators there is no bony deformity – therefore no point – or procedures that involve implants like Bristow with its attendant Cx
— Extent of ST injury should be assessed preoperatively, frequently need to repair Bankart, and may need a capsular shift

9.3.5   Key Points: Anterior Dislocations

■ Bankart not always the "essential lesion", many other possibilities:
— HAGL lesion
— Capsular rupture
— Glenoid fracture or bony erosion
— Capsular stretch/plastic deformation
— Rotator interval insufficiency (lost negative pressure)
— Large Hill Sachs lesion

9.3.6   Pearl

■ Shoulder stability depends equally on static and dynamic stability, thus even after Bankart/capsular shifts, rehabilitation of cuff and scapular muscles are equally important

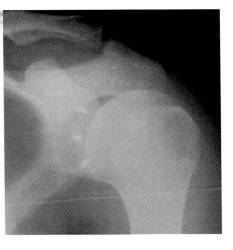

Fig. 9.6 This postoperative radiograph after Bankart repair reviews the position of the suture anchors

9.3.7   Posterior Dislocations

- Differences from anterior dislocations
  - Clinical – apprehension is uncommon, although posterior joint line tenderness may occur. Pain and discomfort in *adduction* forward flexion and internal rotation (IR), and certain clinical situations make it more likely. Clinical Dx more subtle since humeral head is not usually medialised: use jerk test/posterior drawer test
  - X-ray – light bulb sign on AP and axillary view helpful

Pathology – only 10% have the so-called "reverse Bankart" lesion, an occasional one may have hypoplastic glenoid with different glenoid version, or abnormal retroversion of the proximal humerus

  - Arthroscopic method: no large series, more advisable may be the posterior capsular procedures and tackling any strategic lesions if they are found. Bigliani favours open methods such as posterior capsular shift

9.3.8   Pearl

- Beware of the subgroup with HAGL lesions – can cause severe posterior instability

9.3.9   Is It Multi-directional or Voluntary Instability?

- Really "voluntary" dislocators, but not all cases have psychological elements or are intentional. Some are "positional", others are "muscular". Muscular types treated by biofeedback; positional types may need operative Rn
- Multidirectional instability patients mostly have obvious sulcus signs, ligamentous laxity is common. To Dx multi-directional instability (MDI), patient needs to be symptomatic in ≥ two directions

9.3.10   Dx of Multi-directional Instability

- Clinical: Bigliani suggests that after inspection and palpation, always check for sulcus signs, since if other provocative tests are carried out first, there may be too much tensing up of the muscles

- A common positive case has sulcus signs suggesting inferior instability (pathologies may include rotator interval lesions) and anterior instability (in abduction and ER; ± can do the Jobe's relocation tests). Rotator interval (RI) lesions are associated with inferior instability
- Mainstay of Dx of MDI is Hx and P/E, does not always need expensive Rn. Typical symptom: pain not always instability and at mid-range instead of end range. May or may not have a significant traumatic episode
- X-ray may not be positive
- Scope – drive-through sign a common finding
- Open surgery – Bigliani believes that inferior shift is important to shrink the capsular volume in three planes – anterior, posterior and inferior. Thus inferior instability, if present, must be tackled

9.3.11   Appendix on Multi-directional Instability

- If use arthroscopy → tackle
  - Anterior band of inferior glenohumeral ligament (IGHL)
  - Posterior band of IGHL
  - Close rotator interval
- 50% of patients still think they are loose postoperatively
- Pathology: excess capsular volume, other possibilities (labral split/ Bankart can occur in MDI; labral/chondral erosions, capsule or synovial stripping)
- The drive-through sign may be found intraoperatively with arthroscopy; Warner's method to use scope to assess capsule laxity is as follows: with the arm in abduction + ER – humeral head should not go over the glenoid rim (Warner et al. 2005)

9.3.12   A Word About Arthroscopy

- Recurrence rate reported to be 5–50%
- In the best hands, arthroscopic Rn recurrence rate approaches that of open surgery, but not in the presence of bony lesions (e.g. Hill Sachs lesion) or normal variants like pear-shaped glenoids
- Causes of failure of arthroscopic Rn:

- Inadequate technique
- Capsular laxity
- Thin ligament–labrum complex
- Inadequate sutures
- Failure in patient selection process: good candidate = discrete Bankart lesion, no bony glenoid/large Hill Sachs lesion, no capsular ruptures, ± no rotator interval insufficiency
- Often, besides tackling Bankart, capsular shift may be needed to address anterior/inferior laxity

9.4   Fractured Clavicle

- 10% of all fractures, very common
- Most occur at middle third, the normal clavicle mainly functions as a strut, and as suspension to the shoulder
- Most are closed fractures, open fractures are uncommon, as are stress fractures, although these are reported in overhead sports
- The deformity frequently involves shortening, angulation and medial rotation
- Recent literature casts doubt on the old literature, which claimed a low non-union rate for middle third fractures. Recent figures put the rate of non-union with conservative Rn to be > 15%. The fracture does not seem to heal in adults as well as in the paediatric age group
- On the contrary, lateral third fractures have long been known to have a significant non-union rate

9.4.1   Pathomechanics

- Most fractured clavicles are sustained by falling on the point of the shoulder, direct blows rare. Those with high-energy injuries need to rule out brachial plexus injury, pneumothorax and vascular injuries
- The sternomastoid lifts the medial fragment, while pectoralis major gives an adducting/rotating force
- Middle third fractures are most common because it represents a region of transition in bone curvature and cross-sectional anatomy

- In fact, non-unions are not uncommon at this site, partly because of less vascularity from less muscular attachment

9.4.2   Fractured Clavicle Classification
- Popular classification:
    - Group I refers to middle third fractures
    - Group II refers to lateral third fractures, which in turn are divided into three types – see below
    - Group III refers to medial third fractures

9.4.3   Classification of Lateral Third Fractures
- Type 1: CC ligament intact
- Type 2: CC ligament torn, with high riding fractured end of clavicle (Fig. 9.7)
- Type 3: Intra-articular fracture, extending to involve the ACJ

9.4.4   Conservative Treatment: Majority of Patients
- Usually involves either a figure-of-eight bandage or arm sling
- Disadvantages: figure-of-eight bandage frequently causes pain through direct pressure on common middle third fractures and needs periodic tightening
- Medial third fractures may also benefit from figure-of-eight bandages

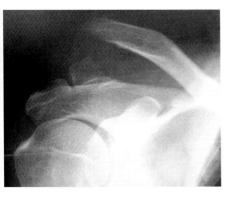

Fig. 9.7 This patient has type 2 variety of group II fractured clavicle

- Lateral third fractures, type II, difficult to be held by the same method, may need Howard Kenny bracing, but even this frequently fails – may need surgery

9.4.5   Operative Indications
- Floating shoulder
- Open fractures
- Associated neurovascular injury
- Skin impingement
- Increasing trend to fix widely displaced fractures. The extent of the fracture displacement (e.g. shortening > 15–20 mm in the younger, high-demand patient) and presence of any somersaulted fragments can be better seen with added X-ray views with 45° cephalic tilt
- Segmental fractures

9.4.6   Reason for the Trend Towards Fixing Displaced Clavicular Fractures
- Recent studies suggest that non-union rates with conservative Rn of mid third fractures is a handsome 15–20%
- Not uncommon functional deficit after conservative Rn: shoulder drooping, shoulder girdle protraction, from shortening of the bone, overhead activities can be rendered difficult
- Non-union is found to occur more likely with extent of fracture displacement, comminution, and shortening > 2 cm, and injury severity, as reported in J Bone Joint Surg Br
- Lower non-union rates reported recently after ORIF with improved operative techniques and fixation methods

9.4.7   Choice of Fixation
- Plate and screw most popular – avoid weak plates such as one-third tubulars (use LC-DCP) placed on the tension side (superior). Avoid the use of k-wires, and cerclage. Also, need to avoid unnecessary periosteal stripping, neuroma, and need to protect the neurovascular structures during drilling. Proper plate contouring is essential
- Intramedullary devices – not too popular and lack rotational control, and danger of migration, although more cosmetic. Seldom used

9.4.8   Choice of Fixation of Lateral Third Fractures

- Trans-articular methods are falling out of favour (e.g. k-wires and tension bands) – risk migration of implant and later joint arthrosis. Avoid distal fragment excision
- Fixation of the medial fragment towards a strong bony point such as the coracoid: e.g. coraco-clavicular screws, cerclage (Fig. 9.8) usually performed
- Others: traditional plate fixation usually rendered difficult by the short distal fragment; use of special plate to insinuate under the distal fragment/acromion while having screw fixation of medial fragment risks shoulder impingement and is not very popular

(P.S. Not all type 2 non-unions need treatment, many are asymptomatic)

9.4.9   Weaver-Dunn Procedure

- For (usually old) symptomatic type II non-unions:
  - Distal fragment excised
  - Proximal fragment stabilisation by transferring a detached CA ligament from the acromion
  - CC also usually needs repair

9.4.10   Complications

- Non-union
- Neurovascular injuries

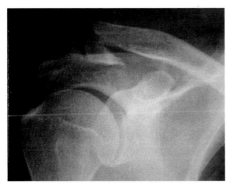

Fig. 9.8 The same patient postoperatively after cerclage of the fractured distal clavicle

- Skin impingement/injury
- Fracture shortening, with resultant ptosis of ipsilateral shoulder and shoulder girdle protraction
- Cx related to ORIF: neuroma, sepsis, hardware problems, etc.
- Cosmesis problem (if huge callus)

9.4.11   Treatment of Non-unions
- Middle third fractures: most require bone graft and rigid plate fixation, while preserving the supra-clavicular nerves
- Lateral third fractures:
  - May need to stabilise the medial fragment by ligament transfer ± resection of the distal fragment

9.5   Fractured Scapula and Glenoid

- Classification of scapula fractures: (usually refers to anatomic region involved, i.e. anatomic classification)
  - Scapula body most common (Fig. 9.9)

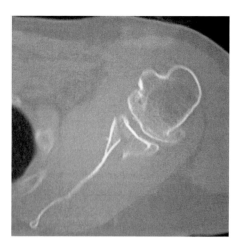

Fig. 9.9 CT film showing fracture of the scapula

- Glenoid neck
- Glenoid fossa
- Acromion
- Coracoid
- Complex (more than one region fractured)

9.5.1 Ideberg Classification of Glenoid Fractures

- Type I: avulsion of the anterior margin
- Type II: transverse fractures exiting inferiorly
- Type III: oblique fractures through the glenoid that exits superiorly ± associated ACJ injury
- Type IV: transverse fractures exiting at medial scapula border
- Type V: combination of types II and IV

9.5.2 Rn of Scapula Body Fractures

- Most are undisplaced
- Conservative Rn: armsling and early motion
- Healing usually not a problem because of good vascularity
- Consider operative intervention only if significantly displaced

9.5.3 Rn of Extra-Articular Glenoid Fractures

- ORIF indicated for displaced and angulated fractures: e.g. angulation of 45° and >1 cm displaced
- Untreated, e.g. displaced glenoid neck fractures will disturb the biomechanics of the shoulder, and influence the rotator cuff mechanics

9.5.4 Rn of Glenoid Intra-articular Fractures

- Ideberg I: consider ORIF if involve > 20–30% of the rim, to prevent instability. Grafting may be required if fracture is too comminuted
- Other Ideberg types: consider ORIF if there is humeral head subluxation and/or articular step-off

9.5.5 SSSC Concept (J Orthop Trauma 1993)

- SSSC = superior suspensory shoulder complex

- A biomechanical concept to aid tackling of complex combined frac
tures in the shoulder girdle area, e.g. concomitant fractured clavicle
and glenoid neck, and in other situations of "floating shoulder"

9.5.6   SSSC and Floating Shoulder (After Goss 1993)

- Contents of the shoulder suspensory complex ≥ two bone struts
(clavicle and scapula spine), ring (coracoid, CA ligament, AC liga
ment, acromion and glenoid neck/fossa region)
- Instability is likely if breaks at:
    - Two bone struts
    - Two articulations
    - One bone strut (e.g. clavicle) and bone of the ring (e.g. glenoid
    neck) – "floating shoulder", etc.

9.5.7   Concomitant Fractured Clavicle and Glenoid Neck

- This combination creates the usual "floating shoulder"
- Although ORIF of the fractured clavicle may reduce the displaced
glenoid, ORIF of the glenoid fracture may be required if residual dis
placement occurs

9.6   Lateral Scapula Dissociation (Closed Traumatic Fore-quarter)

- Severe injury usually with traction element
- X-ray: scapula lateralised
- Need angiogram as high incidence of brachial plexus and vascular
injuries
- Much ST injury found at operation, both to muscles and ST as well
- Rare

9.7 Fractured Proximal Humerus

9.7.1 Introduction

- The proximal humerus is the second most frequently fractured upper limb bone
- Peak after fifth decade
- Most are in women, 80% are undisplaced, which can be treated by conservative means
- In the remaining 20% displaced fractures, incidence of two-part fractures > three-part and four-part
- Neer's classification most popular

9.7.2 Neer's Classification

- Nomenclature depends on the surgeon's assessment of: number of fragments, degree of displacement, any dislocation
- Definition of displacement: > 1 cm from anatomic position, > 45° angulation (Fig. 9.10)

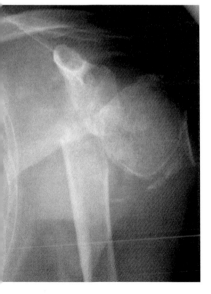

Fig. 9.10 Radiograph showing displaced fracture of the proximal humerus

- Notice that the above definition of 1 cm and 45° was in fact arbitrary (requested by JBJS) before Neer could publish his classic paper
- All undisplaced fractures = one part, irrespective of the number of fracture lines
- Two-part fractures: four possibilities – anatomical neck, surgical neck, greater tuberosity, lesser tuberosity
- Three-part fractures: two possibilities – surgical neck and either greater or lesser tuberosity
- Fracture dislocations: can be two, three or four parts. Need to mention direction of dislocation
- Articular fractures: include
  - Head splitting fractures (may need CT to Dx)
  - Impression fractures (more often seen with chronic dislocation)

9.7.3   Criticism of Neer's Classification

- Low inter- and intra-observer reliability
- Definition of what constitutes displacement was in fact arbitrary
- Quoted Kappa coefficient for Neer's classification: 0.65 for intra-observer and 0.58 for inter-observer

(Kappa reliability coefficient: refers to adjusted level of agreement between and among observers corrected for that which would occur by chance)

- Figures for AO classification also found to be low
- But note that adequate, properly taken X-rays need to be obtained using scapular AP + axillary + scapula-Y before assessment of fracture classification

9.7.4   Other Recent Criticism of Neer's Classification

- Neer's classification was based on Codman's original drawings
- However, some recent criticism pointed out that besides the limited inter-/intra-observer reliability issues, the fracture patterns depicted seem to be oversimplified and some fracture plane combinations were not considered. This led to the development of the more logical

recent system known as "binary classification", as described by Hertel and colleagues

9.7.5 AO Classification

- Type A – lowest AVN risk
- Type B – higher AVN risk
- Type C – most severe, highest AVN risk
- AO classification also has rather low inter- and intra-observer reproducibility and not shown to predict outcome

9.7.6 New Binary Classification (After Hertel)

- The binary system as described by Hertel et al., is based on analysis of fracture *planes* as opposed to fragment number, as in Neer's classification
- It describes five basic fracture planes that can be identified by answering five questions:
  - Any fractures between head and greater tuberosity (GT)?
  - Any fractures between shaft and GT?
  - Any fractures between head and lesser tuberosity (LT)?
  - Any fractures between shaft and LT?
  - Any fractures between GT and LT?
- If the above questions cannot be answered by the X-rays available, further imaging is required
- It is hoped that this classification will have better inter- and intra-observer agreement
- Hertel further showed that the humeral head is likely to retain vascularity if there is lengthy medial metaphyseal head extension, and if there is the presence of a medial hinge

9.7.7 Humeral Head Blood Supply

- Supply to the humeral head is by ascending humeral circumflex, and anterior and posterior humeral circumflex arterial anastomosis
- Also some blood supply at sites of muscle attachment

9.7.8   Associated Injuries

- Gentle exam to check whether the fracture moves in one piece
- Rule out other bony injuries
- Neural exam: incidence of nerve injury: axillary nerve (test regimen batch area and look for deltoid contraction) > others such as ulna nerve, median nerve, radial nerve/anterior interosseus nerve (AIN), musculocutaneous nerve (screen elbow flexion), a few may have brachial plexus injury
- Check limb vascularity:
  - Suspect vascular injury in patients with significant medial displacement of the shaft fracture fragment
  - Suspect axillary vein thrombosis if there is large, diffusely swollen upper limb
  - Look for brachial artery injury in elderly with shoulder fracture dislocation, or dislocation

9.7.9   Work-up

- X-ray: should take at least two views 90° to each other, typically scapula AP and axillary views are most useful. If in doubt, more views are taken
- CT: especially of help in detecting articular, head splitting or impression fractures, and number of fragments. Sometimes need 2-mm cuts
- Others: MRI can be useful in detecting associated soft tissue injuries of shoulder-like rotator cuff injuries (important since they act as points of anchorage in fracture fixation, especially in osteoporotic bones, and if multiply disrupted, may increase compromise of vascularity)

9.7.10   Minimally Invasive Reduction of Proximal Humerus Fractures
9.7.10.1   *Indications*

- Can usually only be considered in the presence of soft tissue bridging of the fracture fragments in order to gain benefit from ligamentotaxis

- Recent works of Hertel et al. show that the vascularity of the humeral head is more likely to be maintained if:
  - There is an intact medial hinge of soft tissues
  - A lengthy metaphyseal head extension is noted on analysing the fracture pattern
- Common indications:
  - Valgus impacted fractured proximal humerus
  - Three-part fractures

9.7.10.2 Advantages of Minimally Invasive Technique

- In the absence of fracture exposure, adhesion within the surrounding gliding surfaces is reduced and the rehabilitation period possibly shorter than open surgery
- Less chance of sepsis
- Less bleeding
- Probably less pain and quicker rehabilitation

9.7.11   Management of Individual Fractures

9.7.11.1 Two-Part Anatomical Neck

- Rare fracture
- High chance of avascular necrosis (AVN) since lack of soft tissue attachments

9.7.11.1.1 Treatment

- Elderly – prosthetic replacement
- Young – ORIF is favoured. It should be noted that attempts are usually made to salvage the young person's humeral head. Previous papers by Gerber on fractured proximal humerus had shown that not every patient with AVN of the humeral head had a poor outcome

9.7.11.2 Two-Part Greater Tuberosity Fractures

- Quite common
- Associated with anterior dislocation
- Require CR ± OR preferably under general anaesthetic

- Although displacement as defined by Neer's classification is 1 cm, here < 1 cm displacement (say 0.5 cm) can produce acromial impingement
- Post-reduction X-ray with axillary view essential to ensure no significant displacement; recheck fracture pattern after reduction to check any other fractures lines not easily seen on the injury film. Finally, also check ER strength after reduction to check the cuff when pain is less
- Method of repair: TBW or screw

9.7.11.3 Two-Part Lesser Tuberosity Fractures

- Rare
- Association with posterior dislocation
- CR may be blocked by the biceps tendon
- Check whether fragment is significantly displaced or not by post-reduction axillary view, since displaced fragment may block IR
- Method of repair: suture or screw

9.7.11.4 Two-Part Surgical Neck

- Even in undisplaced fractures according to Neer's classification, look out for any varus documenting the degree of especially anterior angulation; > 45° angulation may limit forward flexion or abduction
- Significant varus with partial collapse may cause secondary impingement
- In displaced fractures, the shaft fragment is displaced anteromedially by the pectoralis major muscle
- Be careful to rule out vascular injuries in significantly medially displaced shaft fragment
- Method of CR: longitudinal traction, flexion, lateral displacement, then try to lock and/or impact the fragment
- Consider percutaneous pinning if deemed unstable, even if CR successful and fracture not moving in one piece
- Failed CR cases may be due to soft tissue interposition (e.g. periosteum, biceps tendon); consider ORIF

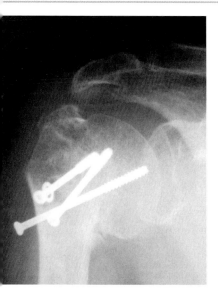

Fig. 9.11 Screw purchase is frequently difficult in the osteoporotic bones of the elderly

9.7.11.4.1 Indication for CR and Pinning

- CR successful
- Good bone stock, often fails in poor bones (Fig. 9.11)
- But the surgeon feels it may re-displace since unstable
- Has been used for two-part and three-part fractures

9.7.11.4.2 Pitfalls with Percutaneous Pinning of Fractured Proximal Humerus and Prevention

- Cx related to the lateral pins:
  - Avoid axillary nerve damage by placing the lateral pin distal enough
  - But avoid placing too low to avoid injuring the radial nerve
- Cx related to the anterior pins:
  - Structures that can be injured include cephalic vein, biceps tendon, musculocutaneous nerve (careful C-arm screening to guard against head penetration recommended)

9.7.11.4.3   ORIF Options
- Double TBW
- Enders nail and TBW
- Enders nail alone
- Locked rigid IM device – frequent cuff problems, shoulder pain or adhesions, and need a design with adequate oblique screw options for proximal locking
- AO newer low profile fixed-angle blades designed for the proximal humerus

9.7.11.5   Three-Part Fractures
- Less common than two-part fractures
- Commonly seen in elderly patients with osteoporosis
- Overall AVN chance 15–25%
- Neural injury more common if associated dislocation (e.g. brachial plexus injury)
- Vascular injury (e.g. axillary artery) needs to be ruled out if marked medial shaft displacement is seen through the surgical neck

9.7.11.5.1   The Deforming Forces
- Three-part fractures involving the greater tuberosity: humeral head may be internally rotated by action of the subscapularis
- Three-part fractures involving the lesser tuberosity:
  – Humeral head externally rotated by the supraspinatus

(In both cases, the humeral shaft tends to be medialised by the pectoralis major)

9.7.11.5.2   Rn Options
- CR and pinning (discussed already)
- ORIF
- Hemi-arthroplasty

9.7.11.5.3   ORIF in Three-Part Fractures
- There are many options for fracture fixation:
  – Double TBW

- TBW + IM rod (or rush pins)
- Traditional AO plating
- Newer locked humeral plating

9.7.11.5.4 Cx of ORIF

- AVN chance ×2 that of closed treatment
- Hardware impingement
- Implant migration and failure
- Pain
- Loss of reduction

9.7.11.5.5 ORIF in Osteoporotic Bones

- The AO locking humeral plate (Fig. 9.12), specifically designed for the proximal humerus, is especially useful in elderly with three-part fractured proximal humerus. Extremely osteoporotic cases may need cement augmentation to better the screw anchorage
- It features:
  - Angular stability

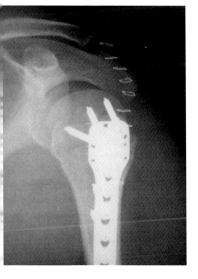

Fig. 9.12 The new LCP is a better option for osteoporotic proximal humerus fractures

- Orientation of screw holes based on anatomic studies to allow optimisation of the number and the direction of screw placement
- Low profile
- Specially designed to suit the local anatomy of the proximal humerus
- Complications with these new implants are beginning to be realised:
- Shoulder impingement is not uncommon
- Postoperative axillary view frequently shows screw penetration to the humeral head since lack of "feel" experienced by the surgeon on inserting screws to very osteoporotic bones

9.7.11.5.6 Who Needs Hemi-arthroplasty?

■ Err on the side of hemi-arthroplasty if:
- Associated dislocation, if present, is indicative of a higher chance of significant trauma
- Poor bone quality
- Advanced age
- Radiologic clues of humeral head vascularity – see below

■ One recent paper describes important X-ray clues concerning vascularity (important as it will affect our decision-making) – humeral head is likely to retain vascularity if there is lengthy medial metaphyseal head extension, and if there is the presence of a medial hinge

9.7.11.6 Valgus-Impacted Four-Part Fracture

■ Here the tuberosities frequently remain at their original height, and the periosteum is usually not torn
■ There is usually still a medial periosteal hinge connection between head and shaft on the medial side
■ The above medial hinge eases reduction manoeuvres to disimpact the impacted humeral head from the metaphysis

9.7.11.7 Other Four-Part Fractures

■ Unlike valgus-impacted four-part fractures, AVN chance is high, >50% and hemi-arthroplasty is usually the option, especially in the elderly

- Here, there is no remaining intact medial periosteal hinge as AVN is even more likely to occur in those fractures associated with dislocation

9.7.11.8 Articular Fractures of the Humeral Head

- Most require the use of prosthetic replacements
- Head splitting fractures are associated with fracture of the tuberosities or the surgical neck. Although ORIF was tried in the past, there is a high chance of re-displacement and need for prosthetic replacements
- Except in those with small impression defects that one can try reduction and a brief period of immobilisation
- Large Hill-Sachs defect may need transfer of the lesser tuberosity to the defect

9.7.11.9 Appendix: Cx of Hemi-arthroplasty for Fractured Proximal Humerus

- Prosthesis and tuberosity malpositioning
- Wrong version
- Migration
- Greater tuberosity detachment
- Prosthetic loosening
- Dislocation
- Glenoid erosion
- Others: sepsis, HO, etc.

9.7.11.10 Possible Improvement in Future: CAOS

- Computer-aided surgery is now coming of age. As shoulder hemi-arthroplasty is commonly associated with complications, and the reported results in many centres did not compare favourably with the initial results of Neer's; it is expected that CAOS will be more popular in the coming future to tackle this problem
- As patients' anatomies are not all the same, a new CAOS technique has recently been shown to allow patient-specific restoration of the shoulder joint based on preoperative CT of the opposite uninjured shoulder

9.7.11.11 Possible Improvement in Future: Fracture-Specific Implant

■ The newer generation of proximal humerus locking plates show the following improvements in design:
  – Can be placed lower and space of 2.5 cm allowance made to prevent cuff impingement
  – Horizontal holes in the proximal head of the plate allow reattachment of tuberosity
  – Less horizontal screw angulation and spacing out the screws both centrally and peripherally
■ Various companies are now manufacturing implants to circumvent the problems associated with hemi-arthroplasty viz:
  – Window in metaphyseal region to allow BG placement
  – Modularity to allow fine adjustment of humeral head offset
  – Better visual positioning guide for correct restoration of version
  – Medialisation of the neck of the prosthesis to ease placement of tuberosities

9.8   Humeral Shaft Fractures

9.8.1   Introduction

■ Previous operative results poor in the old days
■ High level of reported Cx in the past
■ Proper description of the fracture should include:
  – Low- vs. high-energy trauma
  – Associated soft-tissue injury
  – If open fracture, its Gustilo's grade
  – Associated neurovascular injury
  – Other associated injuries

9.8.2   Epidemiology

■ AO type A: 63%, type B 26%, type C 10%
■ Middle third fractures most common
■ Next in frequency are proximal third fractures
■ < 10% are open fractures

- Bimodal age distribution
- Peaks are in third decade and seventh decade

9.8.3   Work-up

- Check injury mechanism – direct vs. indirect
- Clinical signs, including assessing the radial nerve and other nerves – common in Holstein fractures (Fig. 9.13)
- Status of the soft tissue envelope, e.g. compartment syndrome
- Two X-ray views at 90° to each other is essential
- Assess the two nearby joints (shoulder and elbow)

9.8.4   Conservative Rn

- First line of treatment, U-slab and handing cast are mostly used, especially for mid third fractures

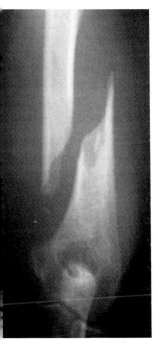

Fig. 9.13 Holstein fracture is sometimes associated with radial nerve palsy

■ Hanging cast:
  – Given for 2–3 weeks, then changed to Sarmiento brace
  – Expect union in 3 months
  – Accepted alignment: 20° anterior angulation, 30° varus, 1 cm in shortening
  – Overall, over 90% of cases unite with conservative treatment i done properly

9.8.5   Operative Indications
■ Failed conservative Rn (Fig. 9.14)
■ Open fractures
■ Neurovascular injury

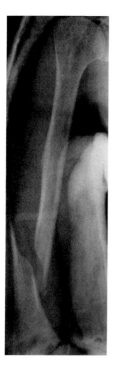

Fig. 9.14 This patient's fractured humerus failed to heal with conservative treatment

- Floating/segmental fractures
- Associated intra-articular fractures that need Rn
- Associated brachial plexus injuries that need Rn
- Poly-trauma or bilateral fractures
- Pathological fractures

9.8.6 Late Operation Needed in Some Scenarios

- Infection (e.g. open fractures)
- Malunion/non-union
- Associated radial nerve injury that fails to improve after adequate period of observation

9.8.7 Radial Nerve Injury and Humeral Shaft Fractures

- Exploration a must if nerve palsy occurs after fracture manipulation/ CR/casting
- For nerve palsy that presents on admission:
  - Incidence reported in literature 2–20%
  - Contused/neuropraxia found in most cases
  - Spontaneous recovery in 70% cases within 3 months
  - EMG little acute value, but can be checked if no recovery after a few months' observation
  - Subtype with Holstein fractures may have lacerated nerve

9.8.8 Main Operative Rn Options

- Plate fixation
- IM nailing
- EF (rarely used, except in some cases of poly-trauma or contaminated open fractures. If used, ensure safe zone of placement, open insertion technique, meticulous pin track care)

9.8.8.1 Common Options

- Plating (Fig. 9.15):
  - Union rate 96% but Cx 3–13%
  - Posterior approach gives access to direct nerve exploration

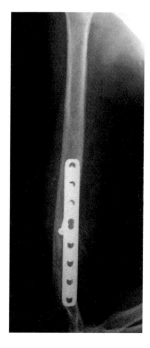

Fig. 9.15 Postoperative radiograph after plating performed for fractured shaft of humerus

- — Remember to record where nerve crosses the plate
- — Wide 4.5-mm DCP usually used, smaller plates in individuals with smaller build. Use a plate of adequate length. Usually use either compression or bridging technique, the latter used to span areas of comminution
- ■ Antegrade nail
  - — Common Cx – adhesive capsulitis, problems with locking
  - — Rotator cuff dysfunction can be problematic
  - — e.g. Siedel nail was found to have such a high Cx rate it was discontinued in some centres (Acta Orthop Belg 1998)
- ■ Retrograde nail
  - — Synthes unreamed humeral nail is an example
  - — Sited 2.5 cm from olecranon
  - — Cx – clumsy proximal locking, periprosthetic fractures

9.8.9 Comparison Between Plating and Nailing

- No significant difference in function, shoulder and elbow scores, pain score, ROM, or time to normal activity shown in recent literature
- But much more impingement after IM nailing, more secondary surgery in nail group (J Bone J Surg Br 2000). Nail mainly reserved for segmental fractures and pathologic fractures
- ORIF with DCP remains the best treatment for unstable fractures of humeral shaft. Most use the triceps-sparing approach as opposed to the triceps split method for exposing distal two-thirds of fractured humerus. Patients with more proximal extension need anterolateral exposure
- IM nail technique demanding, and higher Cx rates (but better in situations with abnormal bone as in pathologic and osteoporotic fractures). To avoid Cx with nailing:
  - Consider the use of newer nail designs that avoid the cuff
  - Do not ream outside the bone, beware especially the radial nerve
  - Do not leave the nail proud that may cause impingement, avoid over-distraction or non-union sets in
  - Carefully document any neurological deficit before nailing

9.8.10 Technical Pearl (with IM Nailing)

- Antegrade: start point just medial and posterior to greater tuberosity through the cuff, meticulous cuff repair needed (some nail designs allow more lateral insertion)
- Retrograde – triceps split approach, prone (or lateral), start point = 2.5 cm proximal to the olecranon fossa – make an oblique oval hole in the bone

9.8.11 What About Flexible Nails?

- E.g. Rush/Enders/Hackethal stacked nails
- All have not infrequent Cx rate
- Main problem: not enough rotatory stability
- May be used in some special situations (e.g. in thin gracile long bones of patients with osteogenesis imperfecta)

9.8.12   Complications

- Non-union
- Malunion
- Neurovascular Cx, e.g. radial nerve palsy
- Iatrogenic shoulder impingement after humeral nailing
- Periprosthetic fractures, e.g. after retrograde humeral nailing

9.8.13   Bring Home the Message

- At present, ORIF remains the Rn of choice in humeral shaft fractures that need operative fixation (J Orthop Trauma 1999)
- Jupiter says the best indication for IM nailing is pathological fractures (or impending fractures). Others feel indicated more in: pathological fractures, severe osteoporosis, and segmental fractures
- Besides higher rate of Cx such as shoulder Cx, shoulder pain, delayed union, fractures around the implant, it is important to remember the *difficulties of reconstruction in case of failures after IM nailing* (J Bone Joint Surg Br 2000). One recent study showed shoulder dysfunction in 33% of cases with antegrade nailing. Plating still remains the gold standard

9.9   Fractured Distal Humerus

9.9.1   Introduction

- Two percent of all fractures, mainly a surgical disease since majority need operation
- Made of two columns and intervening articular surface
- AO classification: divide fractures into
  - A: extra-articular fractures
  - B: partially articular fractures
  - C: completely articular fractures

9.9.2   Alternative Classification

- Extracapsular

- Transcondylar or supracondylar
- Intra-articular

.9.2.1 Extracapsular Fractures
- Include lateral and medial epicondyle fractures
- Consider ORIF if displaced

.9.2.2 Extra-articular Intracapsular Fractures
- Commonly seen in the elderly
- Rn involves CR/OR and internal fixation
- Can be of the flexion/extension type or abduction/adduction variety

.9.2.3 Intra-articular Bi-column Fractures
- Include:
  - T type (involves both columns)
  - Y type (involve both columns with sizable fragments)
  - λ type (sometimes involve only one column)
  - Triplane type (involves an added coronal shear fracture, e.g. of the trochlea)

9.9.3 New Classification of Intra-articular Shearing Fractures (Fig. 9.16) (Ring and Jupiter 2003)
- Type I: capitellum
- Type II: coronal shear
- Type III: coronal shear – two fragments
- Type IV: coronal shear and lateral epicondyle
- Type V: type IV and posterior trochlea
- Type VI: extension to medial epicondyle

9.9.4 Radiological Assessment
- X-ray: in acute fractures, the affected arm is usually held by the patient in a partially flexed position; details of fracture configuration may be masked by routine AP, thus fracture details may be

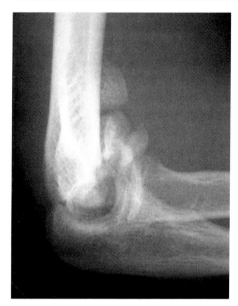

Fig. 9.16 Shearing force is the likely injury mechanism of this articular fracture of the distal humerus

more apparent by tilting the X-ray beam to assess a better AP film (Fig. 9.17)

- Traction X-ray: useful in comminuted fracture assessment, can be done preoperatively or intraoperatively. Sometimes useful to check a contralateral X-ray
- CT: good in assessment of complex fractures like shearing fractures, 3D reconstruction also helps in multi-fragmentary fractures

9.9.5   Treatment Options

- Conservative: mainly a surgical disease. But conservative Rn may be performed in undisplaced fractures, especially in elderly patients. Whether treatment is conservative or operative, always carefully document the neurovascular status, especially for the ulna nerve
- Operative:
  - Main problem is to get adequate rigidity of fixation to allow early ROM

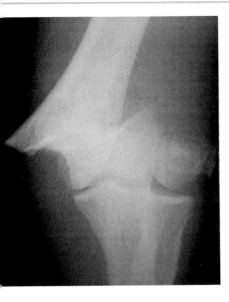

Fig. 9.17 Very distal transverse humerus fracture demands special expertise in fixation

- This is particularly problematic in very distal fractures and in osteoporotic bones
- Goal of surgery: meticulous reconstruction of the intra-articular fragments, rigid multiplanar fixation, early ROM

9.9.6   Operative Pearls

- Most are treated with double plating with the plates placed in two different planes
- Although ulna nerve transposition is not routinely performed, freeing the ulna nerve both proximally and distally is advisable. Freeing is a must if implant impingement detected intraoperatively, especially in fixing very distal fractures
- Trochlea width should be restored and not shortened. Hence, avoid transverse lag screws across the trochlea in the face of comminution
- Meticulous technique if olecranon osteotomy required since Cx common. The chevron cut should point distally to maximise fragment size. Subsequent repair by tension band technique is more reliable than IM screw

9.9.7   Traditional and Newer Implants

- The usual recommendations for the use of plates include: better t use stronger DCP if fracture is not too distal and fixation does nc require too much contouring or plate bending. Very distal (Fig. 9.18 fixation involves more plate bending or contouring (e.g. to partiall cup the capitellum) and reconstruction plates are useful

- Newer plates include pre-contoured plates (Fig. 9.19) and lockin plates. The latter show promise in fixation of these fractures in osteo porotic bones. Also, some of the new locking peri-articular plate can send multiple smaller screws to lock the very distal humeru fractures

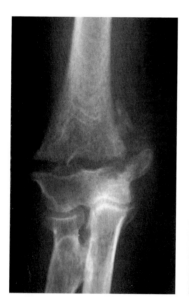

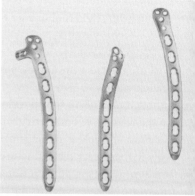

Fig. 9.18 Very distal humerus fractures, as shown here, are even more difficult to fix, but the newer plating systems may help

Fig. 9.19 New low profile pre-contoured plates for treating difficult and distal humerus fractures

.9.8   An Added Option in Osteoporotic Bone

- Severe comminuted distal humeral fractures in elderly with osteo-porosis and poor bone stock (especially in the face of pre-existing osteoarthritis [OA]) make primary total elbow arthroplasty (TEA) a treatment option although Cx rate is of the order of 10–20%
- This partly solves the problem of suboptimal fixation, poor bone stock and comminution
- If TEA is used, the semi-constrained variety is preferred. The litera-ture on this topic by Morrey is worth reading (Cobb and Morrey 1997)

.9.9   Complications

- Non-union
- Elbow stiffness
- Malunion
- Sepsis
- Ulna neuritis – avoid over-traction
- Cx of olecranon osteotomy, e.g. hardware-related impingement, non-union

9.9.10   Management of Non-union

- Prevention is best since difficult to treat
- If ORIF decided rather than other surgical options, fixation must be rigid enough to allow early motion. Stiffness should be avoided at all costs, since a stiff elbow not only causes functional impairment, but macro/micro-motion at the fracture site, predisposing to non-union
- Non-union is very difficult to treat in the face of marked elbow stiff-ness

9.9.11   Non-union and Elbow Stiffness

- Difficult to treat
- May require combination of capsulectomy, triple plating and ulna neurolysis (Jupiter 1992)

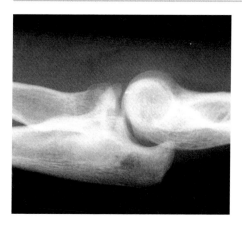

Fig. 9.20 Close-up of an elbow that is subluxated after fracture of the coronoid process

9.10   Fracture Dislocations Around the Elbow (Fig. 9.20)

9.10.1   Introduction
- The high mobility of the human upper extremity depends on the summation of the normal functioning of a chain of mobile joints
- In this kinetic chain, loss of elbow joint function is the least tolerated. As it may affect elbow flexion, extension, or pronosupination which will affect activities of daily living

9.10.2   General Problems in the Elbow Area
- Thin soft tissue envelope: an unfavourable soft tissue situation will affect our surgical timing, approach, and fixation methods
- Relatively complex anatomy involving three joints: ulnohumeral and radiocapitellar articulations, as well as the proximal radio-ulnar articulation
- It is not surprising to find, therefore, that injury to the elbow joint is prone to stiffness. Joint stiffness in turn predisposes to non-union as the micro- or macro-motion will now be at the fracture site (e.g. very distal humerus fractures) rather than the natural elbow articulations. Thus, it is not uncommon to see non-union of the distal humerus

9.10.3 Types of Elbow Dislocation

- Types of dislocation: posterolateral and posterior most common. Dislocations in other directions are either rare or very rare, e.g. anterior, medial, lateral, divergent
- Even in the common posterior dislocation, studies have shown complete disruption of all capsulo-ligamentous structures in most patients
- The soft tissues usually fail in a circular manner: first involves anterior capsule disruption, then lateral ulna collateral, then the anterior band of the MCL fails last although can be intact in some cases (Hori)

9.10.4 Mechanism of Elbow Dislocation

- Elbow hyperextension
- Shawn O'Driscoll showed that an even more common mechanism involves axial loading in a slightly flexed elbow held in valgus and supination (in other words, the outstretched hand is relatively fixed on the ground, and supinates relative to the humerus, which internally rotates with the body)

9.10.5 Method of CR

- Forearm hypersupinated – helps clear the coronoid
- Try flexion from an extended position, with anterior directed pressure at the olecranon
- Check elbow stability after CR, some cases more stable in pronation and immobilised for 2–3 weeks in this more stable position

9.10.6 Concepts of Elbow Instability

- Before we talk about instability, we must know the cornerstone of elbow stability
- Elbow stability depends both on its bony and its ligamentous components viz:
  - Integrity of coronoid
  - Radial head integrity

- Integrity of the olecranon
- Lateral collateral ligament
- Medial collateral ligament

9.10.7 Common Patterns of Elbow Instability

- Posterolateral rotatory instability – most common mechanism of elbow dislocation
- Valgus instability – can result from repeated injury in throwing sports or elbow dislocation; associated with failure of anterior band of MCL of elbow

9.10.8 Spectrum of Posterolateral Elbow Instability (After O'Driscoll)

- Stage 1: subluxation and pivot shift test positive
- Stage 2: coronoid perches on the trochlea
- Stages 3A: dislocation complete with an intact MCL anterior band
- Stage 3B: dislocation complete with MCL disruption

9.11 Elbow Fractures

9.11.1 Ring Concept of the Elbow in Analysing More Complex Elbow Fractures

- Stability of the elbow is also be thought to be dependent on integrity of four columns (Jupiter and Ring)
  - Anterior column: coronoid, brachialis and anterior capsule
  - Posterior column: olecranon, triceps and posterior capsule
  - Lateral column: radial head, capitellum, LCL
  - Medial column: medial condyle, coronoid, MCL

9.11.2 Implications of the Ring Concept

- Helps in the understanding of many complex fracture dislocations around the elbow
- Example: the more columns are at fault after injury, the higher the resultant instability

9.11.3   Clinical Scenario: Lateral Column Injury

- Isolated LCL injury: if the ulna part of LCL is torn, may have degree of posterolateral instability, as evidenced by pivot shift test
- Radial head fractures: after reconstruction or replacement by prosthesis, need to retest for lateral instability

9.11.4   Clinical Scenario: LCL + Coronoid + Radial Head

- Known as the "terrible triad" by Hotchkiss
- The degree of instability depends on the size of the coronoid fracture

9.11.5   Fractured Radial Head + Fractured Coronoid + Olecranon (and Ligaments)

- This case involves loss of the anterior column buttress and medial column, and disrupts the stabilising effect of the triceps
- Rn involves tackling the olecranon and radial head fractures, the frequently associated Regan Type 3 fractures of the coronoid also need fixation in most cases. Retest the stability after fixation and X-ray screening is advised

9.11.6   Added Options in Complex Unstable Elbow Fracture Dislocation

- Hinged fixator: especially useful in the presence of poor soft tissue envelope, and complex elbow fracture dislocations in the elderly with osteoporosis wherein even standard ORIF may not confer adequate stability for early ROM (Stavlas et al. 2004)
- Total elbow arthroplasty: remains a viable option in face of comminution beyond salvage in the elderly elbow reported by Morrey

9.12   Fractured Radial Head (Fig. 9.21)

9.12.1   Mason Classification

- Type I: undisplaced
- Type II: displaced
- Type III: comminuted

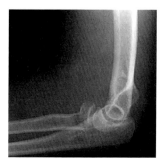

Fig. 9.21 Radiograph illustrating a displaced radial head fracture

9.12.2 Hotchkiss Classification
- Type I: minimally displaced
- Type II: > 2 mm displaced ± mechanical block, more than just a marginal fracture
- Type III: comminuted fracture, with mechanical block and mostly beyond repair

9.12.3 Pathomechanics
- Mostly a result of a fall on outstretched arm, usually with the elbow slightly flexed and the forearm pronated, i.e. axial loading on a pronated forearm

9.12.4 Investigation
- X-ray: standard views and radio-capitellar views
- CT ± 3D imaging if fracture pattern is complex

9.12.5 Management
- Hotchkiss Types 1 and 2 without mechanical block: aspirate haemarthrosis if tense, long arm plaster for 2+ weeks followed by hinge brace and early mobilisation
- Hotchkiss Type 2 with mechanical block and Type 3: ORIF ± metallic prosthetic replacement if beyond repair; avoid excision especially

if young and in situations like concomitant injury to the ulno-humeral axis or Essex–Lopresti lesion

9.13   Fractured Capitellum

- Types:
    - Hahn–Steinthal fractures
    - Kocher–Lorenz fractures
    - Compression fractures
- Treatment:
    - Hahn–Steinthal fractures mostly involve the whole capitellum, treated using Herbert screws
    - In both Kocher–Lorenz fractures and compression fractures; the thin, frequently comminuted shell of bone may need excision. For more sizable ones, vicryl pinning may be tried

9.14   Fractured Coronoid

- Regan Morrey classification is used:
    - Type 1: only the tip avulsed. May well be an indicator of recent elbow dislocation
    - Type 2: < 50% coronoid involved
    - Type 3: > 50% coronoid involved (most Type 3 cases, the fragment is large enough to include the insertion of the anterior bundle of the MCL)
- Although Morrey taught us that a functional elbow may still be obtained with up to 50% of the height of the coronoid lost, it may be wise to assess each patient on a case-by-case basis and under X-ray screening. Sometimes elbow stability is retested after fixing other concomitant injuries

9.15   Olecranon Fracture

9.15.1   Introduction
- Majority are intra-articular fractures
- Majority need operative fixation, unless incomplete or non-displaced
- Majority are hyper-extension injuries
- It is important to restore the extensor mechanism of the elbow joint

9.15.2   Associated Injuries
- Especially need to rule out associated injuries of nearby structures of the elbow, particularly coronoid process and radial head – which, if fractured, can cause marked instability
- Olecranon fractures associated with radial head dislocation are sometimes regarded as a Monteggia equivalent
- Check associated injury to the ipsilateral upper limb (which, if not adequately treated, will affect the function of the kinetic chain)
- Also assess for any neurovascular deficits and injuries elsewhere

9.15.3   Classification
- No single classification in very wide general use
- Most are descriptive
- Better to select those classifications that may to some extent predict outcome
- Two such classifications include: Mayo Clinic classification and the classification by Schatzker

9.15.4   Schatzker–Schmeling Classification
- Transverse fractures – simple (A1), complex ± central impaction (A2)
- Oblique fractures – proximal (B1), distal (B2)
- Multifragmentary – type C, qualify whether there is dislocation
- Association with radial head fractures – type D

9.15.5   Mayo Clinic Classification
- Mayo classification

- Type 1: undisplaced
- Type 2: stable without comminution vs. stable with some comminution
- Type 3: unstable without comminution vs. unstable with some comminution

9.15.6 Olecranon Fracture Management

- Most displaced fractures need fixation to restore joint stability and congruity, and functional restoration
- Even undisplaced olecranon fractures should be monitored for any displacement

9.15.7 Choice of Fixation

- Tension band wiring and parallel k-wires (Fig. 9.22): typically indicated in non-comminuted transverse fractures
- IM screw fixation – an alternative to the use of parallel k-wires in the Rn option above

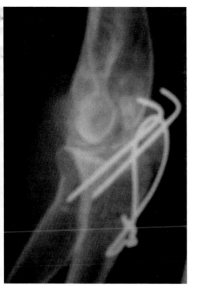

Fig. 9.22 This postoperative radiograph showing tension band wiring to fix a displaced fractured olecranon

- Plate fixation (Fig. 9.23), especially in comminuted fractures and oblique fractures distal to the mid-point of the trochlea notch, e.g. reconstruction plates/one-third tubulars/and DCP have been reported

9.15.8 Added Option in Comminuted Fractures in the Elderly

- Partial resection of the olecranon with reattachment of the triceps is a viable option in the elderly low-demand patient with comminuted fractures (reported by the Mayo Clinic)

9.15.9 Elbow Fracture Dislocation Involving the Olecranon

- Trans-olecranon (anterior) fracture dislocation involves large coronoid fragment and fragmented olecranon; it is not an anterior dislocation of the elbow because the radius and ulna are still associated and displaced anteriorly
- A variant of posterior Monteggia wherein the ulna fracture extends proximally, locating at the olecranon. This pattern can be associated with coronoid fractures, and may even involve the radial head and LCL

9.15.10 Prognosis

- Fracture morphology is an important factor in determining whether arthrosis will occur later (Rommens et al. 2004)
- The accuracy of articular surface reconstruction is also important

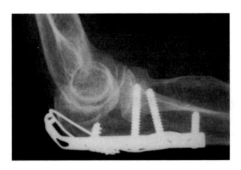

Fig. 9.23 More comminuted fractured olecranons are best treated by plating

9.16   Fractured Forearm

9.16.1   Introduction

- Concept of the forearm bone articulation being viewed as a joint is beginning to be widely accepted
- As such, most displaced forearm fractures merit operative fixation
- As such, anatomical reduction and rigid fixation by the use of plating remains the cornerstone of the treatment of displaced forearm fractures. Intramedullary devices and, rarely, the use of EF were described, but anatomical reduction and plating remain the gold standard

9.16.2   Work-up

- X-ray is essential, not only of the whole forearm, but to include the wrist and elbow. This is important to exclude the not uncommon Monteggia (Figs. 9.24, 9.25) and Galeazzi fracture dislocations
- Assess the status of the soft tissue, rule out compartment syndrome (which can occur, even in open fractures). Document the neurovascular status of the extremity

9.16.3   Principles of Rn

- The importance of the restoration of the radial bowing cannot be over-emphasised

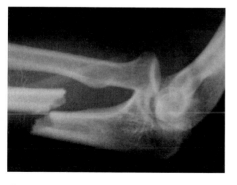

Fig. 9.24 Radiograph showing a Monteggia fracture dislocation

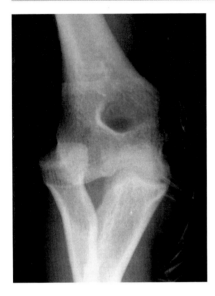

Fig. 9.25 The AP view of the same dislocation

- There are many new developments in shaft fractures of the forearm including:
  - New implants, notably LC-DCP and the PC-Fix, details of which have been discussed in the section on plating
  - It is also important to recognise special fracture patterns like plastic deformation in paediatric patients

9.16.4   Summary of Rn Options
- Conservative – only if undisplaced
- Operative – most cases
  - Plating still remains the gold standard
  - Nailing has been reported but many feel that the forearm (especially the radius) is not absolutely suitable for nailing if restoration of the proper radial bow is so essential for functional return

9.16.5   Operative Indications

- Open fractures (unless severely contaminated, most open fractures can still be Rn by forearm plating)
- Associated neurovascular injury that needs exploration
- Failed conservative Rn
- Displaced fractures of both forearms at presentation
- Segmental fractures
- Poly-trauma

9.16.6   Surgical Approach for Plating

- Fracture distal third of radius: Volar Henry's approach
- Other more proximal radius shaft fractures: both volar and dorsal approaches can be used depending on the situation

9.16.7   Implants of Choice

- Most frequently used implants for plating are the 3.5-mm DCP or the newer LC-DCP
- An occasional patient with small build may consider 2.7-mm DCP
- BG may be needed in open fractures

9.16.8   Complications

- Re-fracture after plate removal is quite common. Newer plates like LC-DCP or PC-Fix may be useful. Some experts try to avoid removal altogether
- Persistent subluxation of PRUJ or DRUJ: a failure to reduce these joints is frequently caused by malalignment of fracture during ORIF
- Malunion: failure of restoration of, say, radial bow may predispose to limitation of pronosupination
- Synostosis: prevented by avoiding dissecting and stripping around the interosseous membrane
- Non-union: rather rare, sometimes seen in open fractures especially if sepsis ensues, delayed presentation or neglected fractures

9.17   Monteggia Fracture Dislocations

9.17.1   Classification
- Monteggia fracture dislocation involves fracture of the proximal ulna shaft and dislocated PRUJ
- Classification:

I – RH anterior dislocation (more in children)

II – posterior dislocation ± RH

III – lateral dislocation (more in children)

IV – anterior dislocation and associated shaft fractures

Monteggia equivalents

9.17.2   Management
- In most cases the dislocated radial head reduces upon proper reduction (open usually) and internal fixation
- In children, beware of plastic deformation of the ulna
- Causes of irreducible radial head: soft tissue interposition (e.g. annular ligament or capsule), ulna fracture not properly reduced
- If there is associated radial head fracture, manage along the usual lines of radial head or neck fractures

9.17.3   Complications of Monteggia
- Nerve palsy: PIN/AIN/ulna nerve palsy
- Recurrent radial head subluxation (Fig. 9.26)
- Non-union
- Synostosis
- Malunion
- Joint stiffness

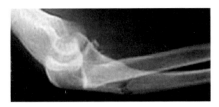

Fig. 9.26 Another patient with a Monteggia fracture dislocation

9.18   Concept of Longitudinal Instability of the Forearm

9.18.1   The Basics
- The forearm axis consists of the elbow joint, PRUJ, radius, ulna, IOM, and DRUJ
- Compression forces transmitted through the radius and ulna are converted to tensile forces in the IOL
- Injury of sufficient force, especially with axial loading, can damage this whole forearm unit

9.18.2   Injury Patterns
- Injury to only one element of the forearm unit
- Or combined patterns, with examples:
    - Elbow injury (e.g. radial head fracture) and forearm (e.g. IOM)
    - Forearm fracture and IOM
    - Elbow injury (e.g. radial head fracture) and IOM and DRUJ
    - Global injuries

9.18.3   Management
- Proper management starts with proper Dx, which depends on the index of suspicion of the treating surgeon
- Example: in treating a patient with concomitant injury with radial head fracture, IOM injury and DRUJ injury, excision of the radial head will magnify the longitudinal forearm instability and marked proximal radial migration may occur

9.19   Fractured Distal Radius

9.19.1   Introduction
- There are three articulations in the region of the distal radius
- They include:
    - Radioscaphoid articulation
    - Radiolunate articulation
    - Sigmoid notch (DRUJ)

- Assessment of all three articulations is important for a more complete assessment
- Associated injuries, e.g. bony (such as carpal injuries) or soft tissue (e.g. median nerve) should be tackled, and attention paid to DRUJ plus PRUJ

9.19.2 Preferred Classification (Jupiter and Fernandez)
- Bending fractures
- Shearing fractures
- Avulsion fractures
- Compression fractures (e.g. die punch)
- Combined

9.19.3 Classification of Intra-articular Fractures (Fig. 9.27)
9.19.3.1 Melone Classification
- Visualises intra-articular distal radius fractures as mostly made of four components: shaft, radial styloid, dorsal medial, palmar medial
- Type 1: undisplaced, minimal comminution

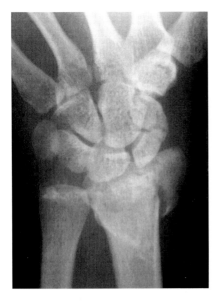

Fig. 9.27 Radiograph showing comminuted intra-articular fracture of the distal radius

- Type 2: (die punch fractures) moderate displacement, comminution of anterior cortex
- Type 3: additional fracture component from the shaft of the radius projects into the flexor compartment
- Type 4: involves transverse split of the articular surfaces with rotational displacement

9.19.3.2 Columnar Classification (Regazzoni)

- Involves dividing the distal radius into:
  - Medial (or ulna) column
  - Intermediate column (i.e. volar or dorsal rim, volar ulna corner of lunate fossa)
  - Lateral (or radial column), i.e. radial styloid, scaphoid fossa
  - Combinations/all columns being injured is possible

(This is the preferred classification for it is very useful clinically [Fig. 9.28])

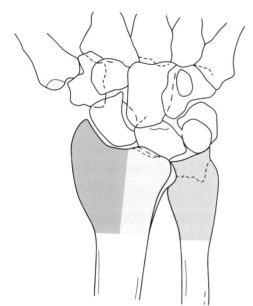

Fig. 9.28 The column classification as depicted here is very useful in planning fracture-specific plating and internal fixation of fractured distal radius

9.19.3.3 Importance of Columnar Classification
- Guides our treatment plan for intra-articular fractures
- Allows fracture-specific treatment

9.19.4 General Work-up

9.19.4.1 Limits of Acceptable Alignment (After Graham)
- Limits of acceptable radiologic alignment in extra-articular unstable bending fractures:
  - < 5 mm radial shortening. X-ray of the contralateral normal wrist can guide assessment of ulna variance in the patient
  - Restoration of normal volar tilt same as normal side (the author here usually allows volar tilt of 0 to 20°, slightly different from Graham's article published in JAAOS 1997)
  - Radial inclination on PA view > 15°
  - To add to this guideline, we may consider adding: restoration of normal carpal alignment (see later discussion)
  - In intra-articular fractures, articular step ≤ 2 mm (Jupiter), and articular incongruency < 2 mm

9.19.4.2 Assessment of the Degree of Comminution
- Method 1: determine percentage of metaphyseal comminution – instability likely present with 30–50% comminution
- Method 2 (Kristiansen): determine the number of intact cortices on AP and lateral X-rays

9.19.4.3 How to Predict Instability?
- The fractured distal radius is more likely to be an unstable fracture if:
  - Cortical comminution (mostly are dorsal)
  - Volar obliquity (e.g. volar barton, volar ulna corner fracture)
  - Failed CR, or displaces while in cast for 2–3 weeks
  - Significant angulation detected in injury film

9.19.4.4 Goal of Reduction (CR or OR)
- Correct radial shortening

- Correct radial inclination
- Correct volar tilt and carpal alignment
- Correct articular step-off
- Have a stable DRUJ

9.19.4.5 Clues to Possible DRUJ Instability

- Presence of basal ulna styloid fractures
- Fracture involving the sigmoid notch
- Avulsion chip fracture arising from the fovea
- Widening of DRUJ
- Dorsal subluxated ulna shaft
- Triangular fibrocartilage complex (TFCC) injury

9.19.5 CR Technique

- Restore radial length by longitudinal traction
- Restore radial inclination by ulna deviation
- Restore volar tilt to normal by palmar flexion, say in fractures with dorsal tilt
- Restore the common supination deformity of the distal fragment by axial pronation

9.19.6 Management: Metaphyseal Bending Fractures

- Aim: restore proper volar tilt and correction of radial length and inclination are the main goals
- The important studies concerning the management of unstable bending fractures (especially common in the elderly) will now be discussed

9.19.6.1 Studies on Management of Unstable Bending Fractures of the Distal Radius in the Elderly (McQueen)

9.19.6.1.1 Prospective Study Comparing Four Treatment Options

- >100 unstable distal radius bending fractures in the elderly, over 80% had premorbid independent ADL, over 60% had metaphyseal comminution
- Four Rn arms:

- — Remanipulation and casting
- — OR and grafting
- — Static spanning EF
- — Dynamic spanning EF
- ▪ Results: initially it was thought that arms 3 and 4 would do better than arms 1 and 2. But this type of unstable bending fracture proved to be quite difficult in terms of achieving good functional and radiological outcome
- ▪ This was because even in the spanning EF groups, there was a significant malunion rate and volar tilt was seldom restored. In all four groups, only 58% patients attained a normal grip (McQueen et al. 1996)

9.19.6.2 Other Findings of McQueen's Study

- ▪ Checking of carpal malalignment is a useful way to assess malunion. It was found that carpal malalignment has significant influence on outcome
- ▪ Carpal malalignment affects restoration of grip strength and range of motion
- ▪ Measurement of carpal alignment: a line drawn along axis of capitate and a line drawn along the long axis of the radius should normally intersect within the carpus. Patients with malalignment frequently have the intersection proximal to the carpus

9.19.6.3 The Case for Non-bridging EF (Fig. 9.29)

- ▪ McQueen then arranged a randomised study comparing bridging and non-bridging EF
- ▪ The non-bridging group had better functional and radiological results in terms of more reliable restoration of volar tilt, better carpal alignment, much better (over 80%) improvement in grip strength, and better flexion range than non-bridging group (McQueen 1998)

9.19.6.4 Current Recommendation for the Use of Different Rn Options

- ▪ Casting: casting alone can be used in easily reduced stable bending fractures

- Percutaneous k-wire and casting: k-wires alone may be able to maintain reduction in the absence of comminution, sometimes with the help of Kapandji intrafocal pinning (Fig. 9.30)
- In the presence of comminution, either EF (preferably non-bridging) or OR + low profile plating ± BG are the choices

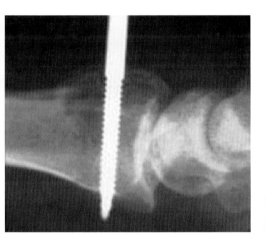

Fig. 9.29 Location of placement of the distal pin in the non-bridging EF

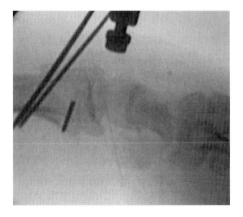

Fig. 9.30 Intrafocal pinning is an intraoperative method of restoring the correct volar tilt

9.19.7   Management: Articular Shearing Fractures (Barton's)

- Volar articular shear fractures:
  - Most need buttress plating. Under-contouring helps to give some degree of compression
  - If there are radial and ulna portions of the volar facet fracture, each of these fragments needs stabilisation. Congruity should be restored
- Dorsal articular shear fractures:
  - Most need buttress, and to restore congruity
  - Use the dorsal 3–4 approach

9.19.8   Management: Avulsion Fractures

- Palmar avulsion fractures:
  - Commonly seen associated with radiocarpal joint (RCJ) dislocation
  - Fixation may be required if fragment sizable
- Dorsal avulsion fractures:
  - Also search for carpal instability as the avulsion is usually a pointer of ligamentous injury to the wrist and treat the instability accordingly

9.19.9   Managing Intra-articular Fractures

9.19.9.1   Investigation of Complex Intra-articular Fractures

- CT scanning is of help for the surgical planning of fixation of displaced intra-articular fractures
- The wrist joint has low tolerance for articular incongruity, and careful preoperative planning is essential

9.19.9.2   Indication of Mini-open Techniques

- Mini-open techniques should be considered if closed reduction fails
- Mini-open is not possible if the intra-articular fracture involves different columns and formal ORIF is required to plate the different columns involved
- For those rather uncommon cases in which CR is successful, a combination of EF + multiple k-wires can be used to provide mainten-

ance of reduction, preferably arthroscopically guided (although large
fragments are best held by plates and screws)

9.19.9.3 Methods of Reduction of Articular Fractures

- It was shown by Jupiter that a 2-mm articular step-off is predictive
  of post-traumatic arthrosis and poor functional result. AVN is rare
  in intra-articular distal radius fractures because of the good blood
  supply, but can occur in high energy injuries
- The methods of reduction include:
  - Open reduction (involves more soft tissue dissection)
  - Mini-open reduction (sometimes mini-incisions for the purpose
    of BG)
  - Small incision to allow placement of newer low-profile fracture-
    specific plates
  - Arthroscopic-assisted reduction

9.19.9.4 Role of Arthroscopy

- Increasingly used in assisting reduction of intra-articular fractures
- Also allows for detection of intercarpal ligamentous injuries not always immediately apparent on plain films. Geissler reported, for instance, in one series of intra-articular fractures a 43% incidence of
  concomitant TFCC injuries

9.19.9.5 Summary of Rn Options for Intra-articular Fractures
of the Distal Radius

- Commonly used treatment options:
  - ORIF – usually plate and screws are used. The key is fracture-
    specific plating
  - Mini-open reduction and internal fixation
  - Arthroscopically assisted reduction and percutaneous fixation
    (e.g. k-wires), i.e. percutaneous subchondral k-wires to restore
    articular surface and EF to tackle the metaphyseal fracture com-
    ponent

9.19.10   Overview of Different Techniques
for Unstable Distal Radius Fractures

9.19.10.1   Comparison of the Use of EF Versus Different Plating
Methods in Unstable Distal Radius Fractures

- Comparison is made between merits and demerits of the following implant options:
    - External fixation
    - Volar plating
    - Dorsal plating
    - Double plating
    - Bi-planar bi-column plating

9.19.10.2   External Fixation (Fig. 9.31)

- Advantages:
    - Technique mastered by most trainees

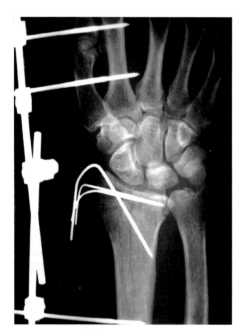

Fig. 9.31 The spanning external fixator is one of the options for treating distal radius fractures

- Recent studies show better results (compared with ORIF) in terms of pain, healing time, maintenance of reduction, function such as hand grip, SF 36, and return to work issues (OTA 2002)
- Disadvantages:
  - Cannot by itself correct volar tilt (Fig. 9.32)
  - Cannot alone correct articular step-off
  - Cannot be reliably used to treat volar shearing fractures
  - Pin track problems
  - Rarely reduce a dislocated DRUJ
  - Joint stiffness with prolonged immobilisation
  - Other Cx: median nerve paresis with, e.g. excessive hyperflexion, over-distraction, reflex sympathetic dystrophy (RSD), etc.
  - Refer to the use of non-bridging EF discussed in Sect. 9.19.6.3

9.19.10.3 Volar Plating

- Advantages:
  - Volar plating can be used for unstable fractured distal radius, including intra- and extra-articular fractures, and whether the fracture is dorsally or volarly angulated
  - Does not have the disadvantages of EF

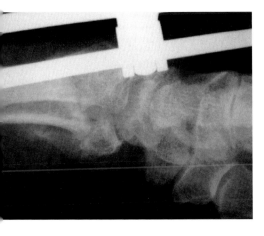

Fig. 9.32 Notice that it is difficult to restore proper volar tilt by a spanning external fixator alone

- Newer implants with subchondral support may aid in fine tuning extra-articular reduction
- Newer implants may obviate the need for BG

- Disadvantages:
  - Cannot see into the joint, need arthroscopy or dorsal arthrotomy to ascertain articular fragment alignment. Never incise the important wrist ligaments in an attempt to see the joint volarly
  - C/I (if used alone) in severe comminution involving distal 25% of metaphysis

9.19.10.4 New Volar Plates

- Fixed angled volar plating
  - Good for osteoporotic bone
  - Even in young patients, the implant is strong enough for early mobilisation and earlier return to work
  - Some newer systems can provide subchondral supports not adequately catered for by traditional AO T-plates
- Pre-contoured screw plates

9.19.10.5 Dorsal Plating

- Advantages:
  - Unlike volar approach, can see into the joint
  - Does not have the disadvantages of EF
  - Can tackle fractures that also involve the dorsal ulna corner
  - Can fix concomitant fractures of the carpal bone or perform ligamentous repair
  - Newer 3D implant system stronger than traditional 2D plates or EF; hence, safer to allow early ROM
- Disadvantages:
  - Extensor tendon attrition and ruptures
  - Entails more dissection (more chance of adhesions) and ± removal of Lister tubercle ± EPL re-routing
  - Since patient likely to have tendon-related problems, plate removal not infrequently required

19.10.6 Newer Dorsal Plates

Low-profile plates are advisable if dorsal plating is indicated to prevent extensor tendon rupture

Dorsal plates are useful if the distal fragment length is small and helps stabilises the rim

19.10.6.1 General Features of Dorsal Plates

Low profile

Can be contoured

AO group product made of titanium to be used in dorsal distal radius

Previous standard AO small fragment plates not designed specifically with problems of the dorsal distal radius anatomy in mind

19.10.6.2 Dorsal Plate Design

The pre-contoured distal limb of the plate adheres to the curvature of the dorsal aspect of the distal radius and tilts to match the radial inclination of the distal radius

The distal juxta-articular limb help confines articular comminution while providing numerous holes through which either 2.4-mm screws or 1.8-mm buttress pins are recessed into the plate and have cribriform heads inside to minimise their profile to lessen the chance of extensor tendon irritation

There are two thin proximal limbs of the plate that help resist shortening and extra-articular bending stress

These limbs are secured to the plate by 2.7-mm self-tapping screws to the distal radius and the heads of the screws are recessed into the plate

Biomechanically, the bending stiffness is comparable to other plates such as the T-plates

19.10.6.3 Indications for Dorsal Plate

Complex comminuted IA distal radius fractures

Distal radius fracture with significant dorsal comminution

9.19.10.6.4   Advantages of the Dorsal Plate

- Anatomically designed for use in the distal radius and pre-cor toured
- David Ring reported almost no plate failures, no loss of reduc tion, non-union or sepsis in a series of 22 patients followed fc 14 months
- Average wrist motion was 76% and grip strength 56% of the opposi side

9.19.10.6.5   Disadvantages of the Dorsal Plate

- Extensor tendon synovitis
- Extensor tendon rupture

9.19.10.7   Double Plating (Fig. 9.33)

- Advantages:
  - Can be used in very comminuted distal radius fractures involv ing the distal 25% of the metaphysis
  - May provide adequate support even in the face of comminutio so as to allow early ROM
- Disadvantages:
  - Have disadvantages of both dorsal and volar plating combined

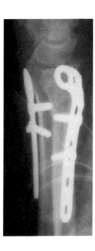

Fig. 9.33 This radiograph shows double plating with more traditional AO T-plates for fractured distal radius

- Joint stiffness more likely due to added dissection, take care to have adequate pain relief and release any concomitant carpal tunnel syndrome (CTS) lest respiratory distress syndrome (RDS) sets in
- Double plating with the use of traditional plating systems may not be adequate to control small subchondral articular fragments

9.10.8 Bi-columnar Plating

Advantages:
- Unlike traditional implant systems, it has built in modularity
- These newer plate systems help capture of radial styloid fractures, and small subchondral and articular fragments (Fig. 9.34, 9.35) – fixation of the latter by screws can be difficult, but in this system fixation can be by the use of tines
- Recent studies have shown it to be stronger than T-plate and Pi-plate

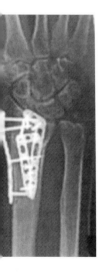

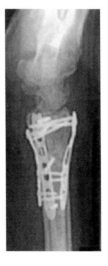

9.34 This postoperative radiograph serves to illustrate the use of low profile plates suitable to be used in conjunction with our principle of fracture-specific plating

Fig. 9.35 The lateral view of the same patient. Notice the low profile of this new plating system

- Modularity not only makes provision for fracture-specific fix ation; but allows the use of mini-incisions (since only placed strategic wrist columns that are fractured) in selected cases minimise surgical trauma
- At last, provision made for low-profile implant fixation of t ulna column to restore the sigmoid notch
- Lower profile lowers the usual Cx of tendon injuries
- Disadvantages:
  - Usual drawbacks of plates such as sepsis, surgical dissection, e

9.19.11   Operative Decision-Making
- The final method used depends on:
  - Fracture configuration and personality
  - Availability of implants
  - Surgical expertise

(Example: volar barton fractures extending into the joint are mos treated by AO T-plate via a volar Henry's approach. However, volar ul corner fractures (which can cause incongruity in the radiolunate jo and the sigmoid notch) are best treated by a small plate and using t interval between the flexors and the ulna neurovascular bundle)

9.19.12   Complications After Distal Radius Fractures
9.19.12.1   Malunion
- Most common Cx
- This can result in dorsal (DISI) or volar intercalated segment instal lity (VISI) changes of the carpal row, or midcarpal instability
- Corrective osteotomy can be performed preferably early on inste of waiting for the malunion to be remodelled
- The aim of the osteotomy is to re-orient the articular surface, a normalise the force transmission across the wrist, and prevent se ondary altered biomechanics of the carpal rows

9.19.12.2   Osteoarthritis
- Quite commonly seen
- But Gelberman found that despite the not uncommon OA chang noted, the number of patients requiring osteotomy is relatively few

OA can occur at the radiolunate articulation (especially in fractures involving the lunate facet) or the DRUJ (especially with increased loading resulting from radial shortening and/or the fracture involving the sigmoid notch). Isolated OA of radioscaphoid articulation is rare, most cases associated with diffuse involvement of RCJ

9.12.3   Resultant DRUJ Problems
Instability – acute vs. chronic
Incongruity – painful restriction of motion
Ulna impingement
Painful non-union of the ulna styloid
Iatrogenic radio-ulnar impingement after distal ulna resection procedures

9.12.3.1   Relevant Anatomy
Any fractures involving the sigmoid notch can cause resultant pain and subsequent OA if there is an articular step and/or notch deformity
The current thinking is that the PRUJ and DRUJ forms two parts of one joint (Hagert)
Disruption of the DRUJ can affect pronation and supination motion of forearm

9.12.3.2   Determinants of DRUJ Stability
The primary stabilisers include: dorsal and volar radio-ulnar ligaments. Normal dorsal translation constrained by dorsal, and volar translation by volar radio-ulnar ligament respectively
Secondary stabilisers: PQ, IOM, DRUJ capsule, ulno-carpal ligaments, sheath of ECU

sultant DRUJ Instability
sultant DRUJ Instability: Acute
Acute: found commonly in association with

- Fractures involving the sigmoid notch: may need CT for assessment, after distal radius fracture properly fixed

- Fractured base of ulna styloid: large fragment needs fixation, need to retest DRUJ stability afterwards since the fixation of ulna styloid process does not always confer the stability of DR
- Fracture of ulna head or neck: usually tackled by ORIF or with outrigger
- TFCC injury: may need to repair dorsal or volar radio-ulnar li ment

Resultant DRUJ Instability: Chronic

- In the chronic phase, may present with ulna wrist pain, and clunk ± stiffness
- Investigations include X-ray, CT may be useful in assessing cong ity of DRUJ, OA and can compare other DRUJ in supination a pronation
- If no OA; consider repairing TFCC and ligament reconstruction ulna shortening
- If OA sets in, salvage includes Darrach operation, Sauve Kapa hemi-resection, ± arthroplasty

9.19.12.3.3 DRUJ Incongruity

- Extra-articular: abnormally oriented sigmoid notch
- Intra-articular: fracture extending to involve the sigmoid notch
- Both

9.19.12.3.4 Ulna Impingement

- Most are secondary to loss of radial length
- Results:
  - TFCC injury
  - OA of ulno-carpal articulation
  - Chondrosis/arthrosis of the ulna head
  - LT ligament tear

9.19.12.3.5 Painful Non-union of the Ulna Styloid

- If very symptomatic, may need excision

9.12.3.6 Iatrogenic Radio-Ulnar Impingement
Such as after excision arthroplasty of the distal ulna

9.12.4 Soft Tissue Problems
RSD or regional pain syndrome
Nerve entrapment, e.g. carpal tunnel
Extensor tendon injury

9.12.5 Others
Non-union: not so common. Can be caused by over-distraction by EF, or extensive soft tissue stripping (as in double plating), or small distal radial fragment, or leaving large voids after reduction not filled with BG
Missed associated injury: e.g. missed injury of the PRUJ like a radial head or neck fracture

20 Carpal Instability and Perilunate Dislocations

20.1 Definition of Carpal Instability
Carpal injury in which a loss of normal alignment of the carpal bones develops early or late
It represents a disturbance of the normal balance of the carpal joints caused by fracture or ligament damage

20.1.1 Incidence
10% of all carpal injuries resulted in instability
5% of non-fracture wrist injuries had scapholunate instability

20.1.2 General Comment
All wrist dislocations/subluxations, etc. are examples of carpal instability
Not all imply joint laxity – some are very stiff
Not all unstable wrists are painful

9.20.1.3 Kinematics of the Proximal Carpal Row

■ In moving from radial to ulnar deviation, the whole proximal r
moves from flexion to extension

9.20.1.4 Carpal Instability – Pathomechanics

■ The proximal row of the carpus is an intercalated segment with
muscle attachments
■ Its stability depends on the capsular and interosseous ligaments
  − According to Gilford, a link joint, as between proximal and dis
    carpal rows, should be stable in compression and will crumple
    compression unless prevented by a stop mechanism
  − The scaphoid may act as a stop mechanism

9.20.1.5 Aetiology

■ Traumatic
■ Inflammatory
■ Congenital

9.20.1.6 Traumatic Aetiology

■ Fall on outstretched extended wrist
■ If thenar first → supination → DISI
■ If hypothenar first → pronation → VISI

9.20.1.7 Symptomatology

■ Pain
■ Weakness
■ Giving way
■ Clunk/snap/click during use

9.20.1.8 Carpal Instability – Classifications (Dobyns)

■ DISI
■ VISI
■ Ulnar translocation (rheumatoid)
■ Dorsal subluxation (after fractured radius)

0.1.9   Carpal Instability – Classifications (Taleisnik)

Taleisnik: concepts of:

— Dynamic instability – partial ligament injuries with pain but minimal X-ray change
— Static instability – end state; scapholunate dissociation, fixed flexion of scaphoid, fixed extension of lunate

0.1.10   Other Carpal Instability Classifications

Carpal instability, dissociative (CID): interosseous ligament damage
Carpal instability, non-dissociative (CIND): capsular ligament damage
Carpal instability, complex (CIC): CID + CIND
Carpal instability, adaptive (CIA): adaption to extracarpal cause

20.1.11   Carpal Instability – Common Clinical Scenarios

Scapholunate dissociation
Lunotriquetral dissociation
Unstable scaphoid non-union
Extrinsic radiocarpal ligament insufficiency (inflammatory/traumatic/congenital)
Distal radial malunion
Carpal instability complex

20.2   Lunate and Perilunate Dislocations (Fig. 9.36)

20.2.1   Introduction

Lunate dislocation less common since bound by the stronger palmar capsular ligament
Presence of chondral and osteochondral injury not uncommon and may not be seen on X-ray

20.2.2   Anatomy of Palmar Side Ligaments

Two inverted 'V' structures
First centred on capitate = radioscaphocapitate (RSC), and ulnocapitate (UC)

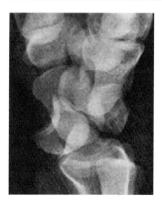

Fig. 9.36 The lateral radiograph of a patient with pe lunate dislocation. It is essential to check the median nerve

- Second centred on lunate = long and short radio-lunate (RL) a ulnolunate (UL)
- "Space of Poirier" – weak point between capitate and lunate – throu which lunate dislocation occurs
- (Radioscapholunate ligament [RSL]) – only a vestigial embryo structure, although it was initially thought that this ligament of T tut was a key stabiliser

9.20.2.3 Dorsal Side Ligaments
- One inverted "V"
- Centred on the triquetrum:
    - Intercarpal dorsal ligament
    - Radiocarpal dorsal ligament

9.20.2.4 Mayfield Stages (Based on Cadavers)
- Based on wrist hyperextension, and varying degrees of ulna devi ion (and forearm supination)
- Postulate failure from the radial side/scapholunate interosseus li ment (SLIL) first
- Four stages – SLIL torn, followed by a sequence of ligament arou the lunate in an ulna direction ± with fracture of the carpal bone

- SLIL – c-shaped, intracapsular ligament, very important ligament of the wrist: controls the rotation of the scaphoid and the lunate without allowing gapping or translation between the two bones (the dorsal portion is the stronger part)

.20.2.5 Mayfield Classes

- Stage 1: SLIL tear with DISI
  - Class a: partial – positive scope
  - Class b: partial – positive stress X-ray
  - Class c: complete – gap seen and ↑ scapholunate (SL) angle
  - Class d: complete – complete and degenerative changes
- Stages 2–4: carpal dislocation ± fracture
- Ulna, midcarpal, or VISI patterns
- Vertical shear injury of the carpus

.20.2.6 Investigation

- Plain X-ray
- Cineradiography
- Stress radiography
- Arthrography
- Arthroscopy

.20.2.7 Radiological Interpretations

- Do not make final comments on AP X-ray alone
- Lateral view is important to DDx lunate vs. perilunate dislocations
- Perilunate cases, look for fractured scaphoid/radial styloid/fractured capitate/#fractured triquetrum/fractured ulna styloid
- After reduction – still look for: Gilula arc, carpal collapse, proximal migration of capitate through the SL interval

.20.2.8 Treatment Principles

- Urgent reduction
- Most will need operation because 60% of cases have loss of reduction after initial reduction and casting is found in previous studies

- 65% with good results after open surgery, most cases with no surgery have a bad result– in summary, too unstable to be left unfixed

9.20.2.9 CR and OR

- Extending the wrist to recreate the deformity and apply dorsal pressure to reduce the capitate into the lunate fossa
- OR and repair of the SLIL and lunotriquetral ligament is indicated in all perilunate and lunate dislocations

9.20.2.10 CR in Lunate Dislocations

- Flex wrist to remove tension from the palmar ligament
- Next, apply palmar pressure over lunate followed by wrist extension to reduce lunate to its fossa
- Flex the wrist to reduce the capitate to the lunate

9.20.2.11 Technical Tip

- A dorsal longitudinal incision, release third extensor compartment and extensor pollicis longus (EPL), elevate fourth compartment longitudinal capsulotomy – exposes SLIL and lunotriquetral interosseous ligament (LTIL) and to reduce the scaphoid to the lunate and lunate to triquetrum
- Repair ligament avulsions with suture anchors, intraoperative X-ray to recheck alignment ± place wire at scaphoid as joystick
- Additionally need k-wires to pin scaphoid to lunate, pin triquetrum to lunate – but avoid pinning from carpus to radius
- A separate palmar approach, especially in lunate dislocations volarly and/or release median nerve
- Rn of lunate dislocations similar to perilunate
- Whichever type, fix associated fractures, e.g. of styloid and scaphoid

9.20.2.12 Delayed Cases

- Long-term pain, weakness, stiffness, OA, carpal tunnel syndrome, attritional flexor injury
- Operation is still advised regardless of time lapse – but nature of operation options differ: open reduction, lunate excision, proximal row

carpectomy (PRC), wrist fusion, etc. – only proper reduction offers the greatest potential for normal wrist mechanics (PRC is reasonable way to go if reduction *cannot* be achieved, provided head of capitate not significantly injured – which alas may require fusion if the head of the capitate is abnormal)

20.2.13 Principle of Rn of Chronic Injury

- Reducible – ligamentous repair
- Fixed – intercarpal fusion (also considered in athletes/manual workers)

20.2.13.1 Options in Late Static Chronic Instability

- Capsulodesis (may stretch out with time)
- Local fusion – adjacent OA
- Total fusion
- Proximal row carpectomy (salvage in scapholunate advanced collapse [SLAC] wrist with old non-union)

20.2.13.2 Overall Management Depends on

- Time of presentation
- Degree of pathology
- Associated carpal injuries

20.3 SL Instability (Fig. 9.37)

20.3.1 Biomechanics of SL Instability

- Relatively normal load distribution: scaphoid:lunate = 60 : 40%
- SL dissociation preferentially loads the scaphoid and unloads the lunate, scaphoid:lunate = 80 : 20%
- SLAC (natural history) left untreated, DISI will progress to degenerative changes; however, timeline still unclear

20.3.2 Sequential Pattern of OA Changes

- Tip of radial styloid and scaphoid
- Remainder of scaphoid and scaphoid fossa
- Capitate/lunate joint

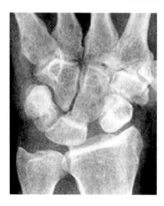

Fig. 9.37 Terry Thomas sign shown here is typical of SL instability

9.20.3.3 SL Ligament Anatomy

- Dorsal part strong > ventral part (middle part membranous)
- Mayfield article on perilunate instability:
  - Stage 1: SL injury
  - Stage 2: SL and RSC affected
  - Stage 3: above and LT ligament injury
  - Stage 4: above and dorsal radiocapitate – palmar lunate dislocated

9.20.3.4 Clinical Exam

- Pain, snapping, weakness
- Pain at dorsal aspect of SLJ, positive scaphoid stress test

9.20.3.5 Radiological Assessment

- Terry Thomas sign
- DISI pattern
- Earliest cases may need arthroscopy for Dx
- Early cases may show up on stress X-rays
- Arthrogram: not all positive cases have symptomatic instabilities. Less used nowadays
- MRI – not yet ideal

Arthroscopy – becoming the gold standard, but not needed if X-ray is diagnostic, yet can offer direct view, and staging of chondral damage/wear)

9.20.3.6 Treatment Options

- Observation (in mildest of cases, one cadaver study claims an incidence 28%, i.e. many asymptomatic)
- Arthroscopic debridement – remember not all tears are part of a carpal instability (e.g. strong portion can be intact)
- Arthroscopic reduction and pinning – better if done in acute phase
- Blatt dorsal capsulodesis
- Tenodesis (by flexor carpi radialis [FCR])
- Limited carpal fusion – scaphotrapeziotrapezoid (STT)/scaphocapitatum (SC)
- OR and repair ligament – still debated
- Bone-ligament-bone – no long-term result, many donors have been reported

9.20.4 LT (Lunotriquetral) Instability

9.20.4.1 Clinical Features

- Thought of as "reverse perilunate injury" pattern
- Pathomechanics – fall on a palmar flexed wrist
- VISI can develop
- But no clear pattern of degenerative changes like the SLAC wrist counterpart

9.20.4.2 Goal of Treatment

- Less pain
- More strength
- Prevent static VISI

9.20.4.3 Anatomy of LT Ligament

- C-shaped like SL ligament
- Unlike SL dorsal part thin, and palmar thick (just the opposite)

- Middle; membranous, consists of fibrocartilage and not true ligament

9.20.4.4 Physical Assessment
- LT articulation tender
- Click on radial and ulna deviation
- Less grip strength
- LT ballottement test – thumb and finger of one hand grasp pisotriquetral complex and use another hand's thumb and finger to grasp the lunate – estimate AP translation of triquetrum relative to lunate
- LT shear test – one thumb at dorsal lunate and the other thumb on palmar surface of pisiform – then radial (RD)/ulnar deviation (UD) check for click
- LT compression test – apply converging load to scaphoid and triquetrum, with pain in LT area

9.20.4.5 Radiological Assessment
- Look for VISI
- Assess Gilula arcs
- Check ulna variance
- Arthrogram – sometimes false and from ulna impaction
- Tc bone scan – non-specific
- MRI – not too easy to see the lesion
- Arthroscopy – new gold standard, the reader should know the different Geissler stages

9.20.4.6 Treatment Options
- Arthrodesis – not advised
- Ligament reconstruction – technique demanding
- Direct repair – reattach and k-wires
- Percutaneous k-wires
- Isolate injury. Can try conservative
- Goal – realign lunocapitate axis and establish LT stability

9.20.5 Ulna Translocation (of the Carpus): Aetiology, Dx and Rn
- RA – common, from trauma – very rare

- Need *global* ligament laxity (probably including RSC and long RL) to occur
- X-ray: assess – by degree of overhang according to the Gilula method (grip and stress view)
- Rn:
  - Acute – ligament repair and fix
  - Chronic – Chamay (radiolunate fusion) in RA cases. Radioscapholunate fusion if the radioscaphoid joint is osteoarthritic

9.20.6 Axial Instabilities
9.20.6.1 Clinical Types
- Radial column stays behind, ulna side displaced
- Ulna portion stays behind, radial side displaced
- Very rare

9.20.6.2 Clinical Feature
- Uncommon
- Most are crush injuries, e.g. printing presses of industrial type
- Complications – skin, tendon, soft tissue loss, associated carpal fractures
- Rn: open reduction and internal fixation with k-wires
- Stiffness common and <50% good result

9.20.7 DRUJ Injuries and Instability
9.20.7.1 Introduction
- The term TFCC coined by Palmer in 1987
- Function – cushion, gliding, helps connect ulna axis to volar carpus
- Normally 80% load carried at distal radius; can change a lot with differing ulna variance

9.20.7.2 Evolution
- One of the three most important advances after assumption of the bipedal gait
- The other two being higher brain centres and prehensile function
- Forearm rotation allows one to better manipulate the environment, handle tools, and helps in defence (after Lindshield)

9.20.7.3 Anatomy
- The reader is referred to the works of Palmer concerning load transmission across the wrist
- Correlation of the shape of the DRUJ articulation with the ulna variance
- Element of incongruity from differences in radii of curvatures of the two surfaces of the DRUJ – to allow not only rotation, but translation with pronation/supination motions – the trade-off is less stability

9.20.7.4 Primary and Secondary Stabilisers
- Primary stabilisers: especially the dorsal and palmar RUL (radio-ulnar ligament) – they insert not only at ulna styloid, but also fovea of the ulna head (they are the dorsal and volar extents of the TFC)
(Implication – their avulsion from the ulna fovea may occur without ulna styloid fracture. On the other hand, basal ulna styloid fracture is suggestive of injury to these stabilisers, check DRUJ instability)
- Secondary stabilisers – ulno-carpal ligaments, sheath of the extensor carpi ulnaris (ECU) (articular disc)

9.20.7.5 Classes of TFCC Injury by Palmer
- Traumatic
- Degenerative

9.20.7.6 Natural History
- 50–70% of this structure damaged with age according to cadaveric wrist studies

9.20.7.7 Common Clinical Scenarios
- TFCC/DRUJ instability – think of possible TFCC injury
- Patients with significant positive or negative ulna variance may predispose to TFCC injury
- One of the many DDx of ulna wrist pain – "low back pain" of the wrist

9.20.7.8 Physical Assessment
- Area of tenderness at TFCC

- Test ROM of DRUJ and any subluxation
- Stress test
- Degree and direction of laxity
- ECU checked

9.20.7.9 Radiological Assessment

- Ulna variance and any ulna impingement – always check the elbow – can be cause of radial shortening
- Normality of form and tilting of distal radius
- Congruency of the sigmoid notch
- Subluxation/dislocation of distal ulna best seen on true lateral X-ray of the wrist
- Carpal height ratio and Gilula lines
- Look for degenerative changes

9.20.7.9.1 Role of Arthrogram Versus Scope Versus MRI/CT

- Arthrogram still has a role in judging the direction of dye leakage – but beware that the pores may fill up with fibrous tissue with time – less accurate for delayed cases
- Arthroscope – good to see lesions sometimes less well seen by MRI such as cartilage, and can probe joint and test for TFCC tension, can be therapeutic at the same time
- CT – good to assess congruency of the sigmoid notch, and cases with bony deformity
- MRI – can assess soft tissue, non-invasive, less good for cartilage

9.20.7.10 Scenario 1: Acute TFCC Injury and DRUJ Unstable

- If fractured, fix ulna styloid and retest stability of DRUJ
- Either try conservative (plaster cast [POP] in supination) or scope/open repair

9.20.7.11 Scenario 2: TFC Isolated Tear with Stable DRUJ

- Central lesion – debridement
- Peripheral lesion – repair (blood supply is from peripheral just like menisci)

9.20.7.12 Scenario 3: Ulna Styloid Fracture
- Need to treat any non-union or malunion

9.20.7.13 Scenario 4: Chronic TFCC Injury
- Some studies show can still intervene with reasonable results up to < 3–4 months
- DRUJ unstable due to malunited distal radius (sometimes subtle from increased volar tilt) – may need osteotomy and cases where radius obviously shortened – ulna impaction and may need joint levelling procedure, or osteotomy of distal radius
- If sigmoid notch area degenerated – may need salvage, e.g. Sauve-Kapanji

9.20.7.14 Example of DRUJ Reconstruction – Linshield Procedure
- Use half of flexor carpi ulnaris (FCU) as a sling
- Make in a strip
- Sling ulna head back

9.20.7.15 Examples of Procedures to Tackle Length Discrepancies
- Ulna alone – shortening, wafer procedure, and Sauve-Kapanji
- Radius alone – osteotomy
- Both – rarely mentioned in the literature

9.20.7.15.1 Role of Joint Levelling
- Reconstruction procedure alone in the presence of significant length differences (between distal radius and ulna) with no joint levelling may not work
- Restoration of joint congruency is important

9.20.7.15.2 In the Setting of Distal Radius Injury
- Check for clinical DRUJ instability most important – since just relying on X-ray assessment of ulna styloid is not good enough

Category I: Acute Situations
- Associated fractured distal radius: assess integrity of the *sigmoid*

notch, good restoration of radial length and prevention of dorsal tilt is important – hence first ensure that adequate anatomic restoration of distal radius anatomy, then check DRUJ instability; if we find fractured base of styloid – fix it, and recheck for DRUJ instability. DRUJ stability should also be checked even if no associated ulna styloid fracture

Rn of Acute Instability

- Repair of TFCC (if subacute, avoid scope since may need open debridement of the granulation tissue)
- If still unstable, repair the secondary stabilisers
- If irreparable – extrinsic methods, like tenodesis

Category II: Chronic Instability

- Key: check whether there is OA
- No OA: reconstruct the soft tissue – intrinsic vs. extrinsic methods – extrinsic runs the risk of not being anatomical and more ROM limitation
- With OA: if severe needs salvage Sauve-Kapanji, Darrach tries to retain some ulna ST; excision arthroplasty alone risks further de-stabilisation; Cooney says some role of DRUJ arthroplasty

9.21   Scaphoid Injuries

9.21.1   Features Peculiar to Scaphoid

- Most of its surface intra-articular
- Tenous blood supply, main one from the dorsal ridge
- Twisted peanut shape, fracture can sometimes be visualised only by seeing multiple X-ray views

9.21.2   Scaphoid Fractures – Definition of Displaced Fracture

- Definition of displaced/unstable fracture = a fracture gap >1 mm on any X-ray projection
- Extra evidence may be provided by: SL angle > 60°, RL angle > 15°; also intrascaphoid angle > 35°

9.21.3 Presentation of Acute Fractures

- Acute fractures – can be tender at anatomic snuffbox or distal tubercle
- Mostly after a wrist dorsiflexion injury
- Some cases are missed Dx or no fracture can be seen on initial X-ray or delayed presentation because the patient cannot recall any injury

9.21.4 Radiological Assessment

- X-ray:
  - PA – distorted by flexion and normal curvature of the scaphoid
  - PA in ulna deviation better, but does not completely solve the above
  - 45° pronated PA
  - Lateral – can see waist fracture better
  - Others – the distal third best seen on semi-pronated oblique view, the dorsal ridge best seen on semisupinated oblique

9.21.5 Other Investigations

- CT – in the plane of the scaphoid, especially 1-mm cut; good for checking whether there is a fracture, whether fracture is displaced, and in preoperative assessment for, say, malunion to check the intrascaphoid angle
- MRI – good to identify fracture even within 48 h, Dx of occult fracture, and help check vascularity. Expensive

9.21.6 Different Clinical Scenarios

- Undisplaced fractures
- Looks like undisplaced fracture – but in fact displaced
- Displaced fractures – definition and implications
- Delayed presentation cases (> 4 weeks)
- Scaphoid non-union with advanced carpal collapse (SNAC) wrist
- AVN of scaphoid
- Unsure of Dx – what to do
- Malunited fracture

9.21.6.1 Really Undisplaced Fracture

- Refer to definition of undisplaced
- Rn – many studies indicate only 4–5% non-union, even with simple casting
- Methods of casting – long vs. short arm reported in the literature with no statistical difference, some experts like Barton had suggested doing away with thumb spica part – but most surgeons still use the traditional teaching of Bohler, i.e. immobilise the thumb as well during casting
- Duration of casting – proximal pole needs too prolonged casting and chance of AVN/non-union so high (90%) that many choose primary (open or percutaneous) fixation via a dorsal approach
- For the common mid third waist fracture, there is a recent trend towards percutaneous screw fixation. There is as yet no long-term result, but should be appealing for those patients who have to return to their work early (e.g. soldiers), those involved in competitive sports like athletes, and sometimes for financial reasons

9.21.6.1.1 Percutaneous Cannulated Screw Fixation

- Advantages:
  - Earlier return to work
  - No need for prolonged immobilisation
- Disadvantages:
  - Not yet very sure whether non-union rate lower (Fig. 9.38)
  - Cx like sepsis, trapezial erosion
  - Some recent arthroscopic studies show that during passage of the screw, fracture site *distraction* may be caused
  - Technically demanding

9.21.6.2 Labelled Undisplaced Fracture, but in Fact Fracture Is Displaced

- Fracture displacement not easy to detect if hand casted
- Fracture displacement can be subtle and sometimes seen only on CT

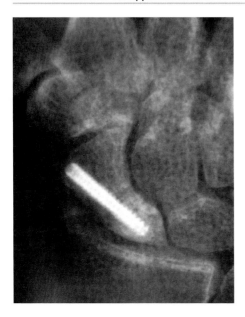

Fig. 9.38 Although cannulated screw is in vogue as treatment of scaphoid fracture, there is still a chance of delayed or non-union

- This difference is important since *non-union rate increases from 5 to 50% with fracture displacement*
- Ease of fracture displacement also depends on fracture configuration, e.g. more likely with vertical oblique orientation

9.21.6.3 Acute Displaced Fractures

- Most use ORIF or percutaneous cannulated screw fixation if reducible
- If any suspicion intraoperatively (of avascularity) can check for punctate bleeding during open reduction (especially for cases with somewhat delayed presentation)
- Screw used mostly is of differential threads, most use headless screws, screw head if present need be countersunk. Placement of screw in the central third essential

9.21.6.4 Summary of Operative Indications for Acute Scaphoid Fractures

- Displaced fracture
- Proximal pole fracture
- Delayed cases (especially > 4 months)
- Perilunate dislocation with scaphoid fracture
- Concomitant scaphoid fracture and fractured distal radius
- ± Possible advantage of fixing acute undisplaced fractures in selected patients has been mentioned

9.21.6.5 Delayed Presentation

- Operate
- VBG (vascularised bone graft) sometimes needed if avascularity sets in
- Mostly volar approach, but dorsal for proximal pole fractures, (since not much more to lose with regard to vascularity). Preserve RSC during volar approach in open reduction

9.21.6.6 Assessment of Any AVN

- Increased radiologic density does not always indicate avascularity of the proximal fragment – two factors, → (new bone forming proximal fragment, and another explanation is relative porosis because of increased vascularity of distal fragment) – these are only tentative explanations
- Gelberman favours intraoperative punctate bleeding as most reliable method to assess any AVN
- Recently, trend to adopt the use of gadolinium MRI to determine any avascularity

9.21.6.7 SNAC Wrist

- Pattern of arthrosis similar to SLAC wrist. Natural Hx of scaphoid non-union is that given time degenerative arthritis will set in although sometimes the time lapse can be as long as > 10 years

- Operative method used depends on stage of disease
- Early non-union cases, especially if no avascularity, screw fixation may need wedge graft to correct humpback
- Late non-union cases probably select among options like limited carpal fusion, PRC, even wrist fusion

9.21.6.8 Unsure of Diagnosis
- Most cases cast for 2 to 4 weeks and repeat X-ray (out of cast)
- Some propose CT if still not sure by then

9.21.6.9 Malunited Fractures
- If untreated, also influence carpal biomechanics, rare
- Clinically, there is loss of extension
- Treatment – operative, frequently need wedge graft to correct hump back and screw fixation
- Malunion rather uncommon

9.22   Hand Fractures and Dislocations

9.22.1   Problems We Face Around this Region
- Small size of the bones
- Compact anatomy
- Yet demanding functional requirements

9.22.2   Concept of Functional Stability in Management of Hand Fractures (Injury 1996)
- Assesses the functional stability – involves both clinical and radio logic assessment – functionally stable if fracture not displaced with active mobilisation, no movement on flexion/extension view or screening under X-ray
- Aim to mobilise early those fractures that are functionally stable. For unstable ones, give adequate stability for early mobilisation via operative means. Traditional very rigid implants like plates and screw not always needed. The exact implant to be used depends on the

fracture geometry and configuration, and the nature of associated injuries. It all boils down to a delicate balance between biology and biomechanics

9.22.3   Usual Reasons for Failure of CR for Fractures

- Resultant significant rotational deformity
- Displaced articular fragment with step-off will not reduce by CR
- Unacceptable angular deformity
- Unacceptable shortening
- Multiple fractures are difficult to control by closed means

9.22.4   General Functional Goal in Operative Surgery for Hand Fractures

- Opposable thumb
- Stable index finger, middle finger for pinch and grasp
- Flexible ring finger, little finger for mobility
- Stable wrist for positioning

9.22.5   General Operative Indications

- Functionally unstable fractures
- Irreducible and significant malalignment present
- Segmental bone loss
- Multiple fractures
- Concomitant soft tissue damage that requires surgery
- Special fracture types that are prone to displacement (e.g. condylar fracture)

9.22.6   General Principles of Finger Fracture Management

- ORIF = if fixable and reducible
- Consider ligamentotaxis and dynamic EF = if reducible but non-fixable
- Severe cases with bone loss – the principle is preservation of bone stock as far as possible in the acute setting, this will ease later reconstructive options, which will be discussed

9.22.7   Options for Peri-articular Hand Fractures with Bone Loss

- Anatomical internal fixation if feasible
- Interpositional arthroplasty
- Arthroplasty with hinged spacer (silicon arthroplasty)
- Surface replacement (e.g. pyrocarbon arthroplasty)
- Osteochondral grafting
- Vascularised toe joint transfer
- Amputation – last resort

9.22.8   How to Choose Among the Options

- If patient's occupation is a labourer, for example, and breadwinner, fusion in functional position and early return to work is a viable option (especially if the other joints in the intercalated chain are preserved)
- If patient's occupation is a pianist, then joint motion preservation is desirable. Options like vascularised joint transfer and arthroplasty can then be considered

9.22.9   The Special Case of Severe Thumb Injury and Thumb Loss

- Since the thumb is of paramount importance in various hand functions such as pinching and grasping; the length of the thumb should be preserved as far as possible
- If injury is severe leaving a shortened stump, the following options can be considered:
  - Thumb lengthening
  - Toe–hand transfer
  - If resultant soft tissue cover a problem, consider wraparound flap from big toe

9.22.10 Priorities in Finger Joint Reconstruction

- For the thumb: carpal-metacarpal joint (CMCJ) > proximal interphalangeal joint (PIPJ) > distal interphalangeal joint (DIPJ)
- Radial-sided fingers: metacarpal-phalangeal joint (MCPJ) > PIP > DIPJ, CMCJ last. Reason = radial side digits need more stability for prehension pinch

■ Ulna-sided fingers: MCPJ ≥ PIPJ > CMCJ > DIPJ. Reason = ulna side digits need more mobility for cupping functions (e.g. holding a hammer tightly)

22.11 Management of Individual Fractures

22.11.1 Feature of the First Ray

■ The thumb or in fact the first ray is much more actively involved in pinching and grasping, and oriented in a different plane from the four digits

■ The above, plus the effect of the moment arm of this mobile first ray, makes first metacarpal base fractures much more commonly seen than first MC shaft or head fractures

22.11.2 Features of Anatomy of the First CMCJ

■ Stability depends on:
  – Articulation: essentially two opposed saddles
  – Capsule: special thickenings confer added stability

■ Four main ligaments:
  – AOL (anterior oblique ligament, strong)
  – Intermetacarpal ligament
  – Dorsoradial ligament
  – Posterior oblique ligament

22.11.3 Metacarpal Base Articulation

■ Second MC articulates with trapezium and trapezoid
■ Third MC articulates with capitate
■ Fourth and fifth MC articulate with hamate

22.11.4 Feature of Second to Fifth MC

■ Second and third MC or in other words CMCJ are much less mobile than the fourth and fifth CMCJ

■ This forms the main reason for accepting much less degree of angulation in cases of second or third MC neck fractures relative to the same fractures occurring in the fourth or fifth MC neck

9.22.11.5 Feature of MCPJ

- Strong box-like structure:
  - Collateral ligament
  - Articular surfaces with cam-like effect of the MC head
  - Capsule
  - Flexor and extensor tendons
  - Volar plate
  - No proximal checkrein (as in PIPJ)
  - Most dislocations are dorsal owing to the strong volar structures

9.22.11.6 Features of Anatomy of Phalanges

- Essentially an intercalated system balanced by opposing forces, e.g. flexor digitorum superficialis, flexor digitorum profundus, hand intrinsics like the interossei
- Fractured distal phalanx mostly undisplaced
- Fractured proximal phalanx usually apex volar
- Fracture pattern of middle phalanx more difficult to predict

9.22.11.7 Features of Anatomy of PIPJ

- Box-like structures stabilising the articulation:
  - Proper collateral ligament
  - Accessory collateral ligament
  - Volar plate
  - Place for insertion of central slip of extensor
  - Place for insertion of FDS

9.22.11.8 Metacarpal Fractures: Clinical Types

- MC head fractures
- MC neck fractures – common
- MC shaft fractures
- MC base fractures

9.22.11.8.1 MC Neck Fractures

- Common, most involve the fourth or fifth ray
- Usual mechanism involves direct impact with a fist hitting a hard object

- Deformity is apex dorsal from the stronger pull of the hand intrinsics
- Acceptable angulation: 15° in the second and third ray; and 35° at the fourth or fifth ray
- Even small degree of rotational malalignment is not usually acceptable
- CR: Jahss manoeuvre involving pressure at MC head and another point of pressure at PIPJ with the MCPJ and PIPJ of the affected finger flexed to 90°

Rn Options

- Conservative – if within the acceptable angulation
- Operative:
  - Percutaneous pinning
  - Cross pinning to nearby distal MC shaft
  - ORIF using k-wires/TBW or mini-plates

9.22.11.8.2 MC Head Fractures

- Rare
- Intra-articular fractures by definition
- May need oblique X-ray or Brewerton view for proper delineation
- Rn options:
  - Undisplaced fractures: may try conservative, need monitor
  - Displaced fractures: need ORIF with screws, if distal fragment large, consider mini-condylar plate
  - If due to human bite wound: leave open, clean, delayed ORIF

9.22.11.8.3 MC Shaft Fractures (Fig. 9.39)

- Undisplaced fractures especially at non-border digits can be braced
- Err on the side of operative Rn for border (second and fifth ray) digits
- Transverse fractures best fixed with 2.7 mm DCP or even percutaneous pinning
- Spiral fractures spanning a length $\geq \times 2$ diameter of the shaft can be fixed with lag screws alone
- Open/comminuted fractures may need temporary EF ± BG

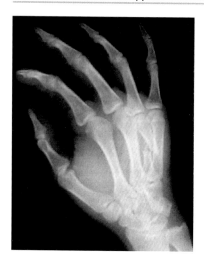

Fig. 9.39 Oblique radiograph showing a displaced metacarpal shaft fracture

- Acceptable alignment: 0° malrotation, dorsal angulation: < 10° in second and third rays, and < 20° in fourth and fifth rays

9.22.11.8.4   MC Base Fractures

- Management of fifth MC base fractures subluxation can be visualised as an analogue of Bennett fracture subluxation, which will be discussed
- Otherwise, most MC base fractures are relatively undisplaced (and many can be treated conservatively) by dint of local strong ligamentous support
- The extent of any associated CMCJ subluxation can be visualised on lateral X-rays

9.22.11.9   Fractures Involving the First Ray
9.22.11.9.1   Clinical Types

- The more common scenarios include:
  - Thumb MC base fractures ± subluxation
  - Thumb MC shaft fractures

9.22.11.9.2   Thumb Base Fractures

- Clinical types:
  - Extra-articular thumb base fractures
  - Bennett fracture subluxation
  - Rolando fracture ± subluxation

9.22.11.9.3   Extra-articular Thumb Base Fractures

- Proximal fragment deforming force is by APL
- Distal fragment deforming force is by adductor pollicis, abductor pollicis brevis (APB), and flexor pollicis brevis (FPB)
- As a result, the distal fragment is frequently flexed, adducted and supinated
- Undisplaced fractures may try CR and spica
- Displaced fractures may need CR and pinning, or ORIF if position not satisfactory

9.22.11.9.4   Bennett Fracture Subluxation

- An intra-articular fracture
- The fragment that stays put is at the volar ulna aspect of first MC base; being held in place by the AOL (anterior oblique ligament)
- The distal fragment subluxates dorsally, proximally and towards the radial side

Treatment of Bennett's Fractures

- Method of CR: by longitudinal traction and some degree of pronation, with the thumb of the surgeon applying a downward pressure on the proximal aspect of the distal fragment
- Stabilisation is via percutaneous pinning, one pin transfixing the first MC to the second MC shaft; the second pin going towards the trapezium
- ORIF is rarely needed since closed reduction internal fixation (CRIF) is usually successful and produces a reasonably good result, but ORIF should be considered if reduction cannot be achieved by closed means, especially with a sizable fracture fragment

9.22.11.9.5   Rolando Fractures

- Essentially a three-part fracture that is Y-shaped or T-shaped ± varying degree of communition
- An intra-articular fracture
- ORIF only possible with sizable fragment
- Options in comminuted fractures include: external fixation ± traction

9.22.11.9.6   Thumb MC Shaft Fractures (Fig. 9.40)

- Displaced fractures require ORIF
- Important to restore the length of the first ray for performance of basic hand functions

9.22.11.10   PIPJ Fracture Dislocation

9.22.11.10.1   Mechanism

- Those associated with volar base fractures of middle phalanx (M/P) due to PIPJ hyperextension and volar plate avulsion. PIPJ dislocated dorsally

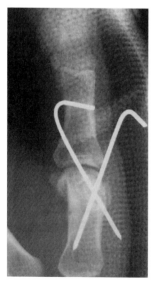

Fig. 9.40 Radiograph showing comminuted fracture of the distal metacarpal of the thumb

- Those associated with dorsal base fractures of M/P due to PIPJ hyper-flexion and central slip avulsion. PIPJ dislocated volarly
- Those pilon-type fractures, base of M/P mostly from axial impaction loading

9.22.11.10.2 Clinical Types

- Acute:
  - Involving volar base of M/P
  - Involving dorsal base of M/P
  - Involving the entire base of M/P
- Chronic PIPJ fracture dislocations

9.22.11.10.3 PIPJ Dislocation and Volar Base Fracture of M/P

- Minor chip fractures and no significant instability: buddy splint, management similar to pure PIPJ dislocation (Fig. 9.41)
- Involves one-third of articular surface, extension block splint

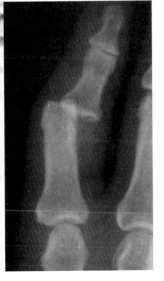

Fig. 9.41 Dislocation of the PIPJ is not uncommon in contact sports

- Involvement of one-third to one half of articular surface: options include ORIF or volar plate plasty ± use of traction device, or even extension block pinning
- Very unstable, >50% articular involvement: ORIF or volar plate plasty, ± BG

9.22.11.10.4 *PIPJ Dislocation and Dorsal Base Fractures of M/P*
- If undisplaced: extension splinting
- If displaced: ORIF by dorsal approach

9.22.11.10.5 *PIPJ Dislocation and "Pilon" Type Fractures of M/P*
- Involves both dorsal and volar bases
- Rn options:
  - Continuous traction device (recommended)
  - ORIF (but usually precluded by tiny fragments)

9.22.11.10.6 *Chronic PIPJ Fracture Dislocations*
- Rn options:
  - Volar plate plasty ± BG
  - Hemihamate osteochondral grafting
  - ORIF/BG

9.22.11.10.7 *Rare Volar PIPJ Dislocation*
- Rare
- Most cases of disrupted extensor mechanism unlike dorsal dislocations (where volar plate or flexor tendon may be entrapped)

PIPJ Volar Dislocation: Management
- CR difficult because torn extensor including central slip holding the P/P out of position
- Many cases need OR to repair the extensor mechanism (CR at most two attempts allowed)
- CR method differs from dorsal dislocation – need to flex MCP and IPJ to relax the lateral band, some wrist extension to relax extensors

■ Postoperative: extension splint – to prevent volar migration of lateral bands and boutonniere

9.22.11.10.8 DIPJ Dorsal Dislocation
■ Also two collaterals and volar plate
■ Also most commonly as dorsal dislocation

9.22.11.11 Miscellaneous Phalangeal Fractures
9.22.11.11.1 P/P Unicondylar Fractures (Fig. 9.42)
■ Most require ORIF since difficult to hold the fracture by conservative means
■ Most use a dorsal approach to fixation

9.22.11.11.2 P/P Bicondylar Fractures
■ ORIF needed for similar reasons, may need TBW or mini-plates
■ Traction will result in fracture rotation instead of proper reduction

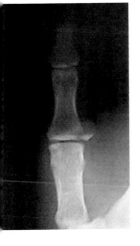

Fig. 9.42 This fracture proved to be a rather sizable articular fragment intraoperatively that requires fixation before early motion can be initiated

9.22.11.11.3 Other Extra-articular Phalangeal Fractures
- These include the usually seen oblique or transverse shaft fractures of the phalanges (Fig. 9.43)

9.22.12 Complications of Finger Fractures
9.22.12.1 General Comment
- One main feature of the anatomy of the hand is that the different structural units are closely packed together (e.g. bony skeleton, tendons, neurovascular structures)
- There is a high chance of stiffness, especially in cases when more than one structural component is at fault, e.g. fractured P/P in association with zone 2 flexor tendon injury

9.22.12.2 Stiffness
- Can be classified as intra- or extra-articular
- Intra-articular causes include OA, adhesions, etc.
- Extra-articular causes are many, common examples include:

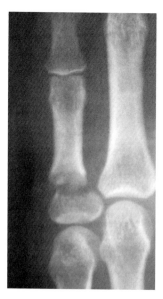

Fig. 9.43 Radiograph showing an extra-articular basal transverse fracture of the middle phalanx

- Capsulotomy and extensor tenolysis can be used to tackle fingers stiff even with passive flexion and extension
- Fingers stiff with passive extension, but can be flexed passively are unlikely to need the above procedures, but may need flexor tenolysis instead, etc.

9.22.12.3 Malunion

- In fractured phalanges, it should be noted that even a small amount of rotational malalignment of 5° can cause obvious deformity and affect function
- Malunion is not uncommonly associated with shortening. Shortening of the thumb should be avoided at all costs since it is important for grasping and pinching
- Corrective osteotomy can be considered to correct rotational and angular deformity

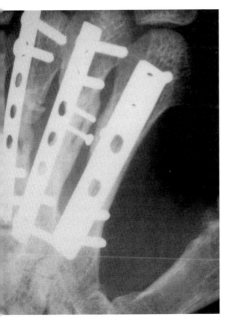

Fig. 9.44 This patient suffered open fractures of multiple metacarpals. Some of the fixed free segments were not viable, requiring subsequent reconstruction

9.22.12.4 Non-union/Delayed Union

- As with Rn of non-union in other areas, strategy depends on the type of non-union, many are results of open fractures in crush injuries (Fig. 9.44)
- Hypertrophic/oligotrophic ones need mechanical stabilisation
- Atrophic ones also require biological stimulus frequently by bone grafting

General Bibliography

1.   Baker CL Jr, Plancher KD (2002) Operative treatment of elbow injuries. Springer New York Berlin Heidelberg
2.   Beredjiklian PK, Bozentka DJ (2004) Review of hand surgery. Saunders, Philadelphia
3.   Perry CR, Court-Brown CM (1999) Master cases: orthopaedic trauma. Thieme, New York
4.   Smith P (2002) Lister's the hand (diagnosis and indications), 4th edn. Churchill Livingstone, London
5.   Warner JP, Iannotti JP, Flatow EL (2005) Complex and revision problems in shoulder surgery. Lippincott Williams & Wilkins, Philadelphia
6.   Watson K, Weinzweig J (2001) The wrist. Lippincott Williams & Wilkins, Philadelphia

Selected Bibliography of Journal Articles

1.   Chapman JR, Henley MB (2000) Randomized prospective study of humeral shaft fracture fixation: intramedullary nails vs plates. J Orthop Trauma 14(3):162–166
2.   Cobb TK, Morrey BF (1997) Total elbow arthroplasty as primary treatment for distal humeral fractures in elderly patients. J Bone Joint Surg Am 79:826–832
3.   Court-Brown CM, McQueen MM (2001) The translated two-part fracture of the proximal humerus. Epidemiology and outcome in the older patient. J Bone Joint Surg Br 83(6):799–804
4.   Goss TP (1993) Double disruptions of the superior shoulder suspensory complex. J Orthop Trauma 7(2):99–106

. Gupta R, Raheja A et al. (2000) Limited contact dynamic compression in diaphyseal fractures of the humerus: good outcome in 51 patients. Acta Orthop Scand 71(5):471–474

. Ip WY, Ng KH et al. (1996) A prospective study of 924 digital fractures of the hand. Injury 27(4):279–285

. Jupiter JB (1991) Fractures of the distal end of the radius. J Bone Joint Surg Am 73:461–469

. Leung KS, Lam TP (1993) Open reduction and internal fixation of the scapula neck and clavicle. J Bone Joint Surg 75(7):1015–1018

. McQueen (1998) Redisplaced unstable fractures of the distal radius. A randomised, prospective study of bridging versus non-bridging external fixation. J Bone Joint Surg Br 80:665–669

0. McQueen MM, Hajducka C, Court-Brown CM (1996) Redisplaced unstable fractures of the distal radius: a prospective randomised comparison of four methods of treatment. J Bone Joint Surg Br 78(3):404–409

1. Neers CS II (1970) Displaced proximal humeral fractures. I Classification and evaluation. J Bone Joint Surg 52:1077–1089

2. Ring D, Jupiter JB (2005) Compass hinge fixator for acute and chronic instability of the elbow. Oper Orthop Traumatol 17(2):143–157

3. Ring D, Jupiter JB et al. (2000) Acute fractures of the scaphoid. J Am Acad Orthop Surg 8:225–231

4. Ring D, Jupiter JB et al. (2003) Articular fractures of the distal part of the humerus. J Bone Joint Surg Am 85:232–238

5. Rommens P, Küchle R, Schneider R, Reuter M (2004) Olecranon fractures in adults: factors influencing outcome. Injury 35(11):1149–1157

6. Rozental TD, Beredjiklian PK et al. (2003) Longitudinal radioulnar dissociation. J Am Acad Orthop Surg 11:68–73

7. Stavlas P, Gliatis J, Polyzois V, Polyzois D (2004) Unilateral hinged external fixator of the elbow in complex elbow injuries. Injury 35(11):1158–1166

8. Tavakolian JD, Jupiter JB (2005) Dorsal plating for distal radius fractures. Hand Clin 21(3):341–346

10 Trauma to the Lower Extremities

Contents

10.1   Hip Dislocation

10.1.1   Introduction

- Mostly the result of high energy trauma
- And poly-trauma in young patients
- It usually requires a large amount of force to dislocate this congruent ball and socket joint (Fig. 10.1)

10.1.2   Relevant Hip Anatomy

- Stable joint – thick capsule
- 70% of femoral head used for load transfer
- Changed force/area relationship can be caused by associated depression/impaction fractures and these must be searched for carefully
- Blood supply to femoral head will be discussed in Sect. 10.3

10.1.3   Diagnosis

- Mostly clinical, e.g.:
    - Hip in abduction and external rotation (ER) in anterior dislocation
    - Hip in adduction and internal rotation (IR) in posterior dislocation

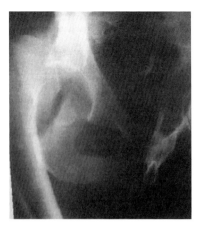

Fig. 10.1 Hip dislocation is associated with high energy trauma, and can be associated with a fracture as in this patient

■ Radiological assessment can aid in assessing position of femoral head, associated fracture on either side of the joint, and even the more subtle impaction injuries

10.1.4   Radiological Evaluation
■ Emergency radiographs
  − AP radiograph both hips – pre-/post-reduction
  − Beware undisplaced femoral neck fractures, and sometimes may see residual subtle subluxation, assess bilateral Shenton's lines and joint spaces
  − Judet views can be useful
■ Other emergency evaluation
  − CT scan mandatory: may show intra-articular fracture fragments, impaction fracture, etc.
  − MRI

10.1.5   Methods of CR Mostly Used
■ Allis method
■ Bigelow method
■ Stimson method

10.1.6   Post-reduction
■ Document neurovascular status
■ Document stability
■ Check post-reduction X-ray
■ CT can detect any intra-articular fracture, joint congruity, detect impaction fracture, etc.
■ Skin/skeletal traction

10.1.7   Common Types of Hip Dislocations
■ Posterior – overall most common
■ Anterior, e.g. after anterolateral approach of total hip replacement (THR)
■ Inferior – rare
■ Obturator – rare

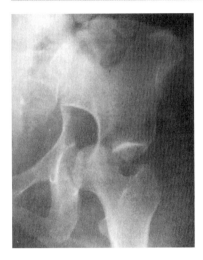

Fig. 10.2 Acetabular fractures are sometimes associated with central hip dislocation

■ Central – usually associated with some types of acetabular fracture (Fig. 10.2)

10.1.8 General Management Principles
■ Rn of associated injuries
■ Immediate reduction – closed ± open
■ Good imaging pre- and post-reduction
■ Ensure hip congruency

10.1.9 Anterior Hip Dislocation
■ 10–18% of all hip dislocations are anterior – superior or inferior
■ Abduction and external rotation injuries
■ Closed reduction is achieved by traction, followed by extension and internal rotation

10.1.9.1 Associated Injuries
■ Femoral head fracture in 22–77%
■ Transchondral fracture – excision/ORIF

- Indentation fracture more common, superior, no specific treatment, prognostic implications
- Osteonecrosis ~10%
- Risk factors: delay in reduction, repeated reduction attempts
- Post-traumatic OA generally occurs with around 4-mm impaction

10.1.10   Posterior Hip Dislocations
- 90% of all hip dislocations
- Flexed knee along the axis of the femur
- CT in all cases post-reduction
- Assessment of stability is essential
- 20–25% of the acetabular wall does not affect hip stability
- Quadratus femoris to prevent injury to the medial femoral circumflex artery
- Osteonecrosis rate 10–50%+ within 2–3 years of injury, but may develop up to 5 years after the injury
- Risk factors for OA necrosis
  - Severity of the injury
  - Delay in reduction – 6–12 h
  - Repeated attempts at closed reduction

10.1.11   Late Posterior Hip Dislocation
- More than 3 weeks peri-articular soft-tissue contracture
- Open reduction is required, but increases the risk of osteonecrosis
- Young patients, ORIF
- In elderly patients, primary prosthetic joint replacement is preferred

10.1.12   Bilateral Hip Dislocations
- High energy trauma
- 1–2% of all hip dislocations
- 50% are bilateral posterior dislocations
- 40% are anterior and posterior dislocations
- 10% are bilateral anterior dislocations

10.1.13   Summary of Common Injuries Associated with Hip Dislocation

- Femoral head fracture
- Acetabular fracture, especially of the posterior wall
- Femoral head impaction injury
- Femoral neck fracture
- Other possibilities: other types of proximal femoral fracture (like pertrochanteric fracture or subtrochanteric fracture), femoral shaft fracture

(P.S. The hip is usually a stable and congruent joint, and many hip dislocations occur in association with high energy trauma, which explains the not uncommon association of fractures)

10.2   Femoral Head Fractures

- Relatively rare
- One trauma centre in UK revealed four femoral head fractures in 10 years
- Because of its relative rarity, literature is rather scarce

10.2.1   Common Mechanism of Femoral Head Fractures

- Force is applied to the flexed knee with the hip adducted and flexed less than 50°
- Femoral head is driven into the postero-superior portion of the acetabular rim, shearing off a fragment

10.2.2   Posterior Dislocations with Femoral Head Fractures

- Associated fracture of femoral head occurs in 10% of all posterior dislocations (Fig. 10.3)
- Epstein type V injury has been further categorised by Pipkin

10.2.2.1   Pipkin Type I

Femoral head fracture below fovea

- 35% of cases

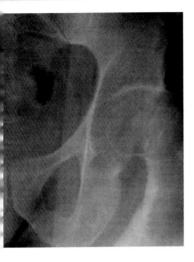

Fig. 10.3 Radiograph of a patient with femoral head fracture accompanying the hip dislocation

- Try closed reduction
  - 4 weeks' bed rest and usually traction
  - 4–6 weeks' protected weight-bearing
- Consider ORIF if CR fails, or joint incongruity, fracture displaced, or instability
  - Bury screw heads in head

10.2.2.2 Pipkin Type II
Femoral head fracture above fovea
- 40% of cases
- Try closed reduction
  - 4 weeks' bed rest and usually traction
  - 4–6 weeks' protected weight-bearing
- Consider ORIF in many cases since fragment is weight-bearing, especially in the presence of joint incongruity or instability
  - Bury screw heads in head

10.2.2.3 Pipkin Type III
Associated femoral head fracture and femoral neck fracture

- 10% of cases, if not sure whether the neck is fractured, perform a CT scan. In many of these cases, the neck fracture may not be displaced at presentation. But if the neck fracture is displaced on presentation, CR is seldom successful and OR is the rule. Note, however, that neck displacement may also be secondary to CR attempts
- Always ORIF, especially in young, fix both fractures
- Elderly: consider primary prosthetic replacement especially if there is hip OA

(Pearl: always look for a subtle fracture of the neck of the femur, especially in high energy hip dislocations)

10.2.2.4 Pipkin Type IV
Associated femoral head fracture and fractured acetabulum

- 15% of cases
- Try closed reduction
- Stability depends on concentricity of reduced joint
- Stress/dynamic views useful especially if >30–40% of posterior wall of acetabulum involved

Consider ORIF if sizable piece, joint unstable, persistent subluxation/dislocation

10.2.3 Reduction of Femoral Head Fractures
- General anaesthetic closed reduction
  - If unsuccessful or non-concentric – then ORIF
- Treatment depends on:
  - Pipkin's type
  - Size of the fracture, and joint stability and congruity

10.2.4 Femoral Head Fracture Complications
- Hip osteonecrosis
- Post-traumatic OA

0.2.5 Prognosis of Pipkin's Types

- Types I and II injuries have the same prognosis as simple dislocations if properly treated with prompt establishment of congruity and stability
- Type IV injuries have the same prognosis as posterior dislocations with acetabular fractures
- Type III injuries have a poor prognosis

0.2.6 Anterior or Posterior Approach

- Meta-analysis done by Swiontkowski seemed in favour of the anterior approach upon follow up at the 2-year mark
- Significant decrease in operative time, blood loss, improved visualisation and fixation with the anterior approach, but more heterotopic ossification (HO). Hip function the same. No AVN
- But searching the older literature there is also support for the posterior approach. Proponents argue that since vascularity is disrupted in these (frequently posterior) hip dislocations, why jeopardise further the femoral head blood supply by an anterior Smith Peterson

0.2.7 Why the Anterior Approach Seemed More Popular

- Supported by meta-analysis in the literature
- The femoral head fragment is often easier to fix by anterior approach using Herbert screws, and there is usually direct vision of the loose fragment
- Fixation by posterior approach more difficult because frequently need extreme IR of the leg to see the fragment, usually less easy to fix fragment than with anterior approach, danger of jeopardising the blood supply to the head

0.2.8 Ganz's Surgical Dislocation of the Hip

- The success of this approach has now been seen in centres other than Bern. It essentially involves a trochanteric flip osteotomy, Z-capsulotomy, and preservation of femoral head blood supply is the key advantage of this approach. Another key advantage is direct visualisation of the hip joint. In the setting of femoral head fracture,

Kregor reported that this approach allows a good visual of the join allows controlled reduction of the hip and can effect a thorough de bridement of the hip joint

10.2.9 Impaction Injury to the Femoral Head

- Described by Lethournel as a localised subsidence of the femora head usually at the superolateral quadrant
- Matta also reported on cartilaginous injury of the femoral head dur ing operation of acetabular fractures. He noted that such injuries ar predictive of a worse prognosis and clinical outcome even if assoc: ated fractures like that of the acetabulum are fixed anatomically

10.3   Femoral Neck Fractures

10.3.1   Relevant Anatomy: Blood Supply

- Medial circumflex posteriorly and lateral circumflex anteriorly to gether form an extracapsular arterial ring at the base of the femora neck
- Ascending cervical arteries arise from this ring, go up laterally/medi ally/anteriorly/posteriorly (lateral ascending cervical supplies mos of head and lateral part of neck)
- The above vessels form another ring – called subsynovial intra-ar ticular arterial ring at the junction between head and neck – vessel that penetrate the head from this second ring = epiphyseal arteries
- Swiontkowski describes the important lateral epiphyseal artery a the terminal branch of medial circumflex supplies the WB area c the head

10.3.2   Relevant Anatomy: The Trabeculae

- Trabeculae system first described by Ward (Ward triangle) – com pression trabeculae are concentrated at medial femoral neck then t superior femoral neck; tensile trabeculae travel from fovea mediall towards the lateral cortex
- Progressive loss of trabeculae with aging and osteoporosis (refer t the Singh Index)

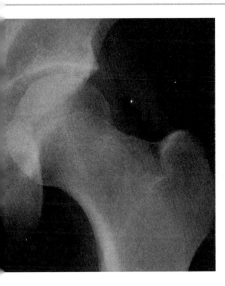

Fig. 10.4 Close-up radiograph showing clearly that trabeculae density is highest in the centre of the femoral head

New study suggested that the densest bone is at centre of head (Fig. 10.4), while surprisingly, posterior inferior is not particularly strong (Crowell 1992). These findings have implications for screw placement

0.3.3 Relevant Anatomy: On Healing of Femoral Neck Fractures

- The common transcervical femoral neck fracture is an intracapsular fracture
- The intracapsular part of the femoral neck has no periosteum and heals only by endosteal union

0.3.4 Garden's Classification

- Type 1 = incomplete fracture
- Type 2 = complete fracture, not displaced
- Type 3 = complete fracture with displacement, posterior retinaculum of Weitbrecht still intact: thus can be treated with CR and IR
- Type 4 = completely displaced fracture and complete loss of continuity

10.3.5　Literature on the Effect of Tamponade

- Beneficial effect of release of tamponade on femoral head vascularity has mainly been supported by animal experiments in the past. Release of tamponade important for both undisplaced and displaced fracture necks of the femur, especially the former where the capsule may not be torn
- Relevant literature mostly in the 1980s viz:
  - Crawfurd et al. (1988)
  - Holmberg and Dalen (1987)
  - Stromqvist et al. (1984)
  - Wingstrand et al. (1986)

10.3.6　General Treatment Principles

- Most do not dispute CRIF ± ORIF ± tamponade release for Garden's classes 1 and 2 (Fig. 10.5)
- Pros and cons of IF vs hemi-arthroplasty for Garden's classes 3 and 4 – still controversial

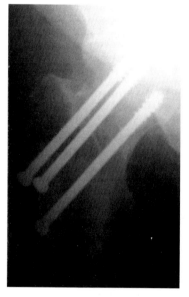

Fig. 10.5 AO screws must be inserted in parallel and care should be exercised to ensure cortical support is obtained

- Example of literature for IF: Injury 1977 – clinical results similar, prosthesis higher mortality
- Example of literature for the use of prosthesis: Br J Surg 1979 – prosthesis better hip score and less Cx

(P.S. proper work-up of these patients with multiple medical co-morbidities is needed, as well as of DVT prophylaxis issues)

10.3.7 Proponents of IF for Femoral Neck Fractures

- In general, risk of death and major Cx are less, and for the 70–75% whose fractures are healed with no AVN – their own femoral head functions as well if not better than prosthesis (J Bone Joint Surg 1994)
- Even in the face of AVN, a well-planned elective THR is a much safer procedure, in THR in an acute setting there is more dislocation and morbidity
- In active patients, a primary THR may not perform as well as an elective one (e.g. more ROM, more dislocation especially for patients with no OA hip to begin with)

10.3.8 Indications for Hemi- or Total Arthroplasty for Femoral Neck Fractures

- Fracture factors: too comminuted, too vertical, failed CR, fractured femoral head, delayed presentation and neck fracture in abnormal hip (RA/OA), and most of Garden's class 4
- Bone: pathologic bone and extreme osteoporosis
- Implant factors: redo of failed screw fixation
- Patient: very elderly, neurologic disease (hemiplegic, parkinsonism), poor general health – likely to tolerate only one operation
- Literature in support of prosthesis over IF, e.g. Lu-Yao et al. (1994), Bray et al. (1988), Sikorski and Barrington (1981)

10.3.9 Unipolar Versus Bipolar

- Literature justification exists for performing unipolar and bipolar hemi-arthroplasty
- Example: JBJS 1996 reported no difference at 2 years; literature in support of bipolars, e.g. Yamagata (1987)

- Bipolar (Fig. 10.6) has theoretical clinical advantage of less acetabular erosion, and more often used for relatively younger patients in case revision to THR is easier in the future. Bipolars are not without disadvantages: high cost, less dislocation, but difficult to reduce if dislocation does occur. Over time, its behaviour may change to resemble monopolars. Low demand in the elderly, who are not quite ambulatory, and tend more to use unipolars

10.3.10 Cement Versus No Cement for Hemi-arthroplasty

- Cement advantages: immediate and secure fixation; better results in some series (Gingras et al. 1980); less thigh pain and loosening in several series
- Disadvantages: sudden death – mechanism: sudden death/cardiac arrest during time of prosthesis insertion from bone cement implantation syndrome – hypotension, hypoxia, arrhythmia, arrest – venous embolisation (of cement) from intramedullary pressurisation suspected (more in cemented total hip arthroplasty [THA])

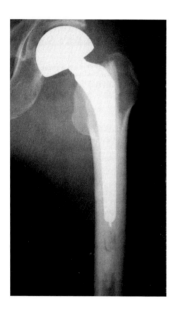

Fig. 10.6 A bipolar prosthesis was used to treat this patient with a fractured femoral neck

■ Summary: cemented ones probably give better results, but use with caution, especially in the elderly with limited cardio-pulmonary reserve (Fig. 10.7)

10.3.11   Newer Literature and Newer Trends
10.3.11.1   Internal Fixation Results:
Displaced Versus Undisplaced Fractures

■ In a recent prospective clinical trial including only those patients who had no cognitive impairment and who were capable of independent living, it was found that:

— There were significantly more complications in patients (treated with internal fixation) presenting with *displaced* fractures on presentation

— Quality of life outcome was significantly worse in those with displaced fractures, even given fracture healing (Tidermark et al. 2002)

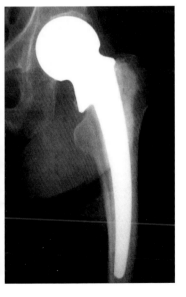

Fig. 10.7 A cemented Thompson prosthesis is another option of cemented hemi-arthroplasty

10.3.11.2 Internal Fixation Versus Hemi-arthroplasty

- A recent prospective randomised multi-centre trial of Garden's class 3 or 4 fractures (excluding those bedridden patients and those with impaired cognition) it was found that:
  - There was a high rate of failure and poor functional outcome after IF (46%) vs arthroplasty (most patients actually had hemi-arthroplasty) in 6% patients
  - The authors recommended arthroplasty for displaced fractures of the neck of the femur in patients over 70 years of age (Rogmark et al. 2002)

10.3.11.3 Internal Fixation Versus THR

- THR was found to be superior to IF with respect to hip function, less need for secondary procedure, and quality of life in the subgroup of hip fracture patients who are healthy and active pre-morbidity (Tidermark et al. 2003), yet the mortality rate was found to be comparable in other studies

10.3.11.4 Disadvantages of THR

- Increased chance of dislocation in acute hip fractures
- Not usually indicated in patients with cognitive problems since cannot follow rehabilitation and high chance of dislocation
- Cementation can pose risk to elderly patients with limited cardiopulmonary reserve, sometimes even sudden death (cement implantation syndrome)

10.3.11.5 Findings from the STARS Study from Edinburgh

- Keating et al. presented the important findings in OTA 2002 concerning this multicentre study in Scotland comparing internal fixation vs bipolar vs THR in displaced neck fractures > age 60. The important findings are as follows:
  - High rate of failure of internal fixation (non-union or AVN) of 37%
  - High re-operation rate for internal fixation group, eight times more
  - Functional outcome highest in THR group

0.3.11.6 Indications for THA in Acute Femoral Neck Fractures (Author's View)

- Abnormal hip to begin with (e.g. RA and OA)
- In some cases of revision of failed IF or hemi-arthroplasty (e.g. with acetabular cartilage erosion)
- Also considered for very active, physiologically young elderly, but they should be cautioned pre-operatively about the higher Cx rate (e.g. rate of dislocation: up to 18% reported in one study)
- For the more sedentary folks, a cemented hemi-arthroplasty will suffice, while uncemented unipolars may be adequate in low-demand elderly with limited mobility, especially if they have poor cardiopulmonary reserve – will benefit from a quick surgery and shy away from cement

0.3.12 Current Trend

- The author concurs with the viewpoint expressed in recent Swedish studies on fractured hip suggesting that future hip fracture research should focus on the best treatment for discrete *subgroups* of patients suffering from fractured hip rather than making too many generalisations (J Bone Joint Surg Br 2005)

0.3.13 Summary of Treatment Recommendation

- If patient active and good projected survivorship = cemented bipolar vs cemented unipolar vs THR
- If not active, low demand, poor projected survivorship and high surgical risk = uncemented unipolar vs IF (if reducible and patient prefers IF)
- Pre-existing abnormal hip = hybrid THR vs cemented THR ± cementless if younger

0.3.14 Complications
0.3.14.1 AVN: Timing and Treatment

- With internal fixation of femoral neck fractures, AVN rate around 22% at 8 years, most present by 2 years; 70% implant survival after 7 years, thus can buy some time (Contemp Orthop)
- Titanium screws advisable since MRI compatible

- Segmental collapse may be treated by well-planned elective THR at a medically safer time

10.3.14.2   Non-union

- Young patients: the principle is to try to salvage the femoral head
  - Improving the local biomechanics, e.g. valgus proximal femoral osteotomy – converts shear forces to that of compression, which promotes fracture healing. Literature reports reasonably good results (Anglen 1997)
  - Improving the biology, e.g. vascularised or non-vascularised grafting, useful for neglected fractures, well-aligned non-union with AVN
- Elderly patients: most receive revision hemi- or total hip arthroplasty. THR in such situations tends to have high dislocation rate (Robinson 2002). It may be useful in such scenarios to avoid posterior approach and consider the use of larger diameter femoral heads

10.3.14.3   Malunion

- Problems that may need to be tackled:
  - Femoro-acetabular impingement
  - Altered hip mechanics
- May need arthroplasty or osteotomy

10.3.14.4   Other Complications

- Periprosthetic fractures (Fig. 10.8)
- Infections – that may necessitate two-stage revision arthroplasty or even Girdlestone (Fig. 10.9)

10.3.14.5   First-Year Mortality

- In a series reported in JBJS 1994, IF resulted in 96% fracture union with low morbidity and mortality, although the same study found increased mortality in male patients
- The reported 1-year mortality of fractured hip varies between 15 and 30%, depending on different series

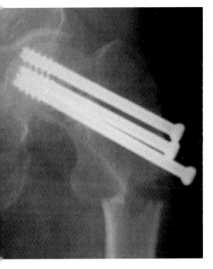

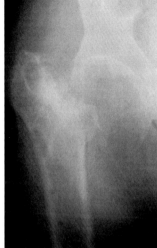

ig. 10.8 AO screws should not be inserted too crowded together or at too low a point of entry to prevent stress concentration and fracture, as is shown ere

Fig. 10.9 The girdlestone is one of the salvage options in infected hip arthroplasty

0.3.15   Appendix 1: Method of Screw Placement

■ Unlike DHS with side-plate, cannulated screw heads buttress against the cortex and threads lock in the head

■ Most important objective in treatment of displaced intracapsular fractures = obtain stable bony support of femoral head on the femoral neck

■ Hodge had shown: even NWB, getting up from sitting posture creates ×3 body weight of forces across the hip

■ Hence:
  — Need to compress the fracture and maintain reduction by neutralising the large forces on the hip

- Neck comminution contraindicates IF
- NWB cannot compensate for poor fixation

10.3.15.1   What Constitutes a Good Reduction?

- A good reduction has the medial femoral head and neck fragment well supported by the medial neck of the femur
- Some use the guidelines by Baumgärtner and Solberg (1997)
- Others use the criteria of Garden's Index (of 160/180 on AP/lateral an expression of the angle of compression trabeculae on AP X-ray angle of the compression trabeculae on lateral X-ray)
- Slight valgus acceptable

10.3.15.2   Goal of Fracture Fixation

- Aim of fixation: prevent posterior and varus migration of the femoral head; adequacy of reduction can be assessed by the method of Lowell (1980)
- The AO screws need to be parallel to maintain bone-on-bone support as the fracture settles over time

10.3.15.3   How to Position the Three Screws

- The first screw: its shaft should rest on the medial femoral neck, with threads fixing the inferior head; this guards against neck varus
- The second screw: placed posteriorly so that it rests on the posterior neck of the distal fragment and at the middle of the head in AP plane
- The third screw: aim at middle of the head level in AP plane, and anterior position on lateral X-ray. In summary, the essence is to obtain cortical support. Lack of cortical support mostly results in varus collapse (Fig. 10.10)

10.3.15.4   Causes of Fixation Failure

- Poor bone quality – general strategies to tackle osteoporotic fractures were discussed in Chap. 5
- Special fracture patterns, e.g. very vertical fractures of the neck of femur (Pauwels type 3) treated by standard AO screws may fail due to the high shear forces

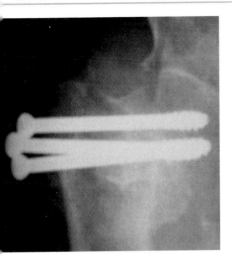

Fig. 10.10 Improperly inserted AO screws for neck fracture will ultimately result in varus collapse, as is shown here

- Poor implant positioning – refer to the discussion on proper positioning of AO screws in neck of femur fracture
- Occult sepsis – remember to culture the non-union during revision surgery

10.3.16 Appendix 2: Prevention of Hip Fracture
- Prevention of falls: discussed in Chap. 15
- Osteoporosis prevention and treatment: discussed in the companion volume of this book

10.4 Concomitant Femoral Neck Fractures and Fractured Femoral Shaft

10.4.1 Alho Classification of Subtypes of Bifocal Injuries
- Subcapital fracture 2%
- Trans-cervical fracture 21%
- Basal neck fracture 39%
- Pertrochanteric fracture 14%

- Inter-trochanteric fracture 24%

(The associated femoral shaft fractures mostly occur near the isthmus area)

10.4.2 Treatment Options

- AO "miss-a-nail" technique (special aiming jig to enable 7-mm cannulated screw placement anterior and posterior to the path of the nail)
- Cephalomedullary nail (Fig. 10.11) with options for proximal locking at the femoral neck
- Fix neck of femur (NOF) fracture with AO screw and ORIF of femoral shaft fracture with plate
- Fix NOF fracture with AO screw and retrograde nailing for femoral shaft fracture

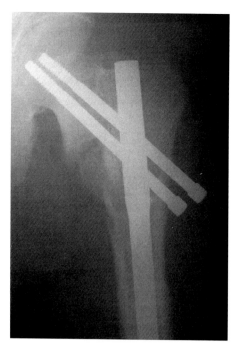

Fig. 10.11 Cephalomedullary nails are one option to treat concomitant neck and shaft fractures of the femur

10.5   Inter-trochanteric Hip Fractures (Fig. 10.12)

10.5.1   Introduction

- Similar in incidence to femoral neck fracture in previous studies in the literature
- But its incidence is expected to climb in those countries where there is an aging population such as in many countries in Asia
- This is because as a person ages, there is progressive loss of the tensile and compressive trabeculae, especially the former. In the senile age group of, say, 90 or over, most of the hip fractures are expected to be of this type. Another predisposing factor is hip OA. There is some suggestion that younger patients with OA changes of their hip tend to suffer inter-trochanteric fractures instead of femoral neck fractures

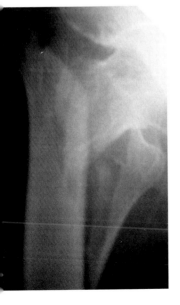

Fig. 10.12 This radiograph illustrates an unstable inter-trochanteric pattern. A lateral device like DHS, if used for this fracture, will be subject to high shear forces

10.5.2 Projected Exponential Rise in Hip Fracture Incidence with Aging

- Studies in the past had documented an exponential increase in hip fracture chance with aging
- Hip fracture is an expensive fracture as it drains lots of manpower and requires a team approach for proper rehabilitation. It also carries with it significant mortality (15–30% at 1 year) and morbidity (hence increasing the length of hospital stay)
- The scope of the problem is going to increase in the coming decades and we expect to see more inter-trochanteric fractures as opposed to femoral neck fractures in countries with a rapidly aging population

10.5.3 Kyle's Classification

- Type 1: stable undisplaced fracture with no comminution
- Type 2: stable with minimal comminution
- Type 3: unstable with large posteromedial comminuted area
- Type 4: with subtrochanteric extension, unstable

10.5.4 Key to Management: Prevention

- Primary prevention measures:
  - Education of the general public
  - Prevention of osteoporosis
  - Suitable exercise, especially Tai Chi exercises
- Secondary prevention measures:
  - Fall prevention programme (discussed in Chap. 15)
  - Treatment of established osteoporosis
  - Home modification
  - Psychosocial support
  - Hip protectors

10.5.5 Treatment Options

- Conservative, e.g. occasionally in incomplete fractures
- Operative:
  - CR + IF: fixation with dynamic hip screw ± trochanteric stabilisation plate (Figs. 10.13, 10.14) or intramedullary device; or valgus osteotomy: not popular nowadays

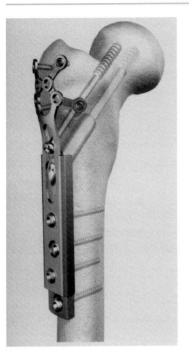

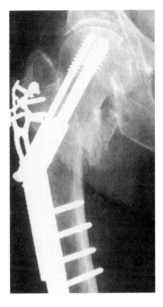

Fig. 10.13 Illustration of the use of a trochanteric stabilisation plate to avoid excessive telescoping in some fractures treated with a DHS

Fig. 10.14 Postoperative radiograph showing the trochanteric stabilisation plate in action

- ORIF if CR fails: may need the use of large bone clamps, bone hooks, cerclage, etc.
- Role of hemi- or total arthroplasty: rarely needed. But may be required in revision, e.g. for failed implants, screw cut-outs

10.5.6 Comparison of DHS Versus Gamma Nail

- A recent prospective randomised comparison reported in JOT 2005 found that:
  - Both implants are equally good in stable fractures (but note that the DHS is significantly less expensive)

- Gamma nail is recommended for unstable fracture patterns
- In particular, Gamma nail or other IM devices are particularly useful in management of reversed obliquity fractures (Int Orthop 2005). This is supported by other studies showing that for this fracture, the revision rate is 11% for DHS vs 0% for PFN (Injury 2005)

10.5.7   Theoretical Advantage of Cephalomedullary Nails over DHS

- Shorter lever arm between the centre of hip rotation and the implant (J Bone Joint Surg 1992)
- Percutaneous fixation, thus less trauma
- Earlier weight-bearing for unstable fracture patterns
- Smaller degree of telescoping than DHS – sometimes screw sliding is excessive with DHS device for some fracture patterns causing altered hip mechanics and limb shortening

10.5.8   Complications of Gamma Nailing

- Recent reports review the following Cx (Arch Orthop Trauma Surg 2004):
  - Trochanteric pain requiring nail removal, some of these patients fracture their femoral neck postoperatively
  - Screw cut-out
  - A few need conversion to THR, which will prove to be technically demanding since there will be a large void at the greater trochanter (GT)
  - Sepsis
  - Fracture around the distal locking bolts (requiring refixation) or between two distal bolts (reported in many other studies)

10.5.9   Comparison of Gamma Nail (Fig.10.15) and PFN (Fig. 10.16)

- In a recent study comparing Gamma nail and PFN reported in Arch Orthop Trauma Surg (2005) the authors found comparable results when either was used in the treatment of unstable inter-trochanteric fractures

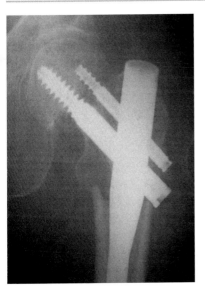

Fig. 10.15 Radiograph showing the Gamma nail used to treat inter-trochanteric fractures of the hip

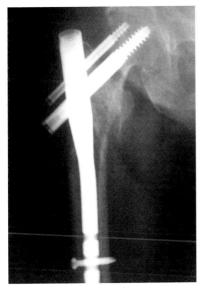

Fig. 10.16 Illustration showing the AO PFN used in nailing inter-trochanteric hip fractures

10.5.10   Newer Implants: Trochanteric Fixation Nail (AO TFN) (Fig. 10.17)

- After the standard PFN, a new version called trochanteric fixation nail equipped with a spiral blade is now on the market and put to clinical use
- Although the Cochrane database of systemic review published in 2005 (Parker and Handoll) showed that there is insufficient evidence to demonstrate important differences in outcome between different nail designs in the treatment of unstable trochanteric fractures, newer designs like TFN are probably a move in the right direction

10.5.11   Summary of Pros and Cons of DHS

- Cons: not suitable for reverse oblique fractures and some other unstable fracture patterns, slightly more blood loss, no early weight-bearing if lack of medial support like posteromedial comminution
- Pros: technique familiar, low cost, easier to revise than a nail, even reverse oblique patterns sometimes may prevent excessive collapse by trochanteric stabilisation plate

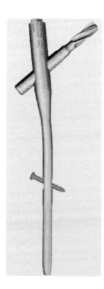

Fig. 10.17 The all new AO TFN, with a spiral blade replacing the PFN screw

10.5.12   Summary of Pros and Cons of IM Nails

▪ Pros: load sharing device, does not disturb the fracture site, more mechanically sound
▪ Cons: high cost, revision more difficult

10.5.13   Postoperative Complications

▪ Screw cut-out: common and will be discussed
▪ Hardware failure
▪ Wound Cx
▪ Malunion: may alter hip biomechanics
▪ Non-union: rare, since large cancellous surface, unless poor bone contact, gap, etc.
▪ Others: excessive telescoping or fracture collapse (Fig. 10.18), peri-prosthetic fractures (Fig. 10.19), deep venous thrombosis (DVT), etc.

10.5.13.1   The Problem of Screw Cut-out (Fig. 10.20)

▪ This is an unsolved problem common to both DHS and cephalomed-ullary nails (Clin Orthop Relat Res 2002)
▪ Screw cut-out is due to stress concentration between the screw threads and the osteoporotic cancellous bone of the femoral head (Clin Orthop Relat Res 1997), or due to jamming of the sliding mechanism of DHS
▪ Possible solution: for some fracture patterns (Fig. 10.21) use of newer devices like the AO trochanteric fixation nail may be useful. For other methods of tackling problems of fixation, refer to Chap. 4

10.5.13.2   Revision Surgery for Screw Cut-out

▪ Since a large column of bone is gone from the head and neck area, re-fixation is usually unreliable in these osteoporotic bones and fre-quently needs:
  − Hemi-arthroplasty, e.g. cemented bipolar (Fig. 10.22)
  − THR (e.g. in the presence of acetabular erosion by the cut-out screw or a pre-existing OA of hip)

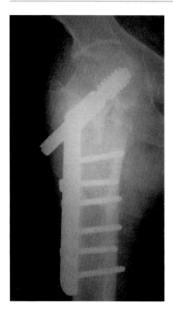

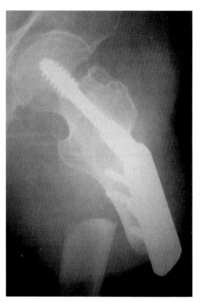

Fig. 10.18 Radiograph illustrating excessive telescoping from marked collapse after DHS performed in a patient with unstable trochanteric fracture. Excessive sliding will affect hip mechanics, and may cause limb shortening

Fig. 10.19 Patient with repeated falls can fracture through an area of stress concentration such as near the end of the DHS implant as illustrated here

— In younger patients with good bone, revision with a fixed angle device aiming at the inferior part of the femoral head (shy away from the cut out screw track) is a common solution

10.5.13.3 Prevention of Screw Cut-out:
Guides to Proper Screw Position

■ TAD (tip-apex distance) proposed by Baumgärtner and Solberg (1997): the distance from the screw tip to the apex of the femoral head on AP view is added to a similar measurement taken from a lateral view. To minimise the cut-out risk, a distance of > 25 mm is not accepted

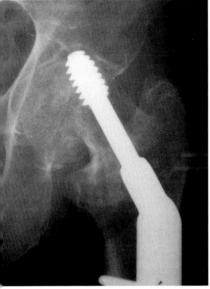

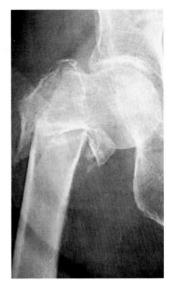

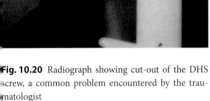

Fig. 10.20 Radiograph showing cut-out of the DHS screw, a common problem encountered by the traumatologist

Fig. 10.21 A typical fracture pattern that allows the use of an adjunctive trochanteric stabilisation plate should a DHS be decided upon

- Garden's Alignment Index

(Besides the above, other important factors include bone quality, and quality of fracture reduction)

10.6 Subtrochanteric Fractures

10.6.1 Introduction

- Definition: the subtrochanteric region spans from the lesser trochanter of the femur to a point 5 cm from the lesser trochanter; i.e. to the junction between the proximal and distal thirds of the diaphysis

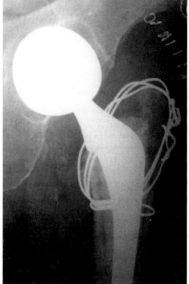

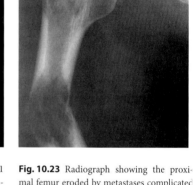

Fig. 10.22 The same patient as in Fig. 10.21 with revision to a cemented bipolar hemi-arthroplasty

Fig. 10.23 Radiograph showing the proximal femur eroded by metastases complicated by subtrochanteric fracture

- It is a region under high tensile and compressive stresses; many pathological fractures occur in this area (Fig. 10.23)
- The lateral cortex is loaded in tension, while the medial cortex is loaded in compression
- In subtrochanteric fractures, the proximal fragment is usually flexed by psoas, externally rotated by short rotator, and abducted by unopposed hip abductors
- For this reason, rigid, especially intramedullary implants should preferably be used for fracture fixation
- The Russell Taylor classification is recommended as it acts as the surgeon's guide to the proper fixation method to be used

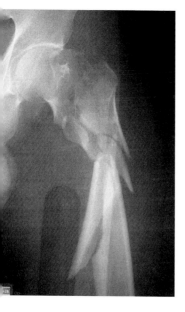

Fig. 10.24 Radiograph showing a comminuted subtrochanteric fracture

0.6.2 General Factors Essential for Stability (After Schatzker)

- Degree of comminution
- Level of fracture
- Fracture pattern

0.6.2.1 Effect of Fracture Comminution (Fig. 10.24)

- Unstable if:
  - Shattering of the medial cortex
  - Presence of segmental comminution

0.6.2.2 Effect of Fracture Location

- The closer the fracture to the LT, the shorter the lever arm and the lower the bending moment
- If GT involved, sometimes difficult to keep the IM nail within the proximal fragment: in these cases it may be better to use a fixed angle device

- If LT involved, necessitates proximal locking at the femoral nec and head. Such as using AO unreamed femoral nail and spiral blad locking

10.6.3 Russell Taylor Classification
- Type I: piriformis fossa not involved
  - Type IA: lesser trochanter not involved
  - Type IB: lesser trochanter involved
- Type II: fracture involved the piriformis fossa
  - Type IIA: lesser trochanter not involved
  - Type IIB: lesser trochanter involved

10.6.3.1 How Does the Russell Taylor Classification Guide Our Management?
- Fractures below the lesser trochanter can be treated by standar locking femoral nail (since this fracture site falls inside the zone c indication)
- Fractures at or above the lesser trochanter, can be treated by cephalo medullary or second-generation IM nails, especially if the piriformi fossa is intact
- Fractures involving the piriformis fossa and greater trochanter ar best treated with an alternative device such as fixed angle blad plates or DCS

10.6.4 Main Treatment Options
- Cephalomedullary IM nailing, e.g. Russell Taylor
- DCS (dynamic condylar screw) (Fig. 10.25)
- Fixed angle device, e.g. angle blade plates (Fig. 10.26), or the newe proximal femoral locking plates

10.6.4.1 Choice of Implant
- The way that the Russell Taylor classification aids in our choice c implant has been alluded to (Sect. 10.6.3)
- If a lateral device instead of an IM nail is used, an initial perio of protected or non-weight-bearing is advisable. It all depends o

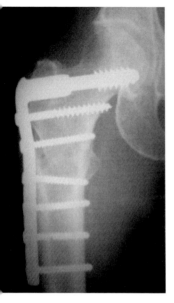 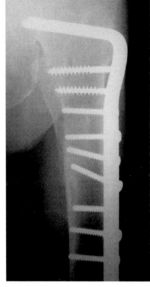

g. 10.25 This subtrochanteric fracture as treated by a DCS (dynamic condylar rew)

Fig. 10.26 Radiograph illustrating the time-honoured angle blade plate used in fixing a subtrochanteric fracture

the stability after fixation, which is best assessed by the operating surgeon

- Angle blade plates are less forgiving an implant than the DCS, but useful in salvaging failed fixations. If a lateral device is used, the tendency nowadays is to use locked plating and biological fixation. An important point is that before using the proximal femoral locked plates, the fracture needs to be reduced first, do not rely on locked plates to do the fracture reduction for the surgeon

0.7   Femoral Shaft Fractures

0.7.1   Introduction

- Most are from high energy trauma

- Although there is an increasing incidence of shaft fracture in low energy injuries in the elderly
- Do not underestimate the amount of blood loss that can occur, adequate fluid resuscitation is essential
- The use of traction by the Thomas splint markedly reduced mortality and blood loss in World War I
- Use of IM nailing came into the arena in the 1970s and has now become the gold standard

10.7.2   Classification

- The reader is assumed to know the common classification system in use:
  - AO classification: good for research and documentation
  - Winquist classification on the degree of comminution
  - Descriptive, e.g. describing the location of the fracture like proximal, middle or distal thirds, etc.

10.7.3   Associated Injuries

- Since most are the result of high energy trauma, associated injuries are common
- These can be divided into:
  - Other bony injuries, e.g. bilateral femoral shaft fractures, floating knee injuries, concomitant neck of femur fractures
  - Associated neurovascular injuries have been documented
  - Injuries to other organs, e.g. severe head injury, severe chest trauma

10.7.4   Work-up

- Diagnosis straightforward, usually with clinical deformity and swelling
- The extent of injury and identification of associated injuries need X-ray and other investigations
- Despite the above, sometimes missed Dx in the acute setting, like in acutely poly-traumatised patient

0.7.5   Treatment Goal

- Restoration of alignment of the lower limb, restoration of proper rotation, and prevention of shortening
- Early weight-bearing
- Early pain relief by fixation with adequate rigidity
- Early return to normal function

0.7.6   Surgical Options

- Traction
- IM nail (Fig. 10.27)
- EF
- Plating

0.7.6.1   Traction

- Sir Robert Jones by using the Thomas splint decreased the mortality rate from 80% to 20% in World War I for compound fractures of the femur

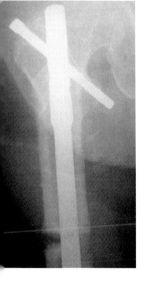

Fig. 10.27 Picture showing the Russell Taylor nail being used to treat a femoral shaft fracture. This nailing system is more commonly used to treat more complex fracture patterns

- It demonstrated that adequate splinting at the earliest possible moment could prevent shock and lower mortality

10.7.6.1.1 Thomas Splint Mechanism

- The Thomas splint helped control the *volume* and thus the haematoma, or amount of blood loss, besides aligning the fracture. A modern version is still very useful nowadays in field treatment of femoral shaft fracture patients, and for transport
- Remember volume $= 4/3 \ \pi r^3$

10.7.6.2 IM Nailing

- Has become the gold standard nowadays for the treatment of femoral shaft fractures
- The newer generations of IM nailing have extended the zone of indication to more proximal fractures. Although the development of distal femoral nails (DFN) via retrograde nailing by different companies

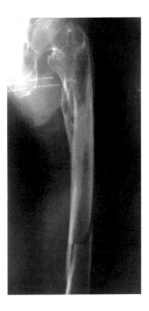

Fig. 10.28 Heed should be taken before embarking on nailing a shaft fracture in the presence of proximal bony deformity or bowing

ies has helped solve the problem in distal fractures, not all femurs can be nailed, e.g. if blocked by a proximal THR implant, deformed proximal femurs (Fig. 10.28), or in situations where part of the medullary canal is not patent

0.7.6.2.1 Advantages of IM Nailing over Other Options Like Plating

- Load-sharing device
- Early weight-bearing (for reamed nailing)
- Offers better mechanical advantage than a lateral device such as plating
- Leave the fracture site undisturbed, hence preservation of soft tissue and local blood supply. Also, less chance of sepsis. The newer nails with a trochanteric starting point have the added advantage of lessening the chance of injury to the vascularity of the femoral head. The initial worry of abductor tendon weakness using the trochanteric start point might be rather excessive thanks to recent gait analysis studies by the Cincinnati group among others

0.7.6.2.2 Reaming Versus No Reaming

- See discussion in the section on IM nailing in Chap. 4

0.7.6.2.3 Complications of IM Nailing

- The general complications of IM nailing will be discussed in the section on tibial nailing (Sect. 10.15.12.2.3)
- But there are several points to note:
  - The danger of reamed nailing in the face of significant pulmonary injury is mainly documented for femoral nailing and less so for tibial nailing
  - Beware of rotational deformities, the prevention of which is by matching the cortical thickness of the proximal and distal segments on X-ray
  - Management of bilateral femoral shaft fractures in a poly-trauma patient may necessitate damage control orthopaedics – see section on damage control in Chap. 2

10.7.6.2.4 Newer Innovations

- The development of newer reamers will further decrease the rate of rise in medullary canal pressure during reaming and hopefully lessen the chance of embolisation
- Many newer IM nails on the market (e.g. AO AFN) have the entry point shifted to the greater trochanter, thus less chance of causing injury to the blood supply of the femoral head
- The advent of virtual fluoroscopy opens the door to better precision and less radiation exposure for the traumatologist. See Chap. 7

10.7.6.3 EF

- Sometimes used in paediatric age group
- In adults, may be considered temporary while awaiting stabilisation if associated with severe pulmonary injury
- In these scenarios, meticulous pin track care is needed to guard against infection since there is a high chance of elective IM nailing later

10.7.6.4 Plating

- Seldom done for adults since it involves opening the fracture site soft tissue damage. However, certain fracture patterns may render a selected case suitable for plating
- Also, we now realise that the perfect anatomical reduction and rigid fixation of the traditional AO approach are not absolutely needed in meta-diaphyseal injuries. If plating is contemplated, most use biologic fixation with locking plates

10.7.7 More Complicated Clinical Scenarios

10.7.7.1 Bilateral Femoral Shaft Fractures

- Require active fluid resuscitation, ×2 more mortality than unilateral shaft fractures, commonly seen in high energy poly-trauma patients
- This is because owing to the much more bulky soft tissue envelopes, bilateral femoral shaft fractures are probably more likely to release more systemic inflammatory mediators than, say, bilateral tibial shaft fractures, which pose extra dangers to poly-trauma patients

- May need to initiate damage control orthopaedics
- If patient in extremis, or borderline; especially with pulmonary injury, can consider EF to tide over and perform elective nailing later. If acute nailing is somehow decided upon, there might be a place for unreamed nailing in the poly-trauma patient. Plating is rarely if ever done. Prolonged traction is not recommended to minimise pulmonary complications, DVT, etc.

10.7.7.2 Combined Fractured Femoral Neck and Shaft

- Just discussed
- Refer to the Alho classification

10.7.7.3 Femoral Shaft Fracture Associated with Severe Pulmonary Injury

- Discussed in the section on high energy trauma in Chap. 2

10.7.7.4 Femoral Shaft Fractures Associated with Severe Head Injury

- Discussed in the section on high energy trauma in Chap. 2

10.8 Fractured Distal Femur

10.8.1 Introduction

- Fractures in this region of the femur are not uncommon, they can be associated with marked osteoporosis (Fig. 10.29), and an occasional fracture with a sharp bony spike can even cause vascular damage (Fig. 10.30) to the nearby popliteal vessels. Many of these osteoporotic patients have knee stiffness from OA, therefore the impact of any external bending moment is borne by the weakened cancellous bone of the supracondylar area. Similarly, fractures can occur if in the presence of stress concentration (Fig. 10.31). Another predisposing factor is anterior notching after TKR, which was discussed in the sections on periprosthetic fractures in Chap. 5. With the findings of dissection studies, the fixation of fractures in this region has gone

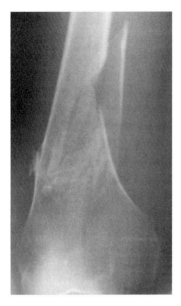

Fig. 10.29 An osteoporotic distal femoral fracture with some degree of comminution

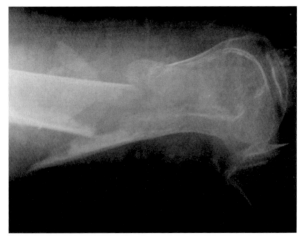

Fig. 10.30 An occasional patient suffers vascular insult from a sharp bony spike impinging on the neurovascular bundle

from wide exposures with traditional implants (Fig. 10.32) to MIPO technique using newly developed implants such as the LISS plate. Isolated femoral condylar fractures (Fig. 10.33) are rare and will not be discussed in detail in this section.

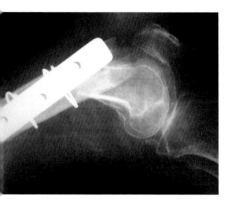

Fig. 10.31 Again, the fracture can be seen just distal to an implant where there is abrupt change in stress or stress concentration

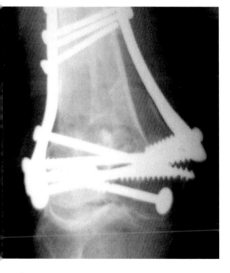

Fig. 10.32 Traditional ORIF involves lots of soft tissue stripping and metals may not be conducive to the local biology

10.8.2 Common Implant Options in this Region

- DCS
- 95° angle blade plate
- Retrograde femoral nail
- Condylar buttress plate
- The newer AO LISS plate or the new Zimmer peri-articular distal femoral locking plate are particularly useful

(There is a general tendency to use angular stable implants like the LISS. The loss of stability in implants that are not angularly stable is due to screw loosening and the windshield-wiper effect between the plate and the screws)

10.8.2.1 DCS

- Good distal angular stability, since fixed angle device and anatomic design and strong, more user friendly than blade plates – use guide-wire and adjustable in sagittal plane
- Significant surgical exposure
- But sacrifice significant amount of distal femoral bone stock
- Less indicated for fractures with multi-fragmentary complex articular involvement
- Usually need significant surgical exposure

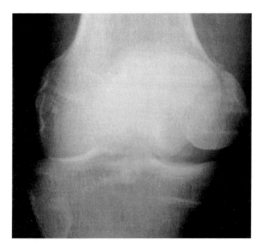

Fig. 10.33 Isolated fracture of a condyle of the distal femur as shown is of rarer occurrence than the usual supracondylar fracture of the distal femur

0.8.2.2 Angle Blade Plate (Fig. 10.34)

- Can be good in revision situation, but cuts out usual in osteoporotic bones
- Fixed angle device with anatomical design, bone sparing
- Can be used as a reduction tool in the setting of indirect reduction
- Needs significant surgical exposure and dissection. Other disadvantages include difficulty in the setting with coronal split (Hoffa), and in the face of multi-fragmentary intra-articular fractures

0.8.2.3 Distal Femoral Nail (Fig. 10.35)

- Made of Ti-Al-Niobium alloy
- Specially developed for fracture of distal femur; mainly used for extra-articular fracture and minimally displaced intra-articular fracture in younger patients
- Can have the choice of choosing either the spiral blade or interlocking bolt for fracture fixation
- The locking mechanism is made angularly stable after the end cap is inserted
- Compared with the condylar plate, DFN showed ×10 higher stiffness under axial load, and ×5 lower stiffness under torsional load

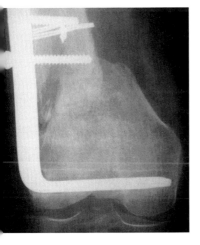

Fig. 10.34 An element of fracture malreduction is not uncommon. The fracture may still heal since this region is full of cancellous bone and rather vascular. Long-standing effects, if any, are dependent on subsequent assessment of joint obliquity, mechanical axis and any subsequent arthrosis

- Has the theoretical risk of injuring the PCL, a longer nail is prefer
  able for there is always a risk of stress concentration and fracture i
  osteoporotic bones (Fig. 10.36)

10.8.2.4 Condylar Buttress Plate (Fig. 10.37)

- Can be used in cases of complex articular involvement and Hoff
  type fractures
- Also in cases with short distal femoral segments
- Mainly acting as a buttress device
- Inherent problems concerning distal screw purchase, screw toggling
  and varus collapse is not uncommon. It is not a fixed angle device

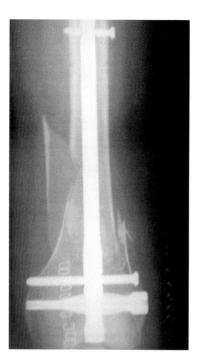

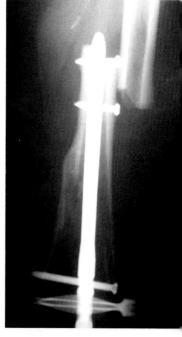

Fig. 10.35 The distal femoral nail is one viable option to treat osteoporotic fractures in
this region

Fig. 10.36 Again, fracture just distal to th
nail is not uncommon in the face of a secon
injury

0.8.2.5 The LISS Plate (Figs. 10.38, 10.39)

- Designed to be used with MIPO technique
- Experiments (with dye injection studies) demonstrated there is a potential cavity underneath the vastus lateralis muscle that allows the passage of the plate and MIPO technique, while preserving the perforating vessels of the femur
- The details of the LISS were discussed in the section on plating in Chap. 4.

0.8.2.5.1 Comparison of LISS with DFN

- LISS has its advantages in severe intra-articular fractures because of free placement of lag screws, and lower risk of additional disruption of the already reconstructed condylar complex

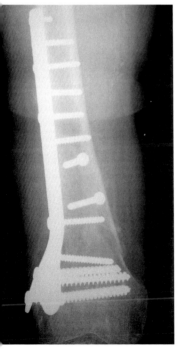

Fig. 10.37 The condylar buttress plate mainly serves a buttressing function

- LISS is possibly better in patients with marked osteoporosis since i provides a larger contact surface area between the implant and the cancellous bone than DFN (even with spiral blade insertion). Essentially, the multiple fixed angle screws are like multiple fixed angle devices. Unlike DFN, distal screw loosening and migration is not a common finding in clinical studies of LISS
- Load distribution on a larger surface decreases the average load on cancellous bone and will lessen the risk of loosening

10.8.2.5.2 Approaches Used in MIPO Cases
- Standard antero-lateral approach
- Lateral parapatellar approach – for cases of multi-plane articular involvement, medial based inter-condylar splits, "Hoffa" fractures, etc

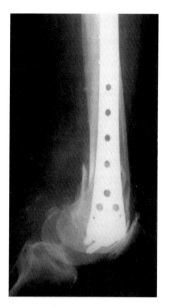 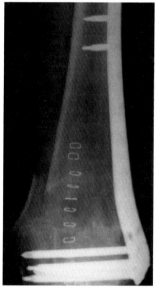

Fig. 10.38 The LISS plate is a good option for fixing fractures in this region in osteoporotic patients

Fig. 10.39 Postoperative AP radiograph after LISS plating, noting the biological fixation of the implant

10.8.3   Aids to Reduction of the Articular Fracture

- Schanz pin
- Large reduction clamps
- Provisional k-wires
- Lag screw insertion

10.8.4   Aids to Reduction of Meta-diaphyseal Components

- If the fracture cannot be fixed early, temporary EF can be used
- Adequate intraoperative muscle relaxation aids reduction
- Supra-condylar towel bumps: can aid in the reduction of the commonly seen hyperextension of the distal femoral fragment. The bump acts as a fulcrum for the vector force of the manual pull
- Manual traction
- Distal femoral condyle Schanz pin
- Whirlybird device can offer corrections in varus/valgus alignment
- Femoral distractor
- Manual pressure
- Other reduction aids under development by the AO group

10.8.5   Complications with LISS

- Poor fracture reduction – fracture not properly reduced before LISS insertion
- Loss of reduction during time of LISS insertion – can sometimes be tackled by fine reduction aids like the whirlybird
- Eccentric screw placement of the diaphyseal screws
- Others

10.9   Acute Patella Dislocation

10.9.1   Introduction

- The knee joint is part of a complex kinetic chain, in which many of the daily motions like kicking need adequate hip motion
- All elements of the kinetic chain need be assessed in P/E
- PFJ is famous for being under high stresses

- Tendency nowadays to view it as mainly a soft tissue joint, and as such, potentially amenable to conservative Rn

10.9.2 Some Features of the PFJ

- Element of intrinsic instability since tubercle lateral to midline of knee and quads pull
- Normally overcome by patella median ridge, lateral slope of the trochlea. The normal patella engages at 30–60° flexion
- High contact pressure

10.9.3 Factors Leading to Instability

- Poor engagement:
  - Patella alta
  - Patella dysplasia
  - Trochlea dysplasia
  - Knee hyperextension
- Fail to stay engaged:
  - Tight lateral structures
  - Lax medially
  - Genu valgum
  - Laterally placed tubercle

10.9.4 Types of Dislocation

- Acute (lateral mostly)
- Chronic
  - Recurrent
  - Habitual
  - Permanent (congenital/acquired)

10.9.5 Clinical Exam

- Knee
  - Look, e.g. any high patella, old scars, squinting of patellae on standing, recurvatum
  - Feel, for infrapatella area tenderness (fat pad), retropatella tenderness, lateral patella tenderness (e.g. retinaculum), size of patella

- Move, e.g. pain/click on early flexion (more likely distal lesion if cartilage lesion present), pain in late flexion (more likely to be proximal lesion)
- Special test, Clark test, glide test, tilt and apprehension sign
- Gait, Q angle

10.9.6   Clinical Examination: Other Areas

- Hip and whole LL axis
- Spine/lordosis
- Ankle/foot, e.g. any foot pronation
- Generalised ligamentous laxity

10.9.7   Investigations

- Merchant's view
- Laurin's view
- Lateral X-ray – Insall/Salvati ratio; trochlear profile
- Note any patella dysplasia, and bipartite patellae
- Other, e.g.
  - CT see tracking (after engagement at 20° flexion), selected cases with suspected excessive femoral anteversion
  - MRI, see cartilage better, search for, e.g. traumatic osteochondral fracture and associated soft tissue injury, e.g. MPFL – injury can be multifocal
- Arthroscopy ± mini-open

10.9.8   Rn of Acute Dislocations

- Current opinion: all worth a trial of conservative Rn
- Except: osteochondral fragments, which require either fixation or excision ± lateral release and medial plication at the same time

10.9.9   Conservative Rn

- Immobilise in extension to allow early ligament healing and minimise swelling
- Consider arthrocentesis if significant to rest the soft tissues and ease their reduction

- After 2 weeks gradual increase in motion and strengthening besides bracing/taping

10.9.10   Where Is the Medial Tear?
- MRI studies in 113 acute patella dislocations:
  - 44% near patella insertion
  - 16% mid-substance
  - 25% femoral epicondyle
  - 26% multiple area (Fithian et al. 1999)

10.9.11   Osteochondral Injury
- 28% medial patella fractures
- 63% contused medial patella/lateral trochlea
- Less in patients with hypermobility (Stanitski)

10.9.12   What About the Predisposed Ones?
- Also had 52–75% good to excellent results
- Can still try conservative first (Cash and Hughston 1988)

10.9.13   Chronic Dislocation Cases
- Rn of instability individualised, no one operation good for every one
- Operative options:
  - Distal realignment
  - Proximal realignment
  - Improving the trochlea

10.9.13.1   Distal Realignment
- Distal transposition: sometimes done in patella alta cases
- Maquet: not suited for patella instability
- Medial transposition (Elmslie/Trillat) as adjunct to distal transposition or if tubercle too lateralised ± in troclear dysplasia
- Anteromedialisation: Fulkerson procedure
- Skeletally immature: Roux–Goldthwait procedure

10.9.13.2 Medial Tightening
- Rarely done alone as adjunct
- Involves plication/tightening by many techniques, e.g. fascia, tendon, imbrication, or advancement of the insertion of distal VMO fibres

10.9.13.3 Lateral Release
- Usually done with tubercle transposition or medial placation – although some workers claim this alone is rather reliable (Dandy)
- Dandy avoids lateral release when: subluxation in extension, shallow trochlea, hypermobility cases
- Beware of the lateral superior geniculate artery during lateral release
- The lateral edge of the patella should be able to be lifted to near vertical post release

10.9.14   Improving the Trochlea?
- Elevating the lateral condyle – technically difficult, no published good results
- Deepens the trochlea – removal of bone from beneath articular surface, or excavation with osteochondral flap replacement

10.10 Patella Fractures

10.10.1   Introduction
- The patella is the largest sesamoid bone in the body
- Besides cosmesis and protective roles, it serves the important function to improve the mechanical advantage of the quadriceps. The details were discussed in the companion volume of this book
- Displaced fracture produces loss of the extensor mechanism and lost ability of the knee to lock in extension

10.10.2   Injury Mechanism
- Sudden violent contraction of the quadriceps

- The weak point of the extensor mechanism (consisting of quadriceps and retinaculae, patella, patella tendon, and tibial tubercle) will fail
- Thus, although patella fracture is a common failure mode; a child may suffer from sleeve fracture (see Chap. 13), and a postoperative patient after a quadriceps snip in TKR may suffer from quadriceps rupture, etc.

10.10.3   Classification
- Mostly descriptive:
  - Transverse fracture
  - Lower or upper pole fracture
  - Comminuted fracture
  - Longitudinal (or vertical) fracture
  - Stellate fracture
  - Osteochondral fracture (as in patella dislocation)

10.10.4 Management
- Undisplaced transverse fracture: casting will suffice if extensor mechanism intact
- Displaced transverse fracture: ORIF by two parallel k-wires and TBW by the tension band principle to effect dynamic fracture compression
- Longitudinal: these are often from direct blows, can mostly pursue conservative Rn since the extensor mechanism usually intact
- Distal pole: if sizable piece, may consider screw fixation, otherwise partial patellectomy can be performed
- Osteochondral fracture: discussed under the section on acute patella dislocation (Sect. 10.9)

10.11   Knee Dislocation (Fig. 10.40)

10.11.1   Introduction
- Most are high energy injuries

- Beware of *spontaneously* reduced knee dislocations – clues include clinical assessment, examination under anaesthesia (EUA), or X-ray clues: residual subluxation, ligamentous avulsions (Fig. 10.41), etc.
- Most important is to check vascular status and not miss the golden period of repair (<8 h)

10.11.2 Classification

- Siliski finds classifying by direction is useful:
  - Can be anterior/posterior/medial/lateral/rotatory, a few are indeterminate
  - Posterior > rotatory, anterior > medial/lateral in a Massachusetts General Hospital (MGH) study
  - Posterior and anterior directions together account for >50% cases
  - These A/P disruptions are sadly the ones most prone to vascular injuries

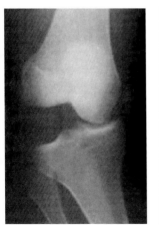 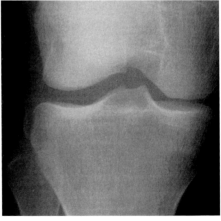

Fig. 10.40 Every patient with knee dislocation, such as this patient, should have detailed vascular assessment

Fig. 10.41 Be on the look out for any tell-tale signs such as second fractures, as shown here, as a hint that there may be associated ligamentous injury

— Medial dislocation: most prone to causing peroneal nerve injury (overall figure 15%, but much higher incidence in medial dislocation)

10.11.3   Why Are A/P Disruptions Most Prone to Vascular Injuries?

- Popliteal artery tethered both below and above the knee: at the fibrous arch of the soleus and the adductor hiatus
- By comparison, the tibial nerve is less tethered and tibial nerve injury *less* common

(Notice: golden time for vascular repair is 8 h before calf muscle necrosis; the amputation rate increases dramatically from 5% < 8 h, to 30–50% > 8 h, note that many also required prophylactic fasciotomy)

10.11.4   More About Vascular Injuries

- Do not waste time obtaining an arteriogram, especially if either not available at night or needs hours before it can be arranged: consider an intraoperative arteriogram in cases of vascular compromise
- Find a vascular surgeon to help if needed
- Many recommend *arteriogram for every knee dislocation:* rationale being if misses the *intimal* tear, delayed thrombosis occurs. If intimal tear present, anticoagulation for at least 1 week is the regimen in large centres like the MGH

10.11.5   Other Clinical Scenarios

- Patients with open wounds: besides surgical exploration, frequently need immobilisation with EF
- Patients with no vascular injury and mild soft tissue trauma, can undergo gentle reduction (confirmed with X-ray) and give extension splint in acute setting
- Cases that are postoperative after vascular repair need immobilisation in 15° knee flexion

10.11.6   Definitive Management

- There are two main schools of thoughts:

- Conservative (Taylor 1972): rationale is that natural history of many of these knees is they get stiff, and more so frequently with operation. Conservative Rx let collaterals heal after 6–8 weeks of immobilisation to at least get some varus valgus stability and then check for instability of cruciates later, especially in lower demand, elderly patients
- Operative:
  - If vascular repair had been done, experts like Siliski tend to reconstruct within about 10–14 days when perfusion stable and no tourniquet. Siliski favours open repair (he uses Marshall's method of cruciate reconstruction and repairs/reattaches the collaterals ± menisci)
  - If vascular status is stable, some experts favour ensuring adequate ROM first, and early repair of posterolateral complex (PLC) and delayed repair of both (anterior cruciate ligament [ACL] and posterior cruciate ligament [PCL]) in one go by arthroscopic means; still others repair PLC first then repair PCL and assess anterior instability on follow-up

10.11.7 Current Recommendations

- There is no controlled comparison between the conservative and operative groups
- Most experts do perform elective reconstructions of these unstable, multiple ligament injured knees via combined use of allografts and autografts arthroscopically, especially in younger individuals. If PLC is injured, however, open PLC repair within 2 weeks, followed by subsequent arthroscopic reconstruction of the other ligaments is advisable

10.12 Floating Knee Injuries

10.12.1 General Features

- High energy injuries
- Most require operative fixation

- High chance of associated bony and soft tissue (especially knee ligament) injuries; as well as injury to other organ systems

10.12.2   Classification (Waddell/Fraser)

- Type I: extra-articular
- Type II: classified according to the knee injury
  - Type IIA: femoral shaft fractures and tibial intra-articular fractures
  - Type IIB: intra-articular distal femur fractures and tibial shaft fractures
  - Type IIC: ipsilateral intra-articular fractures of distal femur and tibial plateau

10.12.3   Work-up

- Locally, despite energy absorbed in the fractured tibia and femur *still* a high incidence of knee ligament injuries
- Also, high chance of associated injuries: fracture or dislocation in nearby joints at ipsilateral limb, fracture of contralateral limb; systemic injuries e.g. head and chest injuries
- Check neurovascular status and search for open fractures and compartment syndrome – all these if present mandate emergency surgery

10.12.4   Timing of Surgery

- Depends on the overall assessment of these frequently poly-trauma patients
- If the patient is in extremis, may need to initiate damage control orthopaedics for extremity fractures, see Chap. 2

10.12.4.1   Management: Type I

- Retrograde nailing of the femur while putting on a pinless fixator for the tibia during femoral nailing
- This is followed by tibial shaft nailing
- However, use antegrade femoral nailing if the femoral shaft fracture is high or subtrochanteric

0.12.4.2 Management: Type IIA
- Use retrograde femoral nailing if possible
- Use same incision (extend somewhat) for ORIF of the intra-articular proximal tibia fracture

0.12.4.3 Management: Type IIB
- Choice of implant to fix the distal femoral fracture (see Sect. 10.8)
- Common choices include DFN and LISS
- Followed by nailing of the fractured tibial shaft

0.12.4.4 Management: Type IIC
- Initial spanning EF
- Followed by elective reconstruction of both the intra-articular fracture of the distal femur and that of the proximal tibia. The midline approach as for TKR is useful

10.13 Tibial Plateau Fracture

10.13.1 Changing Emphasis over the Years
- Previously experts put stress mainly on anatomic articular reduction
- Now, important aspects are manifold:
  - Joint stability (meniscus and ligament injuries common in high energy trauma in young people)
  - Articular congruity (usually important, but in the elderly with degenerative knee, some say even more important to preserve soft tissues and prevent sepsis to make later TKR possible)
  - Restoration of mechanical axis (use of newer plates, minimally invasive and biological fixation especially in the presence of traumatised soft tissues)
  - Soft tissue injury (if severe, may require the use of spanning EF to buy time)
  - Fracture personality
  - Role of arthroscopy (mainly for Schatzker's types 1, 2 and 3 since lower energy trauma; type 1 sometimes entraps the meniscus,

type 3 if occurring in the elderly sometimes conservative if frag ment depressed is small. Otherwise, medial condyle fracture associated with high energy fractures and ligament injuries are common and need proper fixation)

10.13.2   Injury Mechanism

- Associated with high energy trauma like traffic accidents in the young, while plateau fracture in the elderly with osteoporotic bone may just result from a simple fall
- Most fractures involved varus/valgus force together with axial com pression

10.13.3   Associated Injuries

- Meniscus: injured in 20–50% cases, Dx by MRI or arthroscopy, or direct vision in arthrotomy – repair peripheral tears
- Ligaments: injured in 10–30% cases, more in younger patients, some times do pre-operative stress exam; most are medial collateral liga ment (MCL)/ACL. Repair bony avulsions; brace collaterals (many MCL injuries can heal by conservative means)
- Bony injury, e.g. tibia shaft, distal femur, patella

10.13.4   Physical Assessment

- Check soft tissue status
- Check neurovascular status
- Look for compartment syndrome
- Look for associated injuries, the exact mechanism of injury may give a hint on possible associated injury

10.13.5   Investigations

- Knee trauma series: AP lateral obliques and 10–15° caudal views Need to assess: articular depression, rim displacement, shaft exten sion, bony avulsion, tibio-fibular articulation, fibula fracture
- AP traction X-ray: sometimes used in high energy fractures, with assessment of the effects of ligamentotaxis
- CT: (Fig. 10.42) axial cuts especially useful – help plan screw place ment 90° to fracture plane; assess size of depressed fragment, 2D

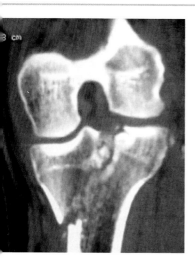

Fig. 10.42 CT views in different planes aid in preoperative assessment of tibial plateau fractures

reformatting – assess amount of articular depression, 3D – usually only done in those with difficult posterior plateau fracture patterns, and comminuted fractures

■ MRI: more used in type 1, sometimes type 4, assess meniscus (ligament) injury

■ Arteriogram – suspected arterial injury and fracture dislocation cases

10.13.6   Schatzker Classification

■ Type 1: split fractures: common in the young, MCL injury common. Beware any entrapment of lateral meniscus that can hinder percutaneous reduction

■ Type 2: split depression fractures – femoral condyle splits the lateral plateau with axial force and then the split fracture depresses off the medial edge of the intact plateau

■ Type 3: centrally depressed fracture: low-energy trauma, commonly seen in the elderly

■ Type 4: medial plateau: high energy trauma – involves medial plateau and tibial spine area, commonly associated ligamentous injuries

- Type 5: bicondylar: split fracture of both plateaus
- Type 6: meta-diaphyseal dissociation and associated proximal shaft fracture of tibia

10.13.7 Clinical Note
- The Schatzker's classification is the most popular classification
- It is important to realise that Schatzker's types 4 to 6 usually indicate high energy trauma and careful assessment of the soft tissue is imperative

10.13.8 Hohl Classification
- Type 1: coronal split
- Type 2: entire condyle – 12% neurovascular Cx
- Type 3: rim avulsion – 30% neurovascular Cx
- Type 4: rim compression – check collaterals and cruciates
- Type 5: four-part fracture – 50% neurovascular Cx

10.13.9 Clinical Note
- Gives an idea of the likely neurovascular compromise with different fracture patterns
- Also looks at some patterns not mentioned in Schatzker's classification

10.13.10 Main Goals of Rn
- Joint stability
- Articular congruity
- Restoration of mechanical axis and axial alignment
- Painless motion with early weight-bearing, and minimise complications
- Preservation of soft tissue and prevention of sepsis, especially important in the elderly

(P.S. Soft tissue status dictates the timing of definitive surgery, while understanding the fracture personality aids preoperative planning of fracture fixation)

0.13.11 Main Rn Options

- Conservative
- Operative
  - Screws only
  - Screws and plates ± locked plates
  - EF (bridging or non-bridging)
  - Combinations of above

0.13.12 The Case for Conservative Rn

- Minimal fracture displacement
- Low functional demand
- Stable to varus/valgus stresses
- < 2–5 mm articular depression (different authors had different criteria here, and criteria looser for lateral plateau)

0.13.13 Operative Indications

- Open fracture
- Vascular injury
- Compartment syndrome
- Most high energy plateau fractures, most medial condylar fractures (medial structural buttress very important), most bi-condylar fractures
- Others: varus/valgus unstable (5–10°), significant articular step-off/depression

0.13.14 Role of Arthroscopy

- Synergistic with intraoperative fluoroscopy
- Can be considered for Schatzker's types 1 to 3
- Avoid in high energy patterns
  - Advantages: good visualisation of intra-articular soft tissues, aid to ensure proper articular congruity, probably the best method to repair posterior meniscal tear
  - Disadvantages: compartment syndrome, increased operative time

10.13.15 Pros and Cons of Arthroscopy

- Cons: increase technical demand and equipment, increase surgical time and arthroscopic Cx, e.g. fluid extravasation and compartment syndrome
- Pros: better visual of intra-articular pathology, confirms fracture reduction, especially good for low energy patterns, high energy one danger of extravasation – here consider mini-arthrotomy instead. Arthroscopically-assisted indirect reduction and IF of split fracture followed by EF or MIPO/LISS

10.13.16 Timing of Surgery

- Previous teaching to postpone around 1 week if significant soft tissue trauma, new trend to wait longer for a more stable soft tissue envelope (if the soft tissue condition unfavourable) before operation say, up to 2 weeks if not more, may need to take down early callus
- Despite the often quoted optimal time for ligamentotaxis to work being within 24–72 h

10.13.17 Fixation Methods in Different Clinical Scenarios

- Good bone stock and simple fracture patterns: two to three percutaneous rafts of screws suffice
- But consider adding antiglide plate if poor bone stock
- Whole condyle fracture and especially if poor bone stock: buttress plate used
- Bicondylar fracture: options include lateral plate and medial EF double plating, spanning EF if poor soft tissue, or selected patient with one-sided locked fixed angle plate and supplementary screws

10.13.18 Commonly Used Plates

- Traditional plates: L-plate (Figs. 10.43, 10.44), T-plate
- Newer: pre-contoured plates
- New locking plates

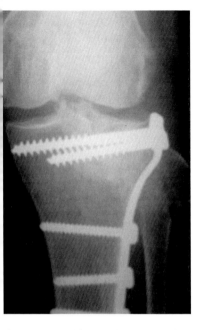 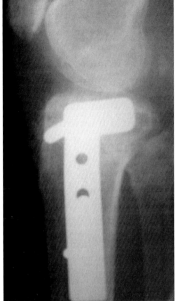

Fig. 10.43 Lateral buttress plating is often done to tackle the commonly seen lateral tibial plateau fractures

Fig. 10.44 Lateral view of the same patient as in Fig. 10.43; note the L-shaped plate

10.13.19 Traditional Versus Newer Plates

- Classic AO ORIF plating is still sometimes needed if fracture fails to reduce by indirect method: requires extensile approach, expect more wound complications and infection for these complex fractures
- Newer locked plates: designed for more biological fixation (after initial reconstruction of the articular surface), depend largely on indirect reduction, preservation of soft tissues

10.13.20 Use of Locked Plates and MIPO

- It should be pointed out again that the fracture must be reducible by indirect reduction method, the locked plates cannot be relied upon to do the reduction for the surgeon

- A mal-reduced fracture treated by these fixed angle plates may well invite delayed or non-union
- Concomitant proper restoration of the articular surface should be performed

10.13.21 Use of EF

- Especially indicated in cases with severe soft tissue injury, or if the proximal fragment(s) are too small to hold the plate, and rarely if comminution at the meta-diaphyseal region is so great as to make stable fixation difficult, or fractures with long diaphyseal extension (neural complication from LISS plate increases using the longer 11–13-hole plates)
- As salvage

10.13.22 EF Limitations and Use of Adjunctive IF Devices/Procedures

- EF uses ligamentotaxis to apply a reduction force, neutralises deforming forces and helps maintain reduction until fracture heals. Some rigid frames like the Ilizarov may allow early weight-bearing
- EF, however, will not reduce impacted articular surface, or have any effect on depressed fragments. These depressed fragments require elevation ± BG; sometimes arthroscopically-assisted techniques for the latter can detect common concomitant soft tissue injuries like the meniscus or collaterals

10.13.23 Complications

- Arthrosis: may need to revise to TKR later (Fig. 10.45)
- Sepsis
- Compartment syndrome
- Malunion
- Non-union
- Neural injury (refer to Hohl's classification, but can be iatrogenic with the increased use of long LISS plate)

(Note: it is easier to tackle arthrosis than joint sepsis, hence handling of soft tissue *equal* in importance to articular reconstruction, especially in the elderly)

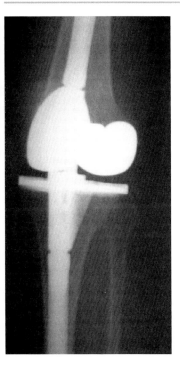

Fig. 10.45 TKR is one possible option in elderly with symptomatic arthrosis after a previous tibial plateau fracture. Higher constrained TKR is needed if there is concomitant collaterals laxity, especially the MCL

10.14 Fractured Proximal Tibia

10.14.1 Problems in this Region

- Much higher rate of complications recorded with IM nailing of proximal tibia than tibial shaft fractures
- Malunion rate varies from 15–30% (Kyro) to over 80% (Lang et al. 1995) reported with resultant disability
- Typical malunion involves valgus angulation in coronal plane and flexion deformity in the sagittal plane ± posterior translation at the site of the fracture

10.14.2 Role of Conservative Rn

- Many displaced proximal tibial fractures need operative treatment

- Occasionally conservative treatment may be adequate for non-displaced fractures especially in the elderly low-demand patient with osteoporotic bones

10.14.3   Aim of Operation

- The aim of peri-articular surgery involves articular reduction with acceptable meta-diaphyseal alignment
- Especially in patients with high energy soft tissue trauma, percutaneous or MIPO techniques are often recommended to minimise soft tissue dissection, disruption of the fractured haematoma, and the often associated bony fragments with tenuous blood supply
- Nailing is not always feasible for every proximal tibial fracture

10.14.4   Problems Encountered with Nailing the Proximal Tibia

- Resultant valgus deformity in coronal plane
- Resultant flexion deformity in sagittal plane

10.14.5   Cause of the Valgus Deformity

- Valgus deformity is caused by a mismatch between the axis of nail insertion in proximal fragment and anatomic axis of distal segment that passes through the medullary canal, i.e. mismatch of the nail-entrance angle and tibial canal (Arch Orthop Trauma Surg 2001)
- A common cause is a starting point that is too medial. Another contribution is from the local anatomy of the proximal tibia, i.e. the AP width of the tibia is narrower on the medial side than on the lateral side and the medial cortex of the tibia then forces the nail laterally (J Orthop Trauma 1997)
- The nature of the attachment of tibial anterior compartment muscles that act in effect as a tether to the lateral proximal tibia also possibly contribute to the final valgus angulation

10.14.6   Cause of the Flexion Deformity

- This can be caused by:
  - Inability to extend the knee during nail insertion may contribute to flexion deformity of the proximal fragment (Clin Orthop Relat Res 1996)

- Exact location of the proximal bend of the tibial nail may be contributory – when the fracture is proximal to the bend, flexion of the proximal fragment and posterior translation of the fracture can occur (J Orthop Trauma 1993)
- Eccentric start point – in the sagittal plane, the start point placement is eccentrically placed at the edge of the articular surface; this position is anterior to the medullary axis and the nail must be initially directed posteriorly in order to gain access to the canal

10.14.7   Prevention of Deformity

- Point of entry: must be collinear with medullary axis and avoid medialisation. Recent studies indicated a safe zone at 9.1 ± 5 mm lateral to the midline of the tibial plateau and 3 mm lateral to the centre of the tibial tubercle (Tornetta)
- Use of Poller screws as popularised by Krettek prior to nail introduction – acts in effect to narrow the canal and as a substitute posterior cortex. Thus, besides AP plane (placed laterally in the metaphysis), a blocking screw is usually placed in the posterior half of the proximal tibia in the sagittal plane
- Use of a small plate ± clamps placed in situ (to prevent fragment alignment) prior to nail insertion
- Use another implant altogether

10.14.8   Ways to Circumvent Problems with Nailing

- Nails equipped with oblique screws
- Use more lateral entry site
- Use of blocking/Poller screws

10.14.9   How to Bail out a Poorly Made Entry Hole

- Blocking screws – sometimes needed in two different planes, and left in situ
- Use another implant other than a nail

10.14.10   Other Operative Options

- Plating
- EF

10.14.11 Role of Locked Plating in Proximal Tibial Fractures: Pros and Cons

- Pros: locked plates allow the performance of MIPO techniques that may decrease devascularisation (biologic plating), minimise soft tissue trauma and infection, may lead to faster healing and lessen the need for BG. Sometimes can do away with the need for double incisions or double plating. Use of pre-contoured plates also eases the performance of submuscular insertion
- Cons: traditional AO plating is bulky and involves much soft tissue dissection and devascularisation. Even with the use of newer locked plates, the fracture must be able to be reduced anatomically (usually via indirect reduction), i.e. the fracture cannot be reduced to the plate, or the plate cannot be relied upon to do the reduction for you. Thus, fracture configurations that are difficult to reduce by indirect reduction alone and depressed fragments may not be well served with such newer plating systems

10.14.12 Choice of Locking Plates

- Implants especially suited for MIPO techniques include the locking plates, where the head of the screw threads and locks into the plate

10.14.13 What About the Use of EF?

- Can be considered in:
  - Paediatric fractures in which nailing is often avoided and healing is rapid, especially with an intact periosteal hinge
  - Open fractures, especially with contamination in which the EF is useful as a temporising device

10.15   Fractured Tibial Shaft

10.15.1   General Problems with Tibial Shaft Fractures

- Fair blood supply, rather prone to non-union and delayed union
- Thin soft tissue envelope, especially at the anteromedial aspects, and also near both the proximal and distal ends of the tibia

10.15.2 Classification

- AO/OTA classification: good for research
- Simple descriptive classification: familiar to most
  - Proximal, middle, distal
  - Transverse, oblique, spiral, segmental, comminuted

(No classification is complete without description of the soft tissue, e.g. Tscherne classification. This point is particularly important in tibia fractures)

10.15.3 Conservative Versus Operative Options

- This boils down (as far as the fracture itself is concerned) to the degree of malalignment that can be accepted. A useful guide is considered operative if: coronal angulation >5°, sagittal >10°, rotation >5°, shortening >1 cm
- However, there is as yet *no* concrete evidence based support for the above figures, which should be regarded only as guidelines

10.15.4 Other Operative Indications for Tibial Shaft Fractures

- Open fractures
- Compartment syndrome
- Poly-trauma
- Failed conservative Rn
- Neurovascular injury requiring intervention
- ± Intact fibula (previous studies indicate that this subgroup may have a higher chance of subsequent angulation)

10.15.5 Pros and Cons of Conservative Rn

- Pros
  - Negligible infection risk
  - Few problems of knee pain
  - No need for hardware removal
  - Does not have the other problems related to IM nailing (e.g. implant failure, screw breakage, thermal necrosis)
  - Refer to the works of Sarmiento et al. (1989) and the fracture patterns that may be suitable for functional bracing (Fig. 10.46)

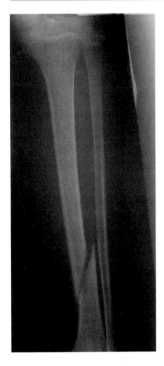

Fig. 10.46 Short oblique tibial shaft fracture is a common pattern included in the study by Sarmiento et al. (1989) on functional bracing

- Cons
    - Hindfoot stiffness is not uncommon
    - More time off work
    - Period of protected weight-bearing
    - Plaster-related complications
    - Joint stiffness

10.15.6   Pros and Cons of IM Nailing
- Pros
    - Literature seems to indicate a low rate of non-union
    - Early return to work and early weight-bearing (reamed nails)
    - Not having cast-related complications

- Cons
  - Knee pain is of common occurrence (Robinson)
  - Implant failure such as screw breakage especially common with the use of unreamed nails (Court-Brown et al. 1990)
  - Embolic complications
  - Other complications: compartment syndrome, malalignment (if performed for fractures outside the zone of indication), thermal necrosis, even nail breakage if the fracture heals slowly or fracture non-union

0.15.7 Pros and Cons of IM Reaming

- Pros:
  - Reaming causes deposition of reamed bone at the fracture site acting as a form of bone graft
  - Reaming stimulates periosteal and extra-osseous blood flow and increases circulation to the forming external callus
  - Reaming allows greater contact between endosteum and nail, thus allowing a bigger and stronger nail to be inserted
- Cons:
  - Systemic complications of reaming:
  - Studies have revealed that the reaming process is associated with inflammatory mediators, may act as a second-hit phenomenon for patients in extremis
  - Reaming is associated with fat and marrow emboli that may cause pulmonary embolism
  - Local complications of reaming:
  - There is necrosis of 50–60% of the cortical bone near the fracture and disruption of the endosteal blood supply plus reversal of centrifugal to centripetal blood flow pattern
  - Theoretically can diminish bone strength by removing bone, but since the outer diameter mainly contributes to the stiffness of the tibia, this effect is not significant

0.15.8 Choice Between Reamed and Unreamed IM Nailing

- It is currently agreed by most experts that:

There is little advantage of the routine use of unreamed nails (Fig. 10.47) since:

- They have been shown to have higher rates of non-union and locking screw breakage
- Whereas studies indicate faster union rate with ↓ need of secondary procedures with reamed nailing
- There is no statistical difference in operative time and blood loss between the two groups (Tornetta)
- Despite ↓ endosteal blood flow after reaming, there is:
- Reconstitution of endosteal flow at 6 weeks
- No difference in blood flow within the callus or in the amount of new bone formed
- Ipsilateral leg perfusion is not affected

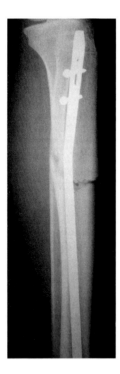

Fig. 10.47 Note the relatively small size of the unreamed nail in a spacious medullary cavity. Unreamed nailing has relatively narrow indications and is more prone to implant breakage and failure

0.15.9 Bring Home the Message

- Literature indicates that reamed nailing is safe, even in up to open type IIIA tibial fractures; it offers the advantage of fewer hardware problems, fewer secondary procedures and better union rates than unreamed nailing
- In closed tibial fractures, reamed nailing is associated with ↓ risk of delayed union and non-union than unreamed nails

0.15.10 Contraindication for Reamed Intramedullary Nailing

- Small canal diameter < 6–7 mm – higher chance of thermal necrosis since requires excessive reaming especially with the use of blunt reamers
- Deformity of the tibial medullary canal
- Grossly contaminated medullary canal
- In the presence of TKR
- Very stiff or ankylosed knee joint

0.15.11 Any Role of Plating and EF

- EF: consider in some tibial fracture patterns in children that are difficult to hold with a cast; type IIIB open fractures; lesser degrees of open fracture with significant contamination; unstable patient with multiple fractures as a temporising measure
- Plating: more indicated in fracture of the proximal and distal ends of the tibia; i.e. beyond the traditional "zone of indication" of IM devices

0.15.12 Complications of Intramedullary Nailing

0.15.12.1 Group A/Intraoperative Cx

- Increased compartment pressure
- Fracture not properly reduced
- Breakage of hardware
- Thermal necrosis

10.15.12.1.1   Fractured Tibia and Compartment Syndrome

- Besides cases presenting with frank signs of compartment syndrome, there are fractures with borderline compartment pressures, which in the process of applying traction to the extremity, reaming the medullary canal and losing additional blood into the soft tissues, can result in a compartment syndrome
- Whenever in doubt, monitoring of compartmental pressure is needed
- Besides functional sequelae of compartment syndrome usually from affection of the flexors, compartment syndrome can also delay the time to union (McQueen)

10.15.12.1.2   Measuring Compartment Pressure in Fractured Tibia

- Measure within 5 cm of the fracture
- As a minimum, measure in both the anterior and deep posterior compartments
- The highest tissue pressure recorded should form the basis for decision to determine need for fasciotomy

10.15.12.1.3   Relation Between Compartment Syndrome and IM Nailing

- Experts like Court-Brown think that intramedullary nailing does not increase the incidence of acute compartment syndrome in tibial fractures
- Many feel that the mere application of significant traction intraoperatively may itself increase the compartment pressure. Reaming with well-designed sharp reamers is recommended, and be gentle
- Delay in nailing may not reduce the risk of raised compartment pressures

10.15.12.1.4   Ways to Prevent Thermal Necrosis

- Avoid the use of nails in patients with a very narrow medullary cavity
- Use sharp reamers
- Use of newer reamers that decrease the rate of rise of medullary pressure

- Avoid the excessive use of pushing force to avoid acute pressure rises
- Avoid the use of tourniquets

0.15.12.1.5   Newer Reamer Designs that May Decrease Pressure Build-up

- Reamer shaft with low friction surface aids rapid debris clearance
- Cutting flute geometry optimised to ensure low-pressure generation
- New AO reamer head equipped with stepped cutting edge – in effect acts like two reamers incorporated into one reamer head. This design produces less clogging of reamed bone at the cutting tip and has less effect as a plunger
- With the newer system, commence reaming with the 8.5-mm diameter reamer

0.15.12.1.6   Breakage of Hardware

- Breakage of hardware like nails or locking bolts mostly occurs post-operatively with delayed union cases or as a result of new trauma
- Intraoperative hardware can still occur, e.g.:
    - Breakage of plastic medullary exchange tube, the method of management was described by the author (Ip 2001)
    - Breakage of frequently distal bolts can occur with forceful "back-slaps" performed pretty much as a routine by some traumatologists

0.15.12.2   Group B/Early Cx

- Fat embolism ± ARDS
- Compartment syndrome
- Sepsis: especially common in cases of open fractures initially treated with EF and left in place for >2 weeks
- Hardware failure

0.15.12.2.1   Ways to Prevent Fat Embolism

- See the aforementioned discussion on tricks to prevent acute pressure increases

- In addition, a vent hole is used by some traumatologists, but more often in femoral nailing
- The majority of emboli during the performance of reamed nails in fact occur during the initial phase of insertion of the guide-wire and reaming. Another rise occurs during nail negotiation into the canal. The latter is part of the reason that emboli can still occur with un-reamed nailing
- Notice also that the reaming pressure tends to be less in reaming a comminuted fracture than a simple, say, transverse fracture

10.15.12.2.2 Nailing and Compartment Syndrome

- According to experts like Court-Brown, there is no concrete evidence that reaming per se will produce a compartment syndrome
- It is possible that significant traction forces to realign the fracture intraoperatively (reducing the fracture shortening and radius of the cylinder) can themselves trigger compartment syndrome. Steps to avoid the acute rise in pressure during reaming was discussed. Remember never to use a tourniquet
- McQueen rightly suggested that whenever possible, the compartment pressure should be monitored in most patients with fractured tibia, preferably by portable monitors

10.15.12.2.3 Early Hardware Failure

- This is uncommon, but not rare
- Examples include, e.g.:
  - Premature breakage of the distal locking bolts in unreamed tibial nailing. A period of protected weight-bearing is advisable
  - The author also reported the premature failure of the distal fixation bolts in IC tibial nails (a nail design with a built-in compression mode) (Ip 2003). Again, the author suggested a period of initial protected weight-bearing after putting fixation bolts in the very distal metaphyseal flare
  - Others, e.g. fixation screws, were scored intraoperatively predisposing to early fatigue failure, etc.

10.15.12.3 Group C/Management of Common Late Cx

- Delayed union
- Non-union: will be discussed in detail
- Non-union with bone loss: refer to the section on bone defects management in Chap. 3
- Infected IM nail
- Malunion
- Hardware failure

10.15.12.3.1 Tibial Non-union: Management Overview

Diagnosis of Non-union

- Dx can be obvious in those with a large gap, or those patients lacking bone bridge across the fracture and pain on weight-bearing on serial follow-up
- Dx can be difficult in other cases, as there is no gold standard to confirm radiologic union
- There are variable reports varying from two to four cortices that are needed to confirm union on orthogonal views. If in doubt, may resort to other imaging like tomogram or CT

Classification

- Relative to vascularity (popular)
  - Atrophic
  - Hypertrophic
- Relative to sepsis
  - Septic
  - Aseptic

Causes

- Biological, e.g. damaged blood supply, sepsis, segmental bone loss and bony comminution, compartment syndrome
- Mechanical, e.g. poorly done internal fixation, fracture gapping, altered mechanical axis, over-distraction, soft tissue interposition, inadequate immobilisation
- Combined

Contributing Factors
- Smoking
- Steroids, non-steroid anti-inflammatory drugs (NSAID)
- Sepsis
- Severely obese

Work-up
- Trace previous records and know the details of previous treatments
- Assess soft tissue envelope
- Assess neurovascular status
- Check full-length weight-bearing alignment films, find the anatomical and mechanical axis, relative limb length. Document deformities in three planes, any translations need to be noted
- Others: stress view X-rays to assess fracture mobility, blood checks and bone scan/MRI ± biopsy if sepsis is suspected

Options for Tibial Non-unions Without Deformity
- Consider the following different case scenarios

Clinical Scenario 1: Previously Treated by IM Nailing
- Avoid IM nailing if there is active or chronic sepsis (nail will act as a foreign body and danger of further spreading the infection)
- Otherwise exchange nailing is an option if other simpler measures like dynamisation fail
- Posterolateral BG (Harmon)
- ± Fibular segmental resection
- ± BM injection, anterior grafting

Clinical Scenario 2: Previously Treated by Plating
- Conversion to IM nailing useful option if no sepsis
- But there may be practical problems encountered in fracture being too proximal or distal, canal malalignment or blockade

Clinical Scenario 3: Previously Treated by EF

- Conversion to IM fixation possible, but first make sure no sepsis. Pin track sepsis should be treated before consideration of IM nail, some give a "pin holiday", but not always needed

Options for Tibial Non-unions with Deformities

- Gradual correction with circular fixators like Ilizarov – especially if there is concomitant LLD
- Rigid fixation by tension-band plating, bone grafting, with the help of indirect reduction techniques: better than option 3 since more preservation of soft tissue and vascularity
- Traditional AO plating and BG: option 2 better, and risks further devascularisation if atrophic non-union
- Open nailing and taking down the non-union site: not popular, may be Cx by sepsis, which is even more difficult to treat
- If very mobile, may well be a pseudarthrosis – and the principle of pseudarthrosis Rn is resection to viable bone with any accompanying deformity corrected acutely

Pros of Ilizarov

- Can tackle LLD
- Can effect compression on the non-union
- Concomitant free tissue transfer possible
- May allow early weight-bearing
- Can allow concomitant bone transport

Cons of Ilizarov

- Pin tract infection
- Fracture of regenerate
- Non-union persists
- Psychological impact if young age

Miscellaneous Cases with Special Problems

- Non-union and soft tissue defect: these cases frequently need early flap coverage to bring in vascularity

- Non-union and large bone defects: see the section on management of bone defects in Chap. 3
- Non-union despite multiple previous operations and poor function resistant cases might even need amputation
- Septic non-unions discussed in Chap. 3

Tibial Non-union with Bone Loss

- The following is a common classification used
- For further discussion please refer to the section on bone defect management in Chap. 3

Classification of the Tibia (and Fibula) Status of Bone Defect (May)

- 1 = both T/F intact, (expected period of rehabilitation < 3 months)
- 2 = BG needed (3–6 months)
- 3 = tibial defect < 6 cm, fibula OK (6–12 months)
- 4 = tibial defect > 6 cm, fibula OK (12–18 months)
- 5 = tibial defect > 6 cm, fibula not intact (>18 months)

10.15.12.3.2   Infected Tibial IM Nail

- Infection is a difficult complication since it will hinder fracture healing
- Infection after closed IM nailing has been successfully treated with exchange nailing as reported by Court-Brown and adjunctive antibiotics
- Severe infection in the setting of IM nailing inserted for open tibial fractures may need nail removal, debridement and even resection of the sequestered segment of dead bone and EF. Lesser cases may try some new innovative ideas of Seligson with the use of antibiotic nails
- A separate discussion of septic non-union is to be found in Chap. 3

10.15.12.3.3   Tibial Malunion

- Most tibial malunions occur during the management of proximal and distal tibial fracture, and the ways to prevent malalignment during acute management was discussed. Prevention is always the key

- The reader is referred to the Chap. 3 concerning the general management of malunions

0.15.12.3.4 Hardware Failure

- Late hardware failure are often due to delayed or non-union of the fracture wherein the race between implant failure and bone healing was lost; and the hardware suffers from fatigue failure
- Another common scenario is breakage of the distal locking bolts especially if an unreamed nail was used
- Can be caused by a new trauma, or a small nail used for nailing a heavy build individual with a spacious medullary canal

0.16 Fractured Distal Tibia (Fig. 10.48)

0.16.1 Problems in This Region

- Thin soft tissue envelope

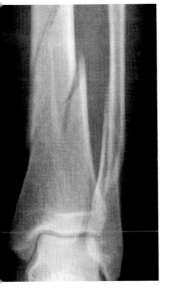

Fig. 10.48 Distal tibial fractures present problems of their own, even given IM nailing, see text for detailed discussion

- Rule out fracture extension into the tibial plafond articular surface
- Chance of malunion if treated by a nail because of small distal fragment

10.16.2 Rn Options

- Conservative/casts
- IM device
- Plating
- EF (mostly for pilon fracture)

10.16.3 Problems with IM Nailing in this Region (Fig. 10.49)

- If standard nails are used, may need to cut short the tip to allow locking
- Better to consider the use of nails specially designed for this region with both AP and ML locking holes near the nail tip
- Owing to the short distal fragment, more prone to malalignment after IM nailing (Fig. 10.50) with resultant malunion and pearls to decrease the chance of malunion will be discussed

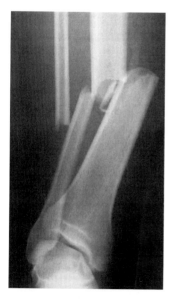

Fig. 10.49 This distal tibial fracture differs from the one illustrated in Fig. 10.48. The fracture in Fig. 10.48 results from torsional forces, while this one results from higher energy bending forces, for the fracture of the tibia and fibula are at roughly the same level

0.16.4 Ways to Circumvent IM Nailing Difficulties of the Distal Tibia

- Nails designed with more distal locking holes
- Must add AP locking besides the medial-lateral locking
- To prevent malalignment: consider distraction device, avoid reaming the distal metaphysis before nail passage, blocking screws, use external reduction aids like a hammer or clamps during nail passage, ensure guide-wire in the midline before nail introduction, sometimes consider plating of associated fibula fractures

0.16.5 Avoiding Malalignment of Distal Tibial Fractures Treated with IM Nailing

- To prevent malalignment:
  - Consider distraction device
  - Avoid reaming the distal metaphysis before nail passage, blocking screws
  - Use external reduction aids like a hammer or clamps during nail passage

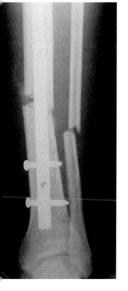

Fig. 10.50 Typical valgus angulation, which is a common problem in nailing these fractures

    — Ensure guide-wire in the midline before nail introduction
    — Sometimes consider plating of associated fibula fractures if present (recommended by some experts)

10.16.6 Any Role for Compression Nails (Fig. 10.51)

- While nailing of distal tibial fractures with nails equipped with hole near the nail tip is useful, there is doubt as to whether a separate compression mode needs to be administered in some newer nailing systems equipped with this compression function
- It has recently been reported by the author that application of compression (even in well-aligned nails) may cause premature screw failure and the author recommended an initial period of protected weight-bearing if the screws are locked in the very distal metaphysis for fear of breakage from four-point bending

10.16.7 Pearls for the Use of Plates in This Region

- Never use large fragment plates

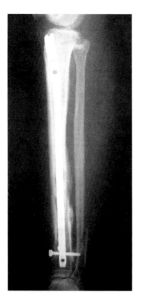

Fig. 10.51 Postoperative radiograph after tibial IC nailing equipped with very distal locking bolts, suitable for use in more distal fractures

- Percutaneous plating is recommended if at all possible
- Use low-profile plates
- Incision must respect the biology of this region

10.16.8   External Fixator
- More often used in comminuted pilon fractures rather than simple distal tibial fractures
- May be considered as a temporary measure in open fractures, especially if contaminated

0.17   Fractured Tibial Plafond (Fig. 10.52)

10.17.1   Relevant Anatomy: Osteology
- Pilon is Latin for "pestle" coined by Destot; plafond in French means "ceiling"
- Anterior portion of plafond is wider than posterior

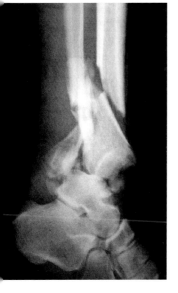

Fig. 10.52 Lateral radiograph showing pilon fracture with comminution

- Hence, margin of the anterior tibia can obscure view of plafond wit a direct anterior approach
- Weight-bearing stress falls mainly on centro-medial area, and this i the area of articular surface that is usually comminuted in explosiv high energy fracture patterns
- Four major syndesmotic structures around the ankle mortise in clude: anterior and posterior tibio-fibula ligaments, transverse tibio fibular ligament, and interosseous ligament (IOM)

10.17.2   Relevant Anatomy: Angiosomes (After Salmon)

- The distribution of cutaneous blood supply from tibialis posterio artery and anterior tibial/dorsalis pedis arteries meet just medial t the tibialis anterior tendon

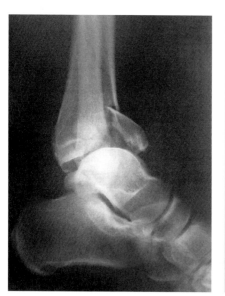

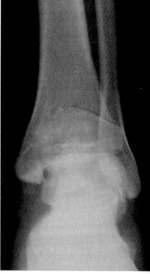

Fig. 10.53 Many pilon fractures are caused by axial loading in dorsiflexion such as in this patient

Fig. 10.54 The AP view of the ankle c the patient in Fig. 10.53.

▪ Incision ideally placed in the inter-arterial location – analogous to the concept of the internervous plane. The anteromedial approach is most often used in open reductions in this region

10.17.3 Mechanism of Injury
▪ Combinations of:
  — Compression – especially important element in explosive types
  — Rotation: many fractures initially reported by Ruedi were of this type
  — + Commonly dorsiflexion (Fig. 10.53, 10.54)– can cause anterior tibial comminution

10.17.4 Typical Fracture Pattern (Explosive Type)
▪ Fibula fractured in 80+% of cases; mostly in the supra-syndesmotic area; (IOM disrupted to level of fibula fracture or even above). Fibula plating helps restore length, lateral column and rotation
▪ Medial malleolus – split off usually at plafond level, there can be a metaphyseal spike – may act as good landmark helping reduction
▪ Anterior tibial margin: can be comminuted if foot was dorsiflexed during the injury
▪ Posterior malleolus: can be a separate fragment
▪ Chaput fragment: important – a means to help stabilise the syndesmosis, and a landmark for proper level of the joint line laterally
▪ Remember that the syndesmosis is usually disrupted to at least the level of the fibula fracture

10.17.5 Ruedi and Allgower Classification
▪ Type 1: fracture undisplaced
▪ Type 2: fracture displaced, not comminuted
▪ Type 3: fracture displaced, comminuted

10.17.6 Comparison: Tibial Plateau Fracture Versus Pilon Fracture
▪ Both regions are difficult to nail, attention to technique is important
▪ Fractures in both regions tend to have poor outcome if significant associated injury, may need to wait till soft tissue envelope quietens down before definitive fracture fixation

- Although post-traumatic arthrosis can occur in both regions, recent studies indicate that the final outcome of pilon fractures does not always correlate well with X-ray appearances, and only a few patients need arthrodesis despite secondary degenerative arthrosis set in at the ankle joint

10.17.7   Physical Assessment

- Assessment of the soft tissue status is most important for pilon fracture. Clinical markers of significant soft tissue injury include:
  - Closed degloving
  - Full thickness contusions
  - Fracture blisters over injury site
  - Severe swelling
  - Poor circulation
  - (Sometimes the real extent of the injury will declare itself after a few days)
- Look for neurovascular injury
- Look for associated injury

10.17.8   Investigation

- X-ray ± traction film (helps assess the effect of ligamentotaxis on the fracture at hand)
- Some points concerning X-ray interpretation:
  - Distal fibula has curvilinear articular surface closely matching the talus – forms sort of an analogue of "Shenton's line of the ankle"
  - Assessing subchondral joint margin landmarks – best assessed by X-ray traction film – may guide us in determining whether articular surface is reconstructable
- CT including 2D (Fig. 10.55) or sometimes 3D (Figs. 10.56–10.58) reconstruction. Axial view especially useful in planning direction of reduction clamps, screws or olive wires

10.17.9   Goal and Methods of Rx

- If follow traditional AO teachings this would include:

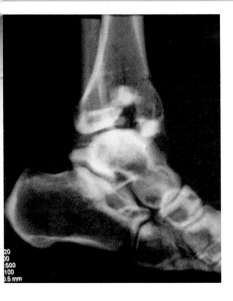

Fig. 10.55 This CT sagittal view shows clearly the impacted articular fragment in this pilon fracture

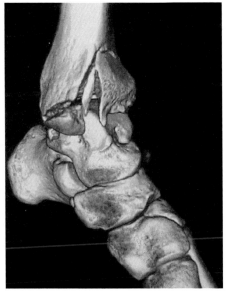

Fig. 10.56 Medial oblique 3D CT of the same patient reviewing the medial malleolar fragment and the medial comminution

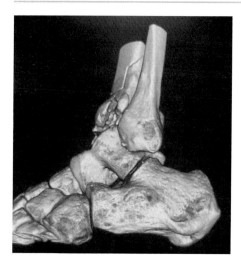

Fig. 10.57 Lateral 3D CT view showing the proximal extent of the same fracture

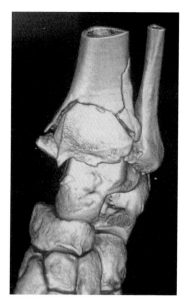

Fig. 10.58 Frontal 3D CT view of the same patient showing the main fragment produced by the dorsiflexion moment

- Anatomic reconstruction of the tibia and fibula needed for good outcome – restore articular surface, length, angular alignment, rotation alignment, bony shape and contour – done via anatomic reduction, and rigid internal fixation, followed by immediate mobilisation

■ Revised goal even among keen AO followers in view of poor result from the use of traditional AO techniques in high energy *explosive* type of pilon fracture: anatomic reduction of articular fracture, but not diaphyseal fracture and stabilisation to withstand the local biomechanical demands – relative stability, preserve blood supply to bone and soft tissue. Initial period of temporising spanning EF to buy time for soft tissues to quieten down. Then, elective fracture fixation (preferably by MIPO) and pain-free mobilisation preventing the development of fracture disease

■ If soft tissue injury too severe (especially in face of a shattered articular surface) the goal is changed to:

■ Aiming at minimal disruption of soft tissue and use of strong EF as the definitive fixation

■ However, reconstruction of the ankle mortise is essential and this often necessitates adjunctive (often percutaneous) internal fixation. Proper alignment of the mortise beneath the shaft is important, although some shortening is acceptable (if it is deemed this will increase chance of union), mobilisation usually has to be delayed for typically around 12 weeks

10.17.10 Rn Options

■ Conservative
■ Operative
  - OR + IF ± BG
  - CR + IF (± MIPO technique)
  - EF (bridging and non-bridging)
  - EF + adjunctive IF (an occasional scenario may even end up in amputation especially in the face of other ipsilateral limb injury, or in the presence of complications)

10.17.11 The Case for Conservative Rn

- Indications:
  - Not commonly indicated except if fracture undisplaced, belongs to low-energy injury, especially in the elderly

10.17.12 Operative Indications

- Most pilon fractures need operation since essentially an intra-articular fracture
- But it is the timing of the operation, and due respect for the soft tissues that are the most important issues

(P.S. Schatzker is of the opinion that a poorly done ORIF is worse than conservative treatment in tibial plateau fractures; it is the view of the author that this statement is even more true if applied to Pilon fractures)

10.17.13 Timing of Operation

- Most high energy injuries need an initial period of EF to maintain length (bone as well as soft tissue), alignment and rotation
- Timing of definitive fixation usually delayed for 2 or more weeks. Early plating of high energy fracture increased sepsis and wound complications
- In situations where plating was not planned, the EF was then used as a definitive buttress device. Elective adjunctive surgery to restore the articular surface (preferably percutaneous technique or mini-incisions) are also usually done when the soft tissue is more stable

10.17.14 Traditional ORIF ± BG

- Traditionally, good results were obtained for rotational type of injuries (as in skiing) as reported by Ruedi, but not for high energy axial compression injuries. Most employ the anteromedial approach
- Wait until soft tissue envelope better, e.g. aspirated blisters had epithelialised, wrinkle sign present. Sometimes this takes several weeks. Impatience is a frequent cause of wound complications, necrosis and sepsis
- Contrary to previous old AO teachings, only small fragment plates are advisable. Examples include one-third tubulars, 3.5-mm DCP. Avoid bulky implants

10.17.15 Role of EF

- Spanning EF: most useful as temporising device, but a much more rigid construct of spanning fixation needs to be made if we plan to use EF as definitive fixation
- Indications for the hybrid fixator:
  - If open reduction not thought to be required, especially if fracture spans large areas
  - The distal fragment can be stably fixed by olive wires

10.17.16 EF Used as Temporary Measure

- Done as urgent procedure usually
- If later plate fixation is planned, can consider fibula plating in the same go to help restore length, rotation, lateral column and articular surface
- Notice fibula plating not always recommended; however, if it is not planned for the patient to have definitive plating, as mild degree of shortening is sometimes allowed if EF is going to be used as definitive fixation

10.17.17 EF Used as Definitive Treatment

- Rationale put forward by proponents for this technique:
  - Minimise soft tissue dissection since soft tissue injury is a major cause of poor outcome
  - EF can help in regaining length and alignment, some shortening is acceptable. The EF also has a buttressing role
  - Reconstruction of the articular surface and mortise is important, but sometimes done electively when the soft tissue quietens down
  - The EF used for this technique must be a strong pin-fixator construct to last for > 12 weeks at least

10.17.18 Complications

- Arthrosis – dependent on restoration of the articular surface, which is not easy in the explosive type of injury. The area commonly affected is the central plafond

- Sepsis – predisposed by poor soft tissue envelope and operating too early. Placement of the pins of the EF too near to the joint may also cause sepsis
- Malunion – early application of the spanning EF helps restore limb alignment and length. If definitive plating of the distal tibia planned, early fixation of the fibula fracture aids restoration of rotation alignment besides reconstitution of the lateral column
- Non-union – adequate BG can be inserted during open surgery for definitive fixation
- Skin breakdown and necrosis – knowledge of the angiosomes of this region help to prevent skin necrosis after open surgery. Use of low profile implants is recommended, as are MIPO techniques
- Neurovascular complications – despite the use of standard published "safe corridors", administration of thin olive wires of the hybrid EF runs the risk of injury especially the neurovascular structures of the anterior compartment

10.18 Ankle: Pott's Fracture

10.18.1 Mechanism
- Most are indirect injuries
- Most common mechanisms being supination external rotation injuries

10.18.2 Neer's Traditional "Ring Concept"
- Neer visualises the tibia, fibula, talus and ligaments form a stable ring in the *coronal* plane
- One break in the ring said not to cause instability
- Two breaks in the ring produces an unstable situation
- This is obviously not entirely true, examples:
  - Maisonneuve fracture: besides medial malleolus fracture (Fig. 10.59), the fractured fibula is located very high up and not in the circle drawn by Neer. Maisonneuve fracture results in mortise instability from significant IOM disruption

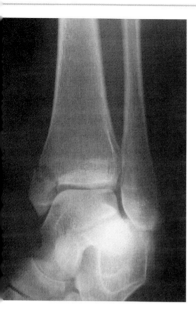

Fig. 10.59 As isolated medial malleolus fractures are not extremely common, sometimes need to rule out an associated proximal fibula fracture and check the mortise view for any diastasis

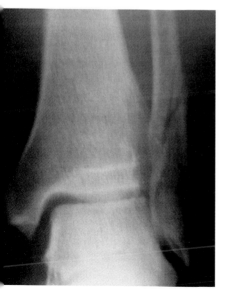

Fig. 10.60 Biomechanical studies showed that even minor degrees of talar shift in, say, fractured distal fibula patients can cause uneven stress distribution over the talus and if present may need fixation. Careful screening is essential before deciding on conservative treatment

— Some displaced isolated fibula fractures have talar shift, which needs operative stabilisation as even minor talar shift (Fig. 10.60) can cause abrupt increase in contact stresses of the ankle

10.18.3   AO Classification (Weber)

- Weber A – infra-syndesmotic lesion
- Weber B – trans-syndesmotic lesion
- Weber C – supra-syndesmotic lesion

(Higher fibular fracture cases tend to have more extensive damage to the tibiofibular ligament, and more likely to have ankle mortise instability, which may require syndesmosis screws)

10.18.4   Lauge–Hansen Classification

- Supination ER injury
- Pronation abduction injury (at syndesmosis)
- Pronation abduction injury (above syndesmosis)
- Pronation ER injury
- Supination adduction injury

10.18.4.1   Supination ER Injury

- Stage 1: anterior tibiofibular complex disruption
- Stage 2: fracture fibula at/above syndesmosis
- Stage 3: posterior tibiofibular complex disruption
- Stage 4: deltoid ligament disruption

10.18.4.2   Pronation Abduction at Syndesmosis

- Stage 1: deltoid ligament complex disruption
- Stage 2: fractured fibula at level of syndesmosis

10.18.4.3   Pronation Abduction Above Syndesmosis

- Stage 1: deltoid ligament complex disruption
- Stage 2: anterior and posterior tibiofibular ligament complex disruption
- Stage 3: fracture of fibula above the syndesmosis

0.18.4.4 Pronation ER Injury (Fig. 6.61)
- Stage 1: deltoid ligament complex disruption
- Stage 2: anterior tibiofibular ligament complex disruption
- Stage 3: fractured fibula above the syndesmosis
- Stage 4: posterior tibiofibular ligament disruption

0.18.4.5 Supination Adduction Injury
- Stage 1: lateral collateral ligament complex disruption
- Stage 2: vertical fracture of the medial malleolus

0.18.5 Some Special Indirect Injury Patterns
- Bosworth fracture
- Maisonneuve fracture

0.18.5.1 Bosworth Fracture
- Involves posterior dislocation of the fibula behind the tibia

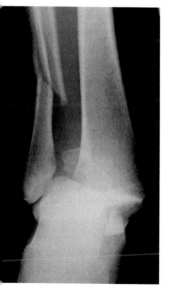

Fig. 10.61 Notice this pronation injury involves fracture of the medial, posterior and lateral malleoli

- Involves seven stages:
  - Anterior tibiofibular complex injury
  - Posterior tibiofibular complex rupture
  - Stretching of anteromedial capsule
  - IOM partial tear
  - Dislocation of fibula behind the tibia
  - Obliquely fractured fibula at level of syndesmosis
  - Deltoid complex injury

10.18.5.2 *Maisonneuve Fracture*

- This injury is important because if Dx is missed, failure to recognis the diastasis and stabilise the syndesmosis can cause widening of th mortise and subsequent OA
- Five stages:
  - Injury of anterior tibiofibular ligament and interosseous ligamen complexes
  - Injury of posterior tibiofibular ligament complex of the syndes mosis
  - Rupture or avulsion of the anteromedial joint capsule
  - PE or SE type fractured proximal fibula
  - Injury of the deltoid ligament complex

10.18.6   Work-up

- Assess associated soft tissue injury and neurovascular status
- The squeeze test may be positive if IOM injured
- X-ray: AP/lateral and mortise should be performed
- Check for any talar shift and subluxation (e.g. Shenton's line of th ankle). In case of doubt, compare with the normal contralateral sid with respect to the medial clear space and the degree of tibiofibula overlap

10.18.7   Pott's Fracture – General Management

- Those with fracture dislocation/subluxation (Figs. 10.62, 10.63 needs urgent reduction to avoid pressure necrosis on the articula cartilage, and restore alignment. Early joint reduction also help t reduce swelling

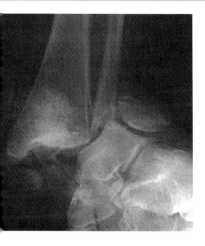

Fig. 10.62 Fracture dislocation of the ankle always needs emergency reduction lest there is pressure necrosis of the cartilage due to impingement by sharp fracture fragments

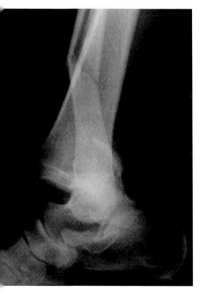

Fig. 10.63 For the same reasoning, urgent reduction is needed for this ankle. The second advantage of early reduction is to prevent excessive soft tissue swelling

■ Undisplaced fractures: casting can be done with NWB ×6 weeks, then gradual weight-bearing. Serial X-ray with mortise view to check alignment

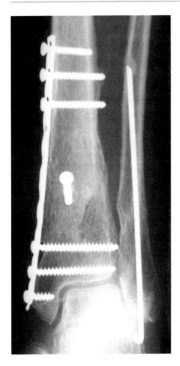

Fig. 10.64 Percutaneous techniques are sometime useful in elderly osteoporotic pilon or Pott's fractures, especially in those with badly traumatised sof tissues or those who have poor vascularity

- Displaced fractures: need ORIF. Syndesmosis screw needed usuall in Weber C and some Weber B. If unsure, intraoperatively stress th syndesmosis with a bone hook and perform dynamic fluoroscopi screening. Percutaneous fixation in the elderly osteoporotic bone i sometimes preferred (Fig. 10.64) especially in the face of trauma tised soft tissues

10.19 Fractured Talus

10.19.1 Osteology
- Anterior wider – DF improves stability

■ Weakest in neck where bone recessed to allow DF
■ Talar neck deviates medially and shortened in medial aspect
■ Medial tilt 25 ± 10°; downward tilt 25 ± 15°
■ 60% coverage by cartilage, no tendon attachment
■ Talar neck – only extra-articular portion
■ Talo-calcaeal ligament important to stabilise talar neck and the distal fragment in talar neck fractures
■ Post T-C ligament usually the last supporting structure before body of talus dislocates from the mortise
■ Os trigonum – congenital non-union of the lateral posterior process and can cause pain in ballet dancers
■ Lateral process acts as a wedge and causes disruption of the acute angle of Gissane in cases of fractured calcaneum

0.19.2   Problems Areas

■ Like the scaphoid, the talus has a tenuous blood supply and AVN can cause problems
■ Assessment of reduction not easy
  – In sagittal plane: use lateral X-ray
  – In the transverse plane (look for any varus ± rotation) using the Canale view
■ Remember the close association of three joints: ankle/subtalar/talo-navicular joint (TNJ). Assess each of these three joints intently in any patient with talus fracture
■ More difficult cases can have rotation element of the distal fragment (as the talo-calcaneal ligament is disrupted) as well as possible varus from medial comminution and association with fractured medial malleolus → reduction of even minor degrees of malreduction important because even minor malreduction causes abnormal peak stresses at the subtalar joint
■ Difficulties with operative exposure

0.19.3   Blood Supply

■ Artery of tarsal canal is major supply (from posterior tibial)
■ Artery of sinus tarsi (from anterior tibial and peroneal)

- Deltoid branch from tarsal artery which enters through the deltoid ligament

(P.S. Anastomotic sling beneath neck of talus from the tarsal and sinus tarsi arteries)

10.19.4   Injury Mechanism

- Hyperdorsiflexion with neck of talus impacting on anterior lip of tibia

(In laboratory experiments: talar neck fractures can be reproduced by neutral ankle position and compressing calcaneus against talus and tibia)

10.19.5   Hawkins Classification

- Type 1: undisplaced fracture
- Type 2: displaced with subtalar joint involvement
- Type 3: displaced with both subtalar and ankle subluxation ± dislocation
- Type 4: type 2 or 3 with talo-navicular joint subluxation

10.19.6   Clinical Setting and X-ray Assessment

- Most in younger patients, and also in aviators (aviator's astragalus)
- High energy trauma
- Associated injuries: medial malleolus (30% Hawkins type 3) and beware of open fractures in Hawkins type 3
- X-ray: AP + lateral + canale view (modified AP)
- Lateral X-ray: check neck displacement, assess congruity of the subtalar joint + ankle joint + TNJ

10.19.7   Use of Canale View in Checking Reduction

- Canale view allows for better profile to assess alignment of talar neck in the transverse plane
- Intraoperative canale view is also recommended to ensure proper talar head alignment

10.19.8 Role of CT

■ Useful to see:
- Talus head fracture
- If not sure about anatomic reduction (sometimes) with talus neck fracture, helps assess talus comminution and usual varus alignment
- Dx: some Cx like non-union
- Talus body fracture assessment and especially assessment of suspected fracture of lateral process (snow-boarder's injury)

10.19.9 Role of MRI

■ Detects AVN 6–12 weeks after injury if titanium screws were used in fracture fixation
■ AVN risks in different Hawkin's classes:
- Type 1 – 0–10%
- Type 2 – 20–50%
- Type 3 – 80–100%
- Type 4 – same as type 3, or higher

10.19.10 Surgical Exposures

■ Anteromedial – from anterior aspect of medial malleolus to dorsal aspect of navicular tuberosity (avoid deltoid ligament) – extensile since can be made posterior to medial malleolus to allow for medial malleolar osteotomy if needed
■ Anterolateral: from tip of fibula to anterior process of calcaneus; retract EDB superiorly – allows irrigation of joint, and more accurate reduction of the talar neck– especially in cases of medial comminution

10.19.11 Goals of Treatment

■ Urgent anatomic reduction – to restore congruency of ankle/subtalar joints to reduce risk of AVN
■ Minimise OA and skin necrosis

10.19.12 Conservative Versus Operative

- Conservative Rn may only be tried in Hawkin's type 1 *if* we are certain there is no fracture displacement and subtalar joint congruence
- Hawkin's type 2 most will operate *even* if CR looks good, if only to avoid ankle equinus contracture secondary to prolonged plantar flexion casting
- Higher Hawkin's grades obviously need surgical treatment

10.19.13 Screw Fixation Pearls (Fig. 10.65)

- Do not use compression screw in the presence of medial comminution
- Mostly use 3.5-mm screws
- Screw countersunk/from posterior towards the head
- Ti screw advisable

10.19.14 Treatment: Hawkins 1

- Undisplaced, stable
- Cast in neutral until X-ray union
- 6–8 weeks short leg then two or more additional protection

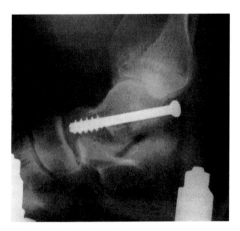

Fig. 10.65 Postoperative radiograph after screw fixation in talar neck fracture. Titanium screws should preferably be used. Intraoperative Canale view is useful alignment checking

- Need to rule out spontaneous reduced Hawkin's type 2 fracture, i.e. those fractures that are likely to displace when ankle placed in neutral position

10.19.15 Treatment: Hawkins 2

- CR that should be immediate via: maximum plantar flexion, traction, and realign talus head with either varus or valgus stress to correct deformity in the transverse plane
- This type features incongruent or dislocated subtalar joint – make sure subtalar joint is properly reduced

10.19.16 Treatment: Hawkins 3

- Real orthopaedic emergency for two reasons:
  - Skin under tension
  - Body of talus pivots upon deltoid ligament twisting the only remaining blood supply from deltoid branches (vessels)
- Rn: immediate ORIF (usually by combined anteromedial/anterolateral approach)
- Look for any associated medial malleolus fractures

10.19.17 Treatment: Hawkins 4

- This type added in the modified Hawkin's classes (by Kanele) – same as type 3 but TNJ involved
- Note: whether to replace a thrown out fragment in open fracture rather controversial: if contaminated may consider removal, followed by spanning EF and elective Blair's fusion. If not, try to preserve fragment

10.19.18 Complications
10.19.18.1 Skin Necrosis/Osteomyelitis

- Debridement and early soft tissue cover ± flap
- Osteomyelitis will require excision of body of talus
- Some authors believe contaminated talar body should not be replaced in the foot if completely extruded

10.19.18.2 Non-union/Malunion

- Non-union not common
- Delayed union common
- Malunion common with incongruent joint and degenerative OA ankle/subtalar articulation
  - Varus most common from medial comminution
  - Some with resultant supination and poor ROM
  - Salvage: triple arthrodesis or talar neck osteotomy

10.19.18.3   Subtalar/Ankle OA/Arthrofibrosis

- Arthrofibrosis very common
- Prevention most important – early ROM following wound healing if rigid IF attained is encouraged
- Some cases of a bad result despite good and early fixation? Due to chondral damage

10.19.18.4   AVN

- Dx:
  - Absence of Hawkin's sign at 6–8 weeks suggestive of but does not guarantee AVN (Hawkin's sign – owing to subchondral osteopenia – is a good sign as it indicates intact vascularity seen in either mortise/AP but not lateral X-ray at 6–8 weeks – do not comment on its presence or absence while in cast)
  - MRI (used if Ti screw used): done at around 6–12 weeks post-injury
- AVN if present, can be complete or partial
- Rn:
  - Use of vascularised BG reported: before there is significant collapse or OA
  - Prolonged NWB
- Prognosis: AVN, although does not universally give poor result; there are case reports of collapse >2 years after AVN post-injury on weight-bearing

10.19.19 Management of Talar Head Fracture

- Dx can be difficult and may require CT

- Healing not a problem since very vascular
- Restoration of articular congruency is our aim

10.19.20 Types of Fractured Talus Body and Rn

- Coronal type – variant of talar neck fracture; more likely to need malleolar osteotomy for exposure
- Sagittal type – also requires anatomic reduction; may additionally need malleolar osteotomy, placement of screws from medial to lateral
- Horizontal fracture – if mixed with a crushed talus high chance of AVN, collapse common despite ORIF
- Acute traumatic osteochondral fracture: anterolateral in position – ankle arthroscopy: excise, or fix if large fragment
- Lateral process – snow-boarder's ankle; present with persistent hindfoot pain after sprain; may miss on plain X-ray – confirms with CT. Rn: excision if pain persists; ORIF if large
- Posterior tuberosity fracture – need to form DDx from OS trigonum. Rn: conservative unless significant involvement of the posterior facet – excise if pain persists

10.19.21 Feature of Talar Body Fracture

- In a recent multiple trauma centre study on fractured talus, it was found that although talar body fractures were less common than fractured talar neck or process; fractured talar body is commonly associated with subsequent degenerative joint disease of both the ankle and subtalar joints and the incidence of permanent disability is high
- Preservation of the talus and reconstruction of the body (if feasible) is preferred to options like primary tibiocalcaneal fusion or external fixation (Foot Ankle Int 2000)

10.20 Fractured Calcaneum

10.20.1 Relevant Anatomy: Osteology

- Four articular facets: anterior and middle hidden by stout TC ligament; posterior facet is the facet that needs to be well visualised intraoperatively in fixing os calcis fractures. The fourth facet is for the cuboid

■ Talus sits medial to the mid-axis superiorly – hence it acts to split the calcaneum in half and shear off the commonly present, important anteromedial fragment (with the attached sustentaculum)

10.20.2   Relevant Anatomy: Trabeculae

■ Understanding trabeculae distribution helps in the design of our screw direction for better fixation. The most dense bone lies just below the articular facets superiorly and the sustentaculum area. Note also the medial wall is significantly thicker than the lateral wall – at some area as thick as 4 mm

■ Four groups of trabeculae – thalamic (continues the pattern of talus, distal tibia), anterior apophyseal (between cuboid and posterior facet), plantar, and posterior group

10.20.3   Trabeculation Density Distribution

■ Superiorly: condensation occurs beneath posterior facet of calcaneum (thalamic portion)

■ Medially: dense at sustentaculum tali

■ Lateral: less dense and thinner cortical shell than medial cortex due to eccentric loading

■ Centre: subthalamic portion sparse trabeculation

■ Anteriorly: quite dense, the anterior part is strong, supporting the lateral foot column

■ Posteriorly: dense bone at the tuberosity

10.20.4   Clinical Correlation

■ Screws should preferably be placed at points of higher trabecular density viz:
  — Superiorly: subchondral area
  — Medially: at sustentacular portion
  — Posteriorly: at tuberosity
  — ± Anteriorly – if calcaneocuboid articulation shattered, may use a longer plate to splint the area of comminution

0.20.5   Location of Primary Fracture Lines

- The primary fracture line is produced by the effect of talus lateral process hitting on the acute angle of Gissane. It is called "primary" because it occurs early in fracture genesis. This will divide the calcaneus into the anterior and posterior portions
- The primary fracture line also splits the posterior facet, then runs anteriorly and dissipates into the body – thus the fracture can extend to anterior/cuboid facets

0.20.6   Other Typical Findings

- Lateral wall crushed outward
- As the talus recoils upwards, it carries with it the superomedial fragment. The split off lateral piece of the posterior facet got buried into the body
- The tuberosity fragment falls into a varus angulation

0.20.7   Main Fracture Fragments in a Typical Case

- Anteromedial fragment
- Tuberosity fragment
- Lateral posterior facet fragment
- Anterolateral fragment

0.20.8   Essex Lopresti Classification

- In pre-CT era, understandably an X-ray classification was used, based mainly on the lateral X-ray
- Classification based on whether fracture is extra-articular or intra-articular, and whether fracture displaced or not
- The "tongue" type included in this classification is so called since the posterior facet fragment is connected to part of the tuberosity and looks like a tongue. This is in contrast to the usual "joint depression" type (Fig. 10.66)

0.20.9   Principle of Roy Sanders' Classification

- Roy Sanders focuses on the number of posterior facet fragments and displacement
- The classification is based on mainly coronal CT images

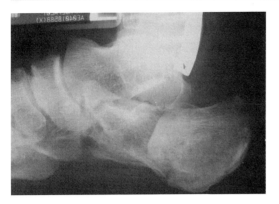

Fig. 10.66 Os calcis fractures that involve the subtalar joint require anatomical reduction, as is true for other intra-articular fractures

10.20.10 Roy Sanders' (CT) Classification
- Type 1: undisplaced fracture
- Type 2: two major posterior facet fragments
- Type 3: three major posterior facet fragments
- Type 4: > three major pieces – i.e. comminuted fracture

10.20.11 Usefulness of Roy Sanders' Classification
- Gives an idea of final outcome
- Type 1: non-operative – 85% good result
- Type 2: if anatomically reduced 85% good result
- Type 3: less good results despite anatomic reduction
- Type 4: as high as 70% had bad result since fracture comminuted and difficult to obtain anatomic reduction

10.20.12 Summary of Problems in this Region
- Broadened hind-foot
- Stiffness of the subtalar joint
- Muscle imbalance
- Peroneal tendon impingement
- Progressive arthrosis

10.20.13 Goal of Surgery

- Proper restoration of the joint. In the usual scenario of joint depression type fractures, restoration of the posterior facet
- Rigid fixation to allow early motion and prevent subtalar stiffness
- Attention to soft tissues to prevent complications like flap necrosis
- Proper restoration of the Bohler's angle and restoration of the normal shape of the os calcis to prevent complications like peroneal impingement, altered mechanics and mechanical advantage of important nearby structures like Achilles tendon

10.20.14 Evidence Supporting the Operative Approach

- Randle in 2000 performed meta-analysis to compare operative vs non-operative treatment of displaced intra-articular fractures of os calcis
- Among 1,845 articles, only six articles made the above comparison
- The statistical summary of the six articles revealed a trend for surgically treated cases to more likely return to same type of work than non-operated cases. The non-operative cases have higher likelihood of severe foot pain than the operated group

10.20.15 The Case for Emergency Operation

- Open fracture
- Compartment syndrome
- Fracture severe soft tissue injury, which may need immediate debridement or coverage

10.20.16 Preoperative Work-up

- Assess bony anatomy: most if not all cases planned for surgery need X-ray and CT scan (Fig. 10.67)
- Assess soft tissue status: affects the timing of operation
- Assess associated injuries: a common injury is collapsed fracture of the lumbar vertebra
- Document neurovascular status

10.20.17 Pearls for Operative Success

- Proper patient selection

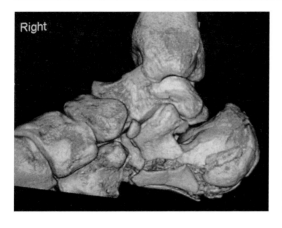

Fig. 10.67 While coronal CT images help us in classification by Sanders' system, 3D CT may be of help in cases with more complex fracture patterns

- Choice of operative approach
- Method of reduction and fixation
- Use of BG

10.20.17.1 *Proper Patient Selection*
- Extra caution should be exercised in patient groups with poor prognosis despite surgery
- Knowledge of who will benefit most from surgery is also important

10.20.17.1.1 *Benefactors of Surgery*
- Younger patients (<30)
- Moderately lower Bohler angle (0–14°)
- Fracture comminution
- Light workload
- Anatomical reduction achieved
- Articular step-off <2 mm

10.20.17.1.2 *Poor Prognostic Factors*
- Workers compensation cases
- Open fractures
- Significant cartilage injury identified intraoperatively

- Significant concomitant soft tissue injury
- Delayed reduction >14 days
- High body mass index
- Smoking

10.20.17.1.3 Recent Prospective Randomised Trial
- In 2002, Buckley reported 309 patients was followed and assessed for a minimum of 2 years
  - Without stratification into groups, the functional results of non-operative and operative groups are comparable
  - However, after unmasking the data by removal of worker's compensation cases; the outcome was significantly better in some groups of surgically treated patients

10.20.17.2 Choice of Operative Approach
- The lateral approach is the most popular
- The medial approach proposed by McReynolds seldom used, the drawback being interference by posterior tibial neurovascular bundle and the cutaneous nerves
- In general, if one approach is used, some type of indirect reduction of the opposite column is needed

10.20.17.2.1 The Medial Approach
- The whole initial idea of McReynolds stems from and stresses the importance of reduction of the anteromedial fragment to the tuberosity fragment *before* proper reduction of lateral wall fragment (harbouring the posterior facet) can occur
- Burdeaux and McReynolds stress that the anteromedial fragment is quite a consistent finding, but fragment size varies, and can be adequately visualised by CT

10.20.17.2.2 The Lateral Approach (Often Used)
- Berniscke is instrumental in proposing the lateral approach – which is essentially a fasciocutaneous flap based on the peroneal artery
- Take care to avoid damaging the sural nerve, especially at the most proximal and lateral extent of the L-shaped incision

10.20.17.2.3   The Case for Minimally Invasive Procedures

- In selected cases with simple fracture patterns (especially if extra-articular) we can consider the use of percutaneous screw fixation ± the help of intraoperative arthroscopy as well as fluoroscopy

10.20.17.3   Method of Reduction

10.20.17.3.1   Pearl 1

- The anteromedial fragment needs to be reduced anatomically, otherwise reduction of the posterior facet will be difficult – done indirectly by distraction or with manipulation by Schanz screw into tuberosity. Once medial wall reduced, can consider temporary k-wire fixation axially directed. Plate used (e.g. one-third tubular, reconstruction plate, AO calcaneal plate, and special Y or W plates). Avoid displacing tuberosity into varus

10.20.17.3.2   Pearl 2

- Reduction of posterior facet needs to be as accurate as possible
- Problem: this can be difficult to assess once it is reduced – use of intraoperative Broden or axial view with X-ray screening is recommended ± use a 2.7-mm arthroscopy light-source to get a better visual

10.20.17.3.3   Pearl 3

- What about assessing the reduction of the anterior and middle facets (which usually remain hidden behind the interosseous talocalcaneal [TC] ligament) and the cuboid facet (with its complex saddle shape making full visual difficult)
- Fortunately, these fractures often reduce indirectly when other components of the fracture have been reduced anatomically

10.20.17.3.4   Intraoperative Pearls

- Intraoperative reduction should be checked to ensure:
  - Restoration of the lateral length and alignment

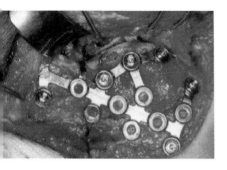

Fig. 10.68 The os calcis plate is specially designed for fixing os calcis fractures, as is shown here

- Accurate reduction of the anterolateral fragment and the acute angle of Gissane
- Anatomical reduction of subtalar congruity and restoration of the overall shape of the calcaneus are important prognostic factors. Most cases can be fixed with the use of the new os calcis plates (Fig. 10.68)
- Before finishing the operation, it is good practice to screen intraoperatively for Bohler angle restoration by fluoroscopy

10.20.17.4 Issue of BG

- Histomorphology revealed that the inferior central region of the calcaneum is normally devoid of trabeculae. Bone grafting to "fill the void of the posterior facet" is not routinely indicated
- At times may be considered to speed healing and support selected very comminuted fracture although clinical data lacking

10.20.18 Role of Primary Subtalar Arthrodesis

- May be considered in very comminuted fractures affecting the posterior facet quite beyond reconstruction
- Not much literature or clinical data available, however

10.20.19 Complications

- Broadened hind-foot

- Stiffness of the subtalar joint
- Muscle imbalance and altered TA mechanics
- Peroneal tendon impingement
- Progressive arthrosis
- Malunion – will be discussed
- Sepsis
- Wound necrosis

10.20.19.1 Malunions
- Should be avoided by proper operative intervention in indicated cases, prevention is important
- In established malunions, Rn options after failed conservative Rn include: lateral wall decompression, subtalar in situ fusion, and sometimes calcaneal osteotomy (along the former fracture line)
- Prevention of other complications discussed already

10.21 Subtalar Dislocation

10.21.1 Classification
- Refers to direction of foot displacement
- Medial dislocation – head of talus prominent dorsolaterally
- Lateral dislocation – the reverse

10.21.2 Diagnosis
- Physical examination: head of talus usually palpated anterior to medial malleolus, foot is shortened, foot deformed, check neurovascular status
- 15% are open injuries, subsequent skin slough common in these cases
- X-ray: order AP/lateral/oblique
- ± CT, e.g. if suspect osteochondral fragment

10.21.3 Common Foot Posture on Presentation
- Most commonly (85%) the foot is displaced medially with the calcaneus lying medially, the head of the talus prominent dorsolaterally

10.21.4   Uncommon Foot Posture

- Less commonly (15%), lateral dislocation occurs. In this case, the calcaneus is displaced lateral to the talus, the talar head is prominent medially, and the navicular lies lateral to the talar neck
- Long-term prognosis appears to be worse with the lateral dislocation

10.21.5   Summary of Management

- Closed injuries: try CR
- Early CR/OR to lessen skin necrosis
- But many cases need open reduction
- CT – check osteochondritis dissecans (OCD) and congruency of reduction post-CR (if open reduction indicated, can check for OCD intraoperatively)
- Rn of associated injuries: fractured talar neck, osteochondral fracture, calcaneus fracture, etc.

10.21.6   Method of Reduction

- Most can be reduced by:
  - Relaxation by general or spinal anaesthesia
  - Flex knee to relax Achilles tendon
  - Firm longitudinal foot traction
  - Reversal of deformity or direct digital pressure
  - Shearing osteochondral fractures from the articular surface in up to 45% of patients

10.21.7   Goal of Surgery

- Congruous reduction and maintain reduction
- CR if successful: cast for 4 weeks if skin satisfactory
- Most need OR, obstacles to reduction include:
  - In medial dislocation: buttonhole of talar head through lateral ST extensor digitorum brevis (EDB), extensor retinaculum, bifurcate ligament)
  - Obstacle to lateral dislocation reduction: tibialis posterior, and occasional case difficult reduction due to osteochondral fragment and fractured talar neck

10.21.8   Operative Method

- Long skin incision over head of talus, remove osteochondral fragment, and retract ST obstacles. Tibialis posterior if ruptured needs repair
- Short leg plaster, 6 weeks NWB
- All pantalar cases need OR. Pinning across TNJ or talocrural joint ± EF needed in severe ST problems

10.21.9   Appendix: Rare Pantalar Dislocation

- High chance of AVN
- Whether to put back depends on time lapse and degree of contamination: ST cover and Rn most important followed by bony procedure
- In acute situation can transfix from calcaneus through talus to tibia, another fixation pin through, say, navicular
- If concomitant comminuted os calcis then situation more complex:
  - If ST bad: spanning EF, but avoid potential flap sites; elective reconstruction later
  - If ST good, and early recovery of a clean talus, then put back, reduce and fix with pins
  - Other possible options – talectomy; or primary subtalar fusion

10.22   Lisfranc Fractures

10.22.1   Relevant Anatomy

- The second metatarsal (MT) can be thought of as the keystone of the Roman arch
- Width of metatarsals dorsal > plantar – hence offers architectural stability
- The second MT is key to reduction in these complex fracture dislocations
- The fourth and fifth MT are much more mobile normally and articulate with the cuboid

- Cuboid-third cuneiform articulation also important for mobility of the lateral complex

10.22.2   Relevant Anatomy (Cont`d)

- Base of first MT stabilised by: capsule + tibialis anterior + peroneus longus
- No interosseous ligament between base of first MT and second MT – but there are strong plantar and dorsal ligaments
- Lisfranc ligament = ligament between the medial cuneiform (under first MT) and second MT (the dorsal and central parts of this interosseous ligament)

10.22.3   Patho-anatomy in Lisfranc Dislocation

- Most dislocations are dorsal. Reason due to the basic bone architecture and the fact that the plantar ligaments and supporting structures are stronger (made up of: plantar fascia, peroneus longus, and intrinsic muscles) – the only time where plantar dislocation (rare) occurs is in some cases of direct crushing
- Look for associated arterial injury => perforating (inter-metatarsal) branch of the dorsalis pedis (from anterior tibial artery) that anastomoses with the plantar circulation

10.22.4   Lisfranc Classification (Quenu and Kuss)

- Homolateral
- Isolated
- Divergent

10.22.5   Association: Arterial Injury
        and Compartment Syndrome

- The anterior tibial artery gives the first dorsal and first plantar MT artery – that are essential to the circulation of the medial portions of the foot
- Disruption of arterial anastomosis can cause significant haemorrhage and compartment syndrome (Fig. 10.69)

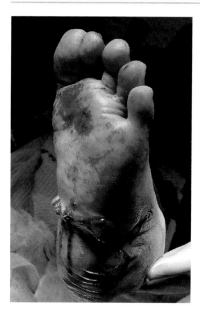

Fig. 10.69 The soft tissue status should be carefully assessed, including assessment for any compartment syndrome and vascularity

10.22.6 Most Essential Reduction to Achieve

- Restore the close relation between the first and second MT and cuneiform to:
    - Allow healing of the important Lisfranc ligament
    - Reduce the stress on the vascular system just described
- Hence, many suggest to aim at <2-mm separation between second MT and the medial cuneiform, some even suggest putting screw from medial cuneiform to second MT base

10.22.7 Mechanism

- Direct (crush) – rare mechanism, may cause the rarer plantarwards dislocation
- Indirect:
    - Axial, e.g. dancers/ballgames
    - Twisting, e.g. horse rider caught in stirrup

10.22.8 Radiological Investigation

- X-ray: AP/true lateral/30° oblique
  - Occasional use of stress films (needs anaesthetic)
  - AP standing (cold case) and compare with the contralateral side

10.22.9 Radiological Assessment

- X-ray, true lateral: proper reduction should see an unbroken line along the dorsum of the first and second MT and the respective cuneiforms
- Fleck sign: at base of second MT – this bony avulsion signifies Lisfranc ligament avulsion
- AP: medial border of second MT should align with medial border of middle cuneiform
- Oblique: medial border of the fourth MT aligns with medial border of cuboid

10.22.10 Dx in Subtle Cases

- Fleck sign
- Clinical suggestion, e.g. pain on pronation or motion of the second MT
- Increased space between second MT and medial cuneiform

10.22.11 Reasons of Failure to Reduce

- Entrapped part of Lisfranc ligament
- Tibialis anterior tendon (e.g. between first and second cuneiform; or between first/second MT) – so-called toe up sign (of Ashworth) of lateral slip of tibialis anterior
- Peroneus longus tendon (can prevent lateral tarsometatarsal joint [TMT] reduction)

(once Lisfranc joint reduced, the remainder of the foot follows since attachments of the interosseous ligament to the lesser MT)

10.22.12 Associated Injuries

- Indirect (abduction) injuries – like caught in stirrup; associated with MTPJ dislocation besides TMTJ dislocations/fracture, sometimes the MT are fractured at the neck or the base

- Abduction injury not uncommonly associated with compression fracture of cuboid
- For those cases that involve the medial complex look hard for injury to the navicular

10.22.13 Rn Goals
- Painless, stable, and plantigrade foot
- Needs early and anatomical reduction

10.22.14 Acute Management
- Index of suspicion
- Assess soft tissue
- Assess foot circulation (compromise of circulation can occur from compartment syndrome or from injury to dorsalis pedis or posterior tibial)
- Assess associated injury
- Assess any compartment
- Assess reduction and need for early operation

10.22.15 Key Tell-Tale Clinical Signs
- Stellate bruise at the plantar aspect (plantar ecchymosis sign with patch in midfoot plantar area if present suggests injury to plantar supporting structures)
- Swelling, forefoot equinus, forefoot abduction, prominence of the medial tarsal, shortened forefoot
- Tender at the Lisfranc joints

10.22.16 Timing of Surgery and Surgical Options
- Urgent reduction suggested by many
- At least early reduction needed since reduction difficult after 4–6 weeks
- Causes of failure of reduction have been discussed

10.22.17 The Case for ORIF

- Experts like Myerson propose OR if closed anatomic reduction fails, although some foot surgeons think that OR is needed in every case
- But OR absolutely indicated if vascular insufficiency not improving after CR

10.22.18 Surgical Approaches

- Extensile dorsal-medial approach ± add a lateral incision
- Dorsal incision between first/second cuneiform ± lateral incision for second/third MT reduction
- Primary arthrodesis can be considered if severe comminution

10.22.19 Surgical Fixation

- K-wires for > 6 weeks (some propose 16 weeks) + short leg cast + NWB 6 weeks + long arch support for 6–12 months
- 3.5 AO screws from MT base to tarsus
- Buzzard suggests screwing from medial cuneiform to second MT as key step (not commonly practiced)
- In general, screws less likely to lose reduction, but lateral joint complex should have some motion and be treated with k-wires

10.22.20 What to Do with Delayed/Missed Cases (Fig. 10.70)

- Sometimes missed in cases of multiple injury, can present with pain after the patient started to walk
- Most of these cases have poor outcome
- May consider arthrodesis (of first to third TMTJ)

10.22.21 Complications

- Deformity
- OA
- Treatment – arthrodesis of all the involved TMTJ except fourth/fifth TMTJ since these two may not fuse reliably and can produce long-term pain

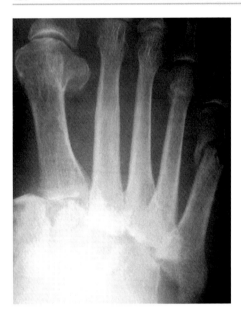

Fig. 10.70 Note the dislocated TMTJ in this patient with previously neglected Lisfranc fracture dislocation

10.23   Navicular Fracture

10.23.1   Types of Navicular Fracture
- Cortical avulsion fracture (dorsum – talo-navicular capsule and anterior deltoid fibres)
- Tuberosity – need to distinguish from accessory navicular
- Body fracture
- Stress fracture

10.23.2   Cortical Avulsion Fracture
- Eversion injury
- Talo-navicular capsule and deltoid ligament attachment
- Two accessory bones, one of talus and other of navicular, may mimic fracture

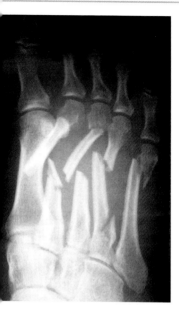

Fig. 10.71 The radiograph of the patient in Fig. 10.70, reviewing multiple metatarsal fractures

0.23.3 Navicular Stress Fracture

- Mostly in young athlete runners
- Dx is often missed
- CT scan recommended
- Early bone grafting needed for delayed cases with sclerotic fracture margins

0.24 Metatarsal Fractures (Fig. 10.71)

0.24.1 Introduction

- Common occurrence
- Several times commoner than Lisfranc injury
- Not uncommon to see fracture of four or more MT in medium- to high energy trauma (e.g. roll over injury of the foot) in which foot compartment syndrome needs to be ruled out

10.24.2   Injury Mechanism
- Direct injury, e.g. forefoot entrapped during sprain injury
- Indirect injury, e.g. foot rolled over by a vehicle

10.24.3   Assessment and Investigations
- Assess local soft tissue injury of the foot
- Assess any neurovascular injury, and any compartment syndrome
- Assess associated bony injuries
- Beware of cases with multiple basal MT fractures need to rule out Lisfranc type TMTJ subluxation or dislocation. If uncertain may need CT to Dx

10.24.4   Classification
- Classify by anatomical region:
  - Head of MT fracture
  - Subcapital fracture
  - Midshaft fracture
  - Basal fracture – rule out subluxation and Lisfranc

10.24.5   Classification of Fracture of Fifth MT
- Zone 1: tuberosity avulsion fracture
- Zone 2: Jones fracture (meta-diaphyseal junction)
- Zone 3: fractured proximal shaft (mostly stress fractures)

(Dameron 1975)

10.24.6   Goal of Treatment
- Even weight distribution of the foot
- Restore the tripod
- Restore the transverse and longitudinal arch

10.24.7   Treatment Options
- Conservative: can be considered if relatively undisplaced fracture, especially in the presence of intact border digits (i.e. intact first and fifth rays)
- Operative: other scenarios

0.24.8   Operative Indications

- Fractured first ray: most displaced fracture of first MT needs fixation. The first ray has important weight-bearing function. Need to restore the tripod action of the foot. Either CRIF or ORIF depends on individual cases
- Fifth ray: indications will be discussed
- Middle rays: err on operative Rn especially if displaced in the sagittal plane (thus affects the pressure distribution of the foot), most use k-wires. Segmental fracture may require plating

0.24.9   Treatment of Zone 1 Fifth MT Fracture (Fig. 10.72)

- Most are avulsions by lateral plantar aponeurosis attachment during inversion injury of the foot
- Displaced fracture may need Rn by k-wires and TBW

0.24.10 Treatment of Zone 2 Fifth MT Fracture

- First described by Sir Robert Jones

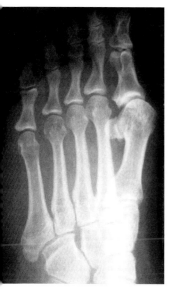

Fig. 10.72 This patient with old avulsion fracture of the tuberosity of the fifth metatarsal went on to heal uneventfully without sequelae

- Occurs in a region of watershed vascularity
- This explains the reason why healing is complicated despite the fact that this region is pretty cancellous. Also the high mobility of the fifth ray adds to the fracture instability
- If healing is slow, consider fixation by medullary screw

10.24.11 Treatment of Zone 3 Fifth MT Fracture

- Most are stress fractures due to cyclic loading, or un-accustomed activity such as marching fracture in soldiers, which is more common in second MT
- Dx sometimes tricky and may need serial X-rays, bone scan or MRI
- Acute undisplaced stress fractures – Rn conservative
- Delayed cases need screw fixation. Subgroup with already medullary sclerosis need additional BG besides internal fixation by plating

10.24.12 Complications

- Delayed/non-union: more often seen in Jones fractures
- Missed fractures, e.g. missed stress fracture
- Metatarsalgia: mostly from altered pressure distribution of the foot
- Sepsis: in cases of open fracture
- Soft tissue Cx, e.g. as in untreated foot compartment syndrome (there are nine compartments in each foot)

10.25 Toe Fractures

10.25.1 General Comments

- Common sprains or even dislocations seen in sports like turf toe and sand toe, as well as sesamoid fractures, have been described in the companion volume of this book
- Most undisplaced fractures can be treated conservatively with buddy splints and heel walking shoe
- Displaced fractures need CRIF or ORIF by miniplates and screws

General Bibliography

1. Helal B, Rowley D, Cracchiolo A III, Myerson M (1996) Surgery of disorders of the foot and ankle. Dunitz, London
2. Perry CR, Court-Brown (1999) Master cases: orthopaedic trauma. Thieme, New York
3. Ricci WM (2004) Tibial shaft fractures. American Academy of Ortho Surgeons, Illinois
4. Robinson CM, Alho A, Court-Brown CM (2002) Musculoskeletal trauma series: femur. Arnold, London

Selected Bibliography of Journal Articles

1. Anglen JC (1997) Intertrochanteric osteotomy for failed internal fixation of femoral neck fracture. Clin Orthop Relat Res (341):175–182
2. Bain GI, Zacest AC, et al. (1997) Abduction strength following intramedullary nailing of the femur. J Orthop Trauma 11:93–97
3. Baumgärtner MR, Solberg BD (1997) Awareness of tip-apex distance reduces failure of fixation of trochanteric fractures of the hip. J Bone Joint Surg Br 79:969–971
4. Bernischke SK, Melder L, et al. (1993) Closed interlocking nailing of femoral shaft fractures. Assessment of technical complications and functional outcomes by comparison of a prospective database with retrospective review. J Orthop Trauma 7:118–122
5. Bone L, Stegemann P, et al. (1993) External fixation of severely comminuted and open tibial pilon fractures. Clin Orthop Relat Res 292:101–107
6. Bray TJ, Smith-Hoeffer E, Hooper A, Timmerman L (1988) The displaced femoral neck fracture. Internal fixation versus bipolar endoprosthesis. Results of a prospective, randomized comparison. Clin Orthop Relat Res (230):127–140
7. Cash JD, Hughston JC (1988) Treatment of acute patellar dislocation. Am J Sports Med 16:244–249
8. Court-Brown CM, McQueen MM, et al. (1990) Closed intra-medullary tibial nailing: its use in closed and type 1 open fractures. J Bone Joint Surg Br 72:605–611
9. Crawfurd EJP, Emery RJH, et al. (1988) Capsular distension and intracapsular pressure in subcapital fractures of the femur. J Bone Joint Surg Br 70:195–198
10. Dameron TB Jr (1975) Fractures and anatomical variations of the proximal portion of the fifth metatarsal. J Bone Joint Surg 57(6):788–792
11. Gingras MB, Clarke J, Evarts CM (1980) Prosthetic replacement in femoral neck fractures. Clin Orthop Relat Res (152):147–157

12. Haidukewych GJ, Israel TA (2001) Reverse obliquity of fractures of the inter-trochanteric region of the femur. J Bone Joint Surg Am 83:643–650

13. Holmberg S, Dalen N (1987) Intracapsular pressure and caput circulation in nondisplaced femoral neck fractures. Clin Orthop Relat Res (219):124–126

14. Ip D (2003) Premature biomechanical failure of the distal fixation screws of the IC tibial nail. Injury 34(10):786–788

15. Koval K, Helfet D (1995) Tibial plateau fractures: evaluation and treatment. J Am Acad Orthop Surg 3:86–94

16. Koval KJ, Kummer FJ, et al. (1996) Distal femoral fixation: a laboratory comparison of the 95 degree plate, antegrade and retrograde inserted nails. J Orthop Traum 10:378–382

17. Krieg JC (2003) Proximal tibial fractures: current treatment, results, and problems. Injury 34 [Suppl 1]:A2–A10

18. Lang GJ, et al. (1995) Proximal third tibial shaft fractures: should they be nailed? Clin Orthop Relat Res 315:64–74

19. Lowell JD (1980) Results and complications of femoral neck fractures. Clin Orthop Relat Res (152):162–172

20. Lu-Yao GL, Keller RB, Littenberg B, Wennberg JE (1994) Outcomes after displaced fractures of the femoral neck. A meta-analysis of one hundred and six published reports. J Bone Joint Surg Am 76(1):15–25

21. McQueen MM, Court-Brown CM (1990) Compartment pressures after intra-medullary nailing of the tibia. J Bone Joint Surg Br 72:395–397

22. McQueen MM, Court-Brown CM, et al. (1996) Acute compartment syndrome in tibial diaphyseal fractures. J Bone Joint Surg Br 78(1):95–98

23. Oh CW, Kim PT, et al. (2005) Management of ipsilateral femoral and tibial fractures. Int Orthop 29(4):245–250

24. Pervez H, Parker MJ, et al. (2004) Prediction of fixation failure after sliding hip screw fixation. Injury 35:994–998

25. Rogmark C, Carlsson A, Johnell O, Sernbo I (2002) A prospective randomised trial of internal fixation versus arthroplasty for displaced fractures of the neck of the femur. Functional outcome for 450 patients at two years. J Bone Joint Surg Br 84:183–188

26. Sarmiento A, Gersten LM, et al. (1989) Tibial shaft fractures treated with functional braces: experience with 780 fractures. J Bone Joint Surg Br 71:602–609

27. Sasaki D, Hatori M, et al. (2005) Fatigue fracture of the distal femur arising in the elderly. Arch Orthop Trauma Surg 125(6):422–425

28. Schenck R (1994) Knee dislocations: initial assessment and complications of treatment. Instr Course Lect 43:127–136

29. Sikorski JM, Barrington R (1981) Internal fixation versus hemiarthroplasty for the displaced subcapital fracture of the femur. A prospective randomised study. J Bone Joint Surg Br 63(3):357–361

0. Stromqvist B, Hansson LI, Ljung P, Ohlin P, Roos H (1984) Pre-operative and post-operative scintimetry after femoral neck fracture. J Bone Joint Surg Br 66(1):49–54

1. Swinotkowski MF, Hansen ST Jr, et al. (1984) Ipsilateral fractures of the femoral neck and shaft. A treatment protocol. J Bone Joint Surg 66:260–268

2. Tidermark J, Zethraeus N, Svensson O, Tornkvist H, Ponzer S (2002) Quality of life related to fracture displacement among elderly patients with femoral neck fractures treated with internal fixation. J Orthop Trauma 16:34–38

3. Tidermark J, Ponzer S, et al. (2003) Internal fixation compared with total hip replacement for displaced femoral neck fractures in the elderly. J Bone Joint Surg Br 85:380–388

4. Tornetta P, Gorup J (1996) Axial computer tomography of pilon fractures Clin Orthop Relat Res 323:273–276

5. Tornetta P, Tiburzi D (1998) Antegrade vs retrograde reamed femoral nailing: A prospective randomized trial. Proceedings of OTA in Vancouver, BC, October 1998

6. Vallier HA, Bernischke SK, et al. (2004) Talar neck fractures: results and outcomes. J Bone Joint Surg Am 86(8):1616–1624

7. Wingstrand H, Stromqvist B, Egund N, Gustafson T, Nilsson LT, Thorngren KG (1986) Hemarthrosis in undisplaced cervical fractures. Tamponade may cause reversible femoral head ischemia. Acta Orthop Scand 57(4):305–308

Fractured Pelvis and Acetabulum

Contents

11.1   Management of Fractured Pelvis

11.1.1   Introduction

- 3–8% of all skeletal fractures
- Associated with high energy trauma
- 10–20% with unstable haemodynamics
- 5–50% reported morbidity and mortality
- Like scapula fractures or fracture of 1st rib, fracture of the pelvis is usually a pointer of high energy trauma, and a careful search is needed for associated injuries

11.1.2   Associated Injuries

- Reported incidence:
  - Head injury (60%)
  - Chest injury (70%)
  - Abdominal injury (60%)
  - Extremities injury (85%)

11.1.3   Clinical Anatomy

- Pelvic ring = two innominate bones and sacrum
- SIJ (sacro-ilial joint) anatomy – stability relies on posterior SI ligaments, mainly interosseous ligaments
- Pubic symphysis – hyaline cartilage on the medial articular aspect of the pubis, surrounded by fibrocartilage and fibrous tissue
- Iliopectineal line: separates true from false pelvis (false pelvis includes iliac wing and sacral ala, nearby abdominal viscera and contains iliacus muscle). True pelvis = pubis, ischium, small part of the ilium, contains true pelvic floor with vagina, rectum, urethra coccyx, levator ani muscle and coccygeal muscle

11.1.4   Normal Stabilisers of the SIJ

- Since it has no intrinsic stability, SIJ is stabilised by the strongest ligament in the body – the posterior SI ligament, which has two portions:

- Short component – runs oblique from posterior ridge of sacrum to posterior superior iliac spine (PSIS)/posterior inferior iliac spine (PIIS)
- Long component – long fibres from lateral sacrum to PSIS (merge with sacrotuberous ligament)
- Anterior SI ligament – from ilium to sacrum
- Sacrotuberous ligament works with posterior SI ligament, offers vertical stability to the pelvis. Runs from posterior sacrum and posterior iliac spine to ischial tuberosity
- Sacrospinous ligament – from lateral edge of sacrum to the sacrotuberous and inserted to ischial spine. Separates the greater and lesser sciatic notches

11.1.5   Other Adjunctive Stabilisers

- Iliolumbar ligament – from L4 and L5 transverse processes to posterior iliac crest
- Lumbosacral ligament – from L5 transverse process to the sacral ala

11.1.6   Structure of SIJ

- Articular portion – located anteriorly, the articular portion is not true synovial joint. This is because there is articular cartilage on the sacral side, whereas there is fibrous cartilage on the ilial side (hence not true synovial joint)
- Ligamentous portion – located posteriorly

11.1.7   Neural Structures at Risk in Fractured Pelvis

- Sciatic nerve sometimes injured at exit of pelvis down to piriformis
- Lumbosacral trunk – associated with fracture of sacral ala and SIJ disruption
- L5 root – easy to injure in anterior approach to SIJ – lies 2 cm medially to the SIJ

11.1.8   Vascular Structures at Risk in Fractured Pelvis

- Superior gluteal artery – most commonly injured in fractured pelvis with posterior ring disruption; also involved in BG harvest and there is danger in some posterior approaches to ORIF (if not careful, the torn artery may retract to the abdomen and need to turn and operate anteriorly)

- Corona mortis – communication between obturator and external iliac systems (arterial link in 30%, venous only in 70%) – if ruptured, may retract inferiorly to obturator foramen and cause serious bleeding

1.1.9 Other Possible Injuries

- Urethra – more fixed in males, more prone to injury than the membranous urethra in females, but bulbous urethra statistically more commonly injured than membranous portion (one Cx of these injuries/urethral ruptures is impotence – due to parasympathetic fibre injury)
- Typical signs of urethral injury – blood at meatus, cannot pass urine, high-riding prostate
- Better to do retrograde urethrogram before inserting Foley catheter, for fear of creating a bigger tear
- Bladder – extraperitoneal rupture can use conservative Rn, intraperitoneal ones require operative Rn

1.1.10 Young and Burgess Classification

- Four types: AP compression, lateral compression, vertical shear, CMI (combined mechanical injury)
- Useful in acute setting as it gives an indication of the likelihood of associated injuries, especially vascular injury: e.g. lateral compression injuries with fewer vascular Cx; open-book injury more urogenital Cx; vertical shear more vascular tears/bleeding and nerve injuries (refer to the section on damage control in Chap. 2)
- By comparison, Tile's classification stresses the direction of instability

1.1.10.1 More Details of Young's Classification

- The hemipelvis is externally rotated in open-book injuries, and internally rotated in lateral compression injuries

- In open-book injuries, diastasis of symphysis >2.5 cm indicates unstable situation, since pelvic floor starts to tear if separation ≥2.5 cm diastasis
- Lateral compression injuries: there are a few subtypes – some impact to sacrum and are stable, some have SIJ subluxation. The ones with SIJ fracture subluxation that sends a fracture line exiting at the ilium is the crescent fracture; finally, some have impaction on one hemipelvis and bucket handle opening of the contralateral hemipelvis
- Vertical instability injuries: involve tearing of the very strong posterior SI ligament, sacrospinous ligament, sacrotuberous ligament (sometimes iliolumbar ligament)

11.1.10.2   Variants of Lateral Compression Injury
- Tilt fracture of pubic rami – can cause vaginal wall impingement
- Locked symphysis pubis – beware urethral or bladder injuries
- (Contralateral) bucket-handle injury
- Crescent fracture (described by Helfet)

11.1.10.3   Crescent Fracture Dislocation of SIJ (Fig. 11.1)
- One type of lateral compression injury
- Ligament disruption of inferior part of SIJ and a vertical fracture of posterior ilium extending from the middle of the SIJ and exiting at the iliac crest (hence "crescent")
- Rotationally unstable but vertically stable (no disruption of the sacrospinous and sacrotuberous ligaments, superior part of SI ligament intact as is the PSIS)
- Operative Rn advised – to avoid Cx like OA, chronic instability, malunion, and chronic pain

11.1.11   Tile's Classification
- Type A: stable (A1 avulsion; A2 undisplaced ring; A3 transverse fractured sacrum)
- Type B: rotationally unstable and vertically stable – B1 AP compression, (<2.5 cm, >2.5 cm, bilateral with posterior injury); B2 one-sided lateral compression (many are impacted), Rami fractures com-

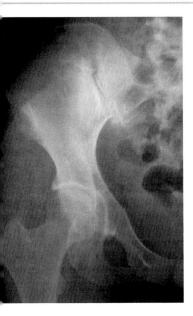

Fig. 11.1 Photograph showing a crescent fracture

mon; B3 lateral compression, contralateral bucket handle, sometimes fracture of all four rami, the bucket rotates anteriorly and superiorly with leg length discrepancy (LLD)

- Type C: both rotationally and vertically unstable – C1: one side, C2: two sides, C3: *any* pelvic fracture associated with acetabular fracture

11.1.12 Physical Assessment

- ATLS protocol: save life first
- Search associated injuries and fractures
- Wounds – e.g. Morel–Lavallee (Hak et al. 1997), and rule out open fracture especially if wound is at posterior SIJ, or at perineum – PR/PV frequently needed
- Contusion – position of bruise may give a hint on the direction of injurious force

- Haematuria – in men suggests urethral injuries, in women, may indicate open fracture
- Neurologic deficit – common with Tile's type C

11.1.13   Local Examination of the Pelvis
- LLD
- LL rotation
- Abnormal motion/crepitus
- Compression can reveal abnormal IR – suggest rotation deformity
- To check for possible vertical (posterior) translation (sometimes under X-ray control), traction by two doctors – one applies traction, the other palpates the iliac crest. Avoid rough handling of the pelvis or having the pelvis examined by different examiners many times

11.1.14   Diagnosis of Instability
- Tile's Type C: usually Dx clinically, rotation unstable if compressed, and translates abnormally both vertically and posteriorly with no firm end point if push-pull applied to the limb (recommend only one examination by an experienced examiner)
- Tile's Type B (partially stable): clinically end point to push-pull, beyond which posterior or vertical translation is not possible

11.1.15   Signs Suggesting Urethral Injury
- Cannot pass urine
- Blood at meatus
- High riding prostate
- If bladder/scrotum/hypogastric area distended and sometimes bruised

11.1.16   Radiological Assessment
- Pelvis X-ray:
  - Inlet (direct X-ray from head to mid-pelvis at an angle of 60° to X-ray table): shows posterior displacement of SIJ, ischial spine can be seen

- Outlet (taken with X-ray beam directed from foot to symphysis at angle of 45° to horizontal): help assess superior migration of iliac crest
- AP view (avulsions of L5, of sacrum and ischial spine, type of pelvic fracture)
- Judet view – useful for assessing associated acetabular fractures

11.1.17 Radiological Findings That Suggest Instability

- \> 1 cm posterior/vertical displacement
- Avulsion fracture of the sacrum or ischial spine (sacrotuberous or sacrospinous disruption)
- Avulsion fracture of the L5 transverse process (iliolumbar ligament disruption)
- SIJ subluxation or dislocation
- Vertical translation of the hemipelvis

11.1.18 Role of CT (Fig. 11.2)

- Good for SIJ assessment
- Fractured sacrum (fine cuts usually needed)
- 3D CT good for complex fracture patterns with associated acetabulum fractures (Figs. 11.3, 11.4)

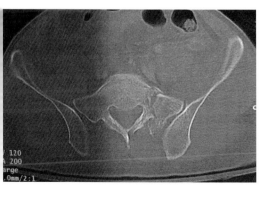

Fig. 11.2 CT film showing a lateral compression trauma

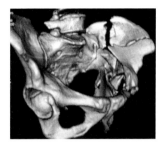

Fig. 11.3 An example of 3-D CT pelvis in assessing more complex fracture patterns

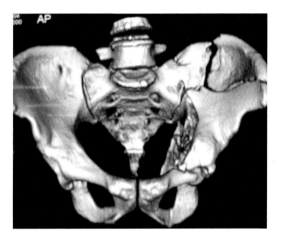

Fig.11.4 The same 3-D re construction can be viewed from different angles

- Congruency of hip relocation
- Any entrapped fragment
- Any impaction fracture on both sides of the joint
- Any associated femoral neck fractures
- Any femoral head fractures

11.1.19 Resuscitation of Shocked Patient with Fractured Pelvis

- See section on damage control for fractured pelvis in Chap. 2
- But the key points need to be highlighted

11.1.19.1 Key Points of Damage Control in Fractured Pelvis

■ Decompress body cavities (e.g. cerebral haematoma, evacuation of haemothorax)
■ Control bleeding, e.g. from the pelvis
■ Repair hollow viscus injury
■ Stabilise central fractures, e.g. pelvic ring disruption

11.1.19.2 Assessing the Severity of Haemorrhagic Shock

■ It was found that parameters like systolic BP are not always accurate since the young poly-trauma patient can tolerate up to 30% blood loss; similarly, haematocrit and Hb level are not useful in the hyper-acute situation
■ Two parameters found to be useful in recent years are:
  — Base excess: if negative BE > 10 mortality 50% (J Trauma 1996)
  — Lactate level: persistent elevation at 48 h after admission only 14% survivorship, if normalised within 24–48 h survivorship rose to 78% (J Trauma 1993). Very high lactate, nearly 10 mmol, also poor prognosis

11.1.19.3 Sources of Bleeding from Fractured Pelvis

■ Venous bleeding and bleeding from cancellous bone are the main sources. In particular, bleeding from pre-sacral venous plexus can be significant
■ Only 10% of cases are caused by arterial bleeding (not all of these can be stopped by embolisation)

11.1.19.4 Does Retroperitoneal Self-Tamponade Exist?

■ The answer is negative
■ Many haemodynamically unstable bleeding patients with fractured pelvis may have ruptured pelvic floor or peritoneum
■ This bleeding can then track downwards to the lower extremities, or upwards, commonly to the chest

11.1.19.5 Ways to Stop the Bleeding

■ Use of sheets or pelvic binder in the accident department

- Use of anti-shock garment
- Use of EF, e.g. C-clamps
- Role of embolisation – only in the less unstable patient, time-con suming
- Packing – if desperate
- Last resort – ligate internal iliac (± aortic clamping) – but save first branch if possible/since supplies gluteal artery
- Rn of associated pathologies – e.g. open fractures, ruptured blad der/urethra

11.1.19.5.1   Anti-shock Garment
- Pros: get more blood to the vital organs, splint-associated fractures ease of transport
- Cons: assessment difficult (e.g. of the abdomen, cannot perform PR PV), can produce or mask compartment syndrome, LL ischaemia can hinder breathing

11.1.19.5.2   Rationale of the Use of EF
- Decrease volume – tamponade
- Provides stability
- Clots formed are useful and prevent further bleeding

Fine Points of EF
- In ER open-book injury, place incision slightly medially to crest and along the crest, for fear of too much tension
- C-clamps useful in posterior SI disruptions
- C-clamp placement: too anterior causes IR, too posterior causes ER too inferior causes sciatic palsy
- Landmark for C-clamp – line between ASIS and PSIS intersects with another line extrapolated from axis of shaft of femur

11.1.19.6   Monitoring of Shock
- Blood lactate levels and base excess are very valuable in monitoring the degree of the haemorrhagic shock
- Severe cases may need transfusions of the order of > 30 units within the first 12 h

1.1.20   Open Pelvic Fracture Treatment

- High mortality – 40%
- Common major vascular injuries, and associated gastrointestinal tract (GIT)/genitourinary (GUT) injuries
- May need colostomy
- Key = aggressive multidisciplinary Rn is needed

1.1.20.1   Aspects of Treatment of Open Pelvic Fractures

- Index of suspicion
- Control haemorrhage
- Debride – faecal diversion may be required
- Fracture stabilisation
- Hemipelvectomy may be needed in severe cases with associated major neurovascular injuries

1.1.21   Morel–Lavallee Lesion

- Soft tissue impaction injury at GT area
- In essence, a closed degloving injury
- Subcutaneous collection up to 1 l of fluid
- Need aspiration/decompression
- High chance of bacterial infection 30–50%

1.1.22   Elective Management

1.1.22.1   Basic Principle 1

- If fracture undisplaced, still possible to have break in one site of the pelvic ring structure
- But if displaced fracture of the pelvic ring is seen, there must be another break elsewhere

1.1.22.2   Basic Principle 2 (Emile Letournel)

- Whatever the type of anterior lesion, the posterior lesion is to be treated first – since its reduction and fixation may reduce sufficiently the anterior lesion to avoid an anterior approach
- The primary fixation of an anterior fracture or disruption seldom if ever sufficiently stabilises a disrupted SI joint (with some exceptions, such as we can adequately treat a partially stable open-book injury

anteriorly if the posterior tension band ligaments are relatively intact)

11.1.22.3 Main Treatment Principles for Fractured Pelvis

- Fixation of anterior ring only cannot be relied upon to stabilise posterior disruption (Emile Letournel), exceptions mentioned
- EF alone can seldom be used as definitive fixation of posterior ring disruption
- Posterior SIJ disruptions mostly need operative fixation
- SIJ subluxation/fracture subluxation can produce chronic pain if uncorrected
- Posterior ring (SIJ) disruptions, if not adequately reduced and heal with malunion, are difficult to correct even with elective corrective surgeries, e.g. 20% complication rate, and may require a staged procedure with complicated release and/or osteotomy

11.1.22.4 How to Handle Cases of Associated Acetabular Fractures

- If patient haemodynamically unstable, priority is always given to the pelvic fracture

11.1.22.5 General Treatment Options for Fractured Pelvis

- Conservative:
    - As in Tile's A fractures, and some stable, relatively undisplaced fractures (e.g. selected AP compression injury with minimal diastasis of symphysis and spared posterior SIJ, etc.)
- Operative:
    - Most Tile's C fractures
    - Tile's B1 fractures with significant diastasis of symphysis ± SIJ involvement, some Tile's B2 fractures, e.g. crescent fractures (Rn discussed below), and most B3 fractures

11.1.22.6 Overview of Methods of Fracture Stabilisation

- Temporary measures:
    - EF mostly used with skeletal traction, especially in vertical shear injuries

- Very unusually, EF used as definitive fixation if patient cannot tolerate major surgery
- Definitive measures:
  - Percutaneous screws, e.g. iliosacral screws, have been described for selected fractures (see below)
  - These can be done with the aid of surgical navigation
  - All other cases ORIF with different implants, e.g. pelvic reconstruction plates, long cortical screws, and a host of different reduction aids and clamps needed

11.1.22.7 Summary of Causes of SIJ Disruption in the Setting of Pelvic Injury

- Associated with vertical shear injury to pelvis, as is advanced AP III
- Some subtypes of lateral compression injury to the pelvis – where there may be SIJ opening up (one type involved fracture subluxation with exit to iliac crest called crescent fracture). Other types can involve impaction into sacrum on one side with contralateral bucket-handle effect on the other contralateral hemipelvis
- X-ray assessment: look for avulsion injury of bony fragment at L5, sacrum, and ischial spine; assess vertical translation by the pelvic outlet view and AP translation in the pelvic inlet view

11.1.22.8 Summary of Rn of SIJ Disruption

- Resuscitation since bleeding can be copious
- Arrest bleeding and check sources of bleeding
- Temporary fixation, e.g. EF can be needed, sometimes with skeletal traction especially if vertical shear injury
- Assess any wounds and rule out open fracture
- Rn of associated injuries, e.g. of bladder, bowel
- Definitive fixation important since untreated SIJ subluxation dislocation is associated with chronic pain ± LLD

11.1.22.8.1 Major Fixation Methods of SIJ

- Extra-articular fixation, e.g. used by Helfet in the fixation of crescent fractures especially if the fragments are large enough

- Intra-articular – e.g. SI screws, or anterior plating (beware L5 root – use two short plates (three-holed)

11.1.22.9   Treatment of Crescent Fracture (SIJ Involved)

- OR needed to achieve a stable fixation with a congruous joint
- Helfet suggested extra-articular fixation without further violating the articular surface with hardware and provide the best potential to maintain mobility of joint and help prevent OA

11.1.22.9.1   Pros and Cons of the Anterior Approach

- Pros: anatomic reduction difficult with posterior fracture since direct visual not easy
- Cons: extensive retroperitoneal dissection, need transarticular fixation, endangering nerve root, indirect reduction of the SIJ
- Helfet uses extra-articular lag screw and neutralisation plate

11.1.22.9.2   Pros and Cons of the Posterior Approach

- Pros: familiar, easier, less dissection, many different implants to choose from, e.g. iliosacral screw, threaded rods spanning both ilia, cobra plates
- Cons: if transarticular used, danger of screw injury of neural structures, vascular (iliac vessel) ± GI as well, but all these are made unlikely if an extra-articular approach is used (make use of the partially intact posterior SI complex as part of the stabilisation construct)

11.1.22.9.3   Methods of Fixation

- Intra-pelvic: e.g. anterior SI plating

(Beware: L5 root, no need to routinely dissect it out, lest injury to structures like the vessels and ureter)

- Extra-pelvic: e.g. sacral bar

(Drawback: does not work if the post iliac prominence is not intact, and is not used if there is ST degloving)

(P.S. percutaneous iliosacral screws: X-ray C-arm to see inlet/outlet true lateral, know the screw positions, usually used for sacral fractures)

lthough sometimes used for SI fixation since anterior SI plating is a
tronger construct

1.1.23   Cx in Fractured Pelvis

- Neurological
- Urological
- HO (heterotopic ossification) – will be discussed
- Malunion – LLD, abnormal gait, sitting, back pain
- Non-union
- Back-pain – more with sacral bars
- How about pregnancy – obstetricians must be informed of the condition when vaginal delivery planned

1.1.24   Risks Factors for HO

- Double approach
- Iliofemoral approach
- Less with Kocher–Langenbeck
- T-fracture
- Hx of HO

1.1.24.1   Brook's Classification

- Type I: Islands of bone <1 cm diameter
- Type II: larger bone islands, leaving at least 1 cm free space between the two bones of the hip
- Type III: free space between the ossification and the pelvis or femur is < 1 cm
- Type IV: apparent ankylosis by bone bridge

N.B. critics say this classification is unreliable since it is 2D, hence the 3D CT classification is preferred)

1.1.24.2   Alonzo CT Classification of HO

- Type I: isolated islands either anterior or posterior to the hip
- Type II: isolated islands both anterior and posterior to the hip
- Type III: ankylosed hip

11.2   Management of Fractured Acetabulum

11.2.1   Introduction
- Commonly associated with high energy trauma, and frequently associated with (especially posterior) hip dislocation
- Although they can also occur with lower energy injuries in the osteoporotic elderly after a fall
- Fractured acetabulum is by definition an intra-articular fracture and as such is a joint threatening fracture (Fig. 11.5) that frequently needs anatomic reduction and fixation, especially in the young

11.2.2   Common Associated Injuries
- Hip dislocation (see section on hip dislocation in Chap. 10)
- Femoral head fracture (discussed in Chap. 10)
- Femoral head impaction injury (discussed Chap. 10)
- Femoral neck fracture
- Other femoral fractures: pertrochanteric fractures, subtrochanteric fractures and femoral shaft fractures

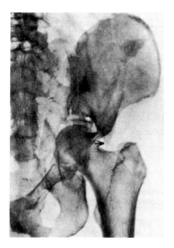

Fig. 11.5 AP pelvis radiograph of a patient with an acetabular fracture

11.2.2.1 Association with Femoral Head Impaction Injury

- It should be noted that femoral head impaction injury alone has a negative effect on prognosis, even given anatomic reduction of the associated acetabular fracture
- Common acetabular fracture patterns associated with femoral head impaction injuries:
  - Associated posterior wall fractures (impinged by ilium)
  - Transverse acetabular fractures (impinged by ilium)

11.2.2.2 Association with Femoral Neck Fractures

- An associated femoral neck fracture is frequently missed, the fracture can sometimes be detected on X-ray screening
- The femoral neck fracture needs to be urgently fixed, especially in the young and tamponade-released. If ORIF needed, most use the interval between TFL and gluteus medius
- Definitive fixation of the acetabular fracture can be done electively after, say, CT assessment via an approach relevant to the fracture at hand

11.2.2.3 Surgical Options for Concomitant Femoral and Acetabular Fractures

- Options include:
  - Fixation of both the acetabular fracture and the fracture of the proximal femur (e.g. pertrochanteric/sub-trochanteric) in one go
  - Or the proximal femur may be fixed first, followed by elective fixation of the acetabular fracture (if it needs fixation)

(Some strategies to avoid the incision for fixing the proximal femur getting in the way when fixing the acetabulum include choosing options like retrograde nailing (of shaft fracture) and plating of the femoral fracture)

11.2.3 Letournel Classification

- Elementary types

- — Posterior wall
- — Posterior column
- — Anterior wall
- — Anterior column
- — Transverse
- Associated types
  - — T-type
  - — Transverse and posterior wall
  - — Posterior column and posterior wall
  - — Anterior and posterior hemitransverse
  - — Both columns

11.2.4 Work-up

- Priority is to exclude any associated life threatening or limb-threatening injuries first
- Most fractures of the acetabulum can be seen on AP X-ray of the pelvis during screening in the acute setting
- When patient is stabilised, obtain standard Judet views ± pelvic inlet/outlet view
- Most fracture patterns can be seen on X-ray alone. There are also some characteristic tell-tale signs like the spur sign (Fig. 11.6) in double column injuries
- Document any associated soft tissue and neural injury
- Arrange for urgent/early reduction of any hip dislocation
- Central hip dislocation, say, in transverse fractures, may need to apply leg traction to diminish chance of impingement of the femoral head cartilage

11.2.5 Examination

- Soft tissue injury (especially Morel-Lavalle lesion), closed soft tissue shear injury around the hip and trochanter – the serosanguinous fluid collection that develops in these cavities is culture-positive in 30% of cases
- May need irrigation and debridement, and operation delayed until these areas are clean

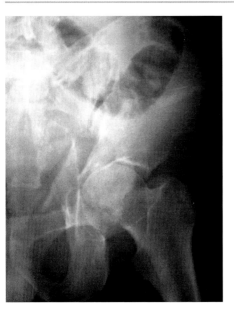

Fig. 11.6 The "spur sign" is indicative of a double column fracture

11.2.6   Associated Conditions

- Sciatic nerve
- Position of hip: subluxation and dislocation
- Femoral head fracture
- Nearby joints
- Vascular status
- Soft tissue status

11.2.7   Radiological Assessment

- According to some experts, proper radiological assessment alone can Dx 90% of acetabulum fractures as well as giving an idea of the type of injury
- Examination candidates should avoid mentioning the use of CT scanning too prematurely when being asked about investigations in the setting of acetabular fractures

11.2.8   Five Standard X-ray Views

- AP view
- Judet views – sometimes hip subluxation only seen in these oblique views
- Pelvic inlet
- Pelvic outlet

11.2.8.1   Things to Look for on X-ray

- Standard AP
  - Weight-bearing dome
  - Iliopectineal line and ilio-ischial line
  - Radiographic U or "teardrop"
- Iliac oblique
  - Posterior column and anterior wall
  - Dome
- Obturator oblique
  - Anterior column and posterior wall
  - Dome

11.2.9   CT Assessment

- Regarded as complimentary to a thorough radiological assessment
- Ideal in looking for:
  - Hip congruency
  - Intra-articular fragments
  - Assess secondary congruency if both columns fractured
  - 3D reconstruction in complex fracture patterns

11.2.9.1   Pros and Cons of CT

- Fractures *in the plane of the CT may be missed* if CT is the only modality used – always interpret in the light of X-ray
- May need to specially request thin-cut CT in areas of interest to the surgeon

11.2.10 Decision-Making and Rn Options

11.2.10.1 Importance of the Weight-Bearing Dome

- Decades ago, Rowe first recognised the importance of displaced fractures affecting the roof of the acetabulum
- Matta followed up this process by describing the roof arc measurements that describe the location of the main-column fracture lines with respect to the roof. These measurements are relevant only if there is no hip subluxation (Matta and Saucedo 1989)
- Three roof arc measurements are made – one in AP, one in each of the Judet X-ray views
- Each arc is generated by measuring the angle between a vertical line from the centre of the non-subluxated femoral head, to a point where the fracture enters the joint
- If the fracture does not enter the joint on one of the views, the angle cannot be measured, and the joint in that view is considered intact. Thus, with larger arcs, the fracture is farther away from the roof, a 90° arc indicates that the fracture is low and not likely to affect the roof

11.2.10.2 Use of Roof Arc as a Guideline in Decision-Making

- The precise area of the acetabulum that must remain intact to allow good function result is not known
- But the minimum roof arc measurement that is required to consider non-operative Rn is now usually taken as 45°

11.2.10.3 Newer Development

- Matta, after describing the radiological roof arcs, later described the CT equivalent of having 45° roof arc measurements in all three views – called the CT subchondral arc – defined as the subchondral ring of the acetabulum 10 mm inferior to the subchondral bone of the roof
- Matta says that according to mathematical calculation, if the fracture does not break this ring, the roof arcs must be > 45°

11.2.10.4 Poor Prognostic Indicators
According to Roof Arc Measurements

- Displacement of the weight-bearing dome at the time of union

- Any roof arc measurements < 45° or
- Broken CT subchondral arc

(These cases are more likely to have early onset OA)

11.2.11   Cases to Argue for Non-operative Rn

- Matta – intact 10-mm CT subchondral arc, intact 45° roof arc measurements on plain X-ray, > 50% of the articular surface of the posterior wall intact on all CT sections; femoral head congruent on AP and Judet views
- Use of fluoroscopic stress test recommended to augment these criteria – stable hips can be treated non-surgically with early mobilisation (Tornetta and Tempelman 2005)

11.2.12   Hip Stability and Role of CT and Stress X-ray

- A fracture pattern that results in hip subluxation *increases the stress on the articular cartilage in the area adjacent to the fracture*
- X-ray: incongruity between head and roof
- Good results in only half the cases with incongruence – two-thirds of which develop OA
- Dynamic instability – subtle, e.g. certain posterior wall fractures may allow dynamic hip subluxation, and cause degeneration. Posterior wall fractures cannot be assessed by roof arcs since outside the plane of measurement

11.2.13   The Special Case of Double Column Fractures with Secondary Congruence

- Matta – results of non-operative Rn for displaced both columns fractures with secondary congruence better than those for other displaced both column fractures affecting the roof
- In both column fractures with *secondary congruence*, the entire articular surface is separated from the intact ilium. The columns rotate away from each other, allowing the femoral head to medialise, but they still maintain a congruent relationship with the head

11.2.14   The Case for Early/Urgent Operation
- Open fracture
- Vascular injury
- Associated irreducible hip (e.g. loose body)
- Hip instability after reduction
- Progressive nerve palsy

11.2.15   Indications for Operative Intervention
- Most displaced (> 2 mm) acetabular fractures
- Hip joint incongruent
- Especially if involve weight-bearing dome
- In fractured posterior wall, mostly hip rendered unstable if > 40% wall affected, consider EUA/stress test for hip stability if between 20 and 40%, cases with < 20% wall affected usually stable

11.2.16   Goal of Surgery
- Restoration of joint congruity
- Anatomical reduction of weight-bearing dome
- Rn of associated injury

11.2.17   Common Problems in Fractured Acetabulum Management: Summary
- Problems in Dx: may need multiple X-ray views for proper Dx and delineation of fracture pattern
- Associated concomitant injuries, either of the soft tissues (e.g. sciatic nerve) or bony (e.g. femoral head or femoral neck fracture)
- Problems in exposure: since no single exposure can fully expose the whole acetabulum easily, and even in the more often used exposures (e.g. ilio-inguinal) the reduction is indirect and a direct visual of the joint cannot easily be attained
- Problems in fracture fixation and reduction: some fracture patterns are more difficult to reduce (e.g. T-fractures) and there are areas of the bony pelvis that are too thin to hold screws. There are also danger areas during screw insertion of the pelvis that need to be heeded

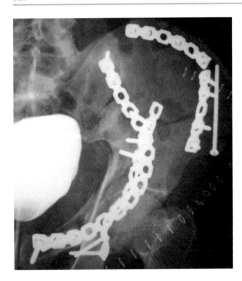

Fig. 11.7 Reconstruction plates as shown are commonly used for fracture fixation of the acetabulum

lest we injure the joint cartilage or other structures like the vessels. Fixation of acetabulum fractures frequently requires the use of properly contoured reconstruction plates (Fig. 11.7)

11.2.18 Quality of Reduction
- Learning curve
- Complexity of fracture
- Becomes very difficult after 3 weeks
- Poor reduction leads to OA (which is very likely to occur in late referrals)

11.2.19 Common Surgical Approaches
11.2.19.1 Basic Exposure
- Kocher–Langenbeck – posterior column and wall (sometimes add trochanteric osteotomy)
- Ilio-inguinal – through four windows, can see pubic rami, quadrilateral plate, iliac fossa through the different windows
- Iliofemoral

11.2.19.2 Variants of Basic Exposure

- Extended iliofemoral = iliofemoral + posterior part, can strip the glutei to get added exposure
- Extended ilio-inguinal = ilio-inguinal + posterior dissection along iliacus to reach SIJ
- Tri-radiate = Kocher-Langenbeck + an added anterior limb

11.2.20 Management of Individual Fractures

11.2.20.1 Posterior Wall

- Common
- Association with posterior hip dislocation
- X-ray: typical Gull's sign (Fig. 11.8). CT appearance can aid in assessing the joint congruency, any subluxation, or loose fragment (Fig. 11.9)
- Fix any sizable fragment with Kocher-Langenbeck approach
- Fixation involves the use of screws or buttress plate
- Pearl: ensure no screw penetration into the joint, ensure no residual hip joint subluxation postoperatively

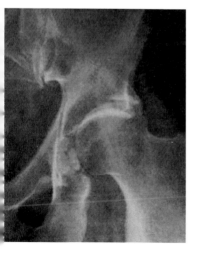

Fig. 11.8 The "gull sign" shown here is suggestive of posterior wall fracture, looking like the wing of the sea-gull

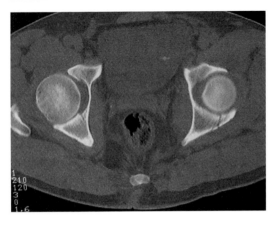

Fig. 11.9 This CT scan shows a patient with posterior wall fracture of the acetabulum

11.2.20.2 Posterior Column

- Ensure ruling out of injury/bleeding from superior gluteal artery in those fractures that exit at the greater sciatic notch
- During reduction manoeuvres, any malrotation must be corrected with the help of reduction aids like the Schanz screw
- Fixation may consider the use of a buttress plate. An occasional case may consider a lag screw from ilio-inguinal exposure if such exposure is used to tackle other concomitant fractures
- Kocher-Langenbeck approach recommended
- Intraoperative assessment of adequacy of reduction, e.g. by the use of a finger palpating the surface of the quadrilateral plate

11.2.20.3 Anterior Wall

- Significantly rarer than posterior wall fractures
- Ilio-inguinal approach
- Fix with reconstruction plate

11.2.20.4 Anterior Column

- Ilio-inguinal approach
- Fix with reconstruction plate

1.2.20.5 Transverse Fractures

- Posterior approach (e.g. Kocher-Langenbeck) if displacement mainly posterior or anterior fracture that is relatively undisplaced
- Anterior approach (e.g. ilio-inguinal) if displacement mainly anterior or posterior fracture that is relatively undisplaced
- Complex cases or delayed presentation: combined or extensile approach

1.2.20.6 T-fractures

- Can be thought of as a transverse fracture with a vertical limb
- Difficult to reduce and fix, may sometimes use cerclage as temporary fixation or as adjunctive definitive fixation
- Most need extended iliofemoral approach or triradiate approach
- Combined approach (e.g. Kocher-Langenbeck + ilio-inguinal) possible, but some experts (e.g. Helfet) do not recommend this combination

1.2.20.7 Posterior Column and Posterior Wall

- Kocher-Langenbeck approach
- In cases of combined posterior column and posterior wall fractures, fix the posterior column first

1.2.20.8 Transverse and Posterior Wall

- Kocher-Langenbeck approach
- Fix the transverse component first

1.2.20.9 Anterior Column and Posterior Hemi-transverse

- Mostly use ilio-inguinal approach
- Anterior column fixation by buttress plate and screw
- Sometimes posterior column lag screw can be inserted via the ilio-inguinal approach

1.2.20.10 Double Column Fractures

- Most need either combined or extensile approaches

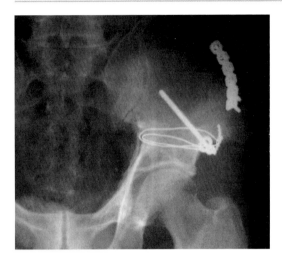

Fig. 11.10 The fixation of double column fractures shown here is sometimes followed by the use of cerclage as well as lag screws and plates

- In the occasional case the ilio-inguinal approach alone may suffice if posterior wall intact and posterior column is a big piece whereby application of lag screw ± cerclage (Fig. 11.10) from the anterior approach is feasible after fixation of the anterior column has been performed

11.2.21   Role of Surgical Navigation in Acetabular Fractures

- It should be remembered that techniques of percutaneous fixation of acetabular fractures have *not* been formally validated in random clinical trials (RCT)
- Percutaneous fixation should be carried out by experts in the field and in carefully selected fractures
- Consent for open surgery should always be obtained since percutaneous fixation may need to be aborted if there is inadequate imaging, inadequate reduction, or inadequate experience

11.2.21.1   Patient Selection

- Fractures like posterior wall fractures of the acetabulum are a *contraindication* to percutaneous technique since the fragment is deep seated and in view of the nearby vital structures like the sciatic nerve

- Situations in which percutaneous fixation may be contemplated include, say, percutaneous lag screw fixation across fractures where there is a convenient palpable bony prominence for insertion of either joystick or guide wire. Example: some relatively undisplaced, high anterior column acetabular fractures

11.2.22 Complications of Fractured Acetabulum

- General: e.g. DVT/PE, unstable haemodynamics from associated injuries like fractured pelvis
- Local complications listed below

11.2.22.1 Neurologic Deficits

- Example: sciatic nerve palsy
- Most common present as foot drop

11.2.22.2 Cartilage Defects ± Later OA

- Can affect either side of the joint
- Matta demonstrated that cartilage injury to the femoral head if visible on gross visual inspection is risk factor for OA – even with a good reduction

11.2.22.3 Heterotopic Ossification

- Higher association with surgical approaches that involve extensive surgical dissection
- Examples: extended iliofemoral approach, triradiate approach, etc.

11.2.22.4 AVN Hip

- Can occur after hip dislocation/subluxation
- Although immediate reduction of the hip decreases AVN risk, the patient is at risk for up to 5 years after the injury (Tornetta)
- Effect of AVN – depends on site and size

11.2.23 Poor Prognostic Factors

- Cartilage injury of either side of the joint with joint surface impaction
- Inadequate restoration of the weight-bearing Sourcil or dome
- Persistent hip joint subluxation or incongruency
- Missed or inadequate Rn of associated injuries, e.g. sciatic nerve injury, fractured femoral head or neck

General Bibliography

1. Tile M (ed) (1995) Fractures of the pelvis and acetabulum. Lippincott Williams Wilkins, Philadelphia

Selected Bibliography of Journal Articles

1. Burgess AR, Eastridge BJ et al. (1990) Pelvic ring disruptions: Effective classification system and treatment protocols. J Trauma 30(7):848–856
2. Hak DJ, Olson SA, Matta JM (1997) Diagnosis and management of closed internal degloving injuries associated with pelvic and acetabular fractures: the Morel–Lavalle lesion. J Trauma 42(6):1046–1051
3. Matta JM, Saucedo T (1989) Internal fixation of pelvic ring fractures. Clin Orthop Relat Res 242:83–97
4. Tile M (1996) Acute pelvic fractures. I. Causation and classification. J Am Acad Orthop Surg 4(3):143–151
5. Tile M (1996) Acute pelvic fractures. II. Principles of management. J Am Acad Orthop Surg 4(3):152–161
6. Tornetta P, Templeman DC (2005) Expected outcome after pelvic ring injury. Inst Course Lect 54:401–407

Contents

12.1   Introduction and Acute Assessment

12.1.1   Goals in the Spine-Injured Patient

- Save life
- Restore and maintain spinal cord function preventing secondary injury
- Realign and stabilise the spinal column
- Prevent medical Cx
- Programmed rehabilitation

12.1.2   Acute Assessment

- Follow ATLS protocol
- Index of suspicion for spinal injury – especially in coma patients and the drunk; particularly the C-spine is assumed injured and unstable until proven otherwise
- Do no harm and good protection of the C-spine. Methods of acute assessment of C-spine will be discussed
- Clinical and X-ray assessment – and check for deformity and step
- Beware of problematic areas, e.g. cervicothoracic junction (CTJ)
- Maintain perfusion and oxygenation

12.1.3   Cervical X-ray Assessment

- Upper limit of ST space: general guidelines
    - Upper C-spine level = half width of vertebra
    - Lower part of C-spine = one vertebral width (retro-pharyngeal space >7 mm, or retro-tracheal space >14 mm; displaced pre-vertebral stripe ± deviation of trachea should be noted)
- Alignment: look for any lordosis, acute kyphosis, torticollis, widened interspace, axial rotation of the vertebrae
- Adult Atlas-Dens interval (ADI) >4 mm abnormal (5 mm in children) narrow/widened disc space, wide facet joint, and look for facet dislocation – unilaterally, can check oblique view if unsure
- The ATLS course teaches that the cervical spine lateral film done as part of the trauma series is 75% sensitive. This means we will be missing 25% of injuries. Furthermore, most cervical lateral X-rays

taken in casualty are of poor quality. Some centres nowadays prefer not to waste time doing pull-shoulders or swimmers in these hectic situations, and order C0–T4 CT (or at least to CTJ), especially in severely traumatised, obtunded patients, claiming a sensitivity of over 95%, if not more

■ Having said that, with properly taken X-rays, four important lines should be checked (anterior and posterior vertebral lines, spinolaminar line, spinous process line); contour of vertebra and position of spinous process (if deviates to one side implies rotation), distance between spinous processes. Never perform flexion/extension X-ray in acute settings. (If the patient is obtunded, there is a chance of causing or increasing the neural deficit, if the patient is conscious the muscle guarding makes the exam unreliable and only causes the patient more pain)

12.1.4 Neural Assessment

■ Spinal shock: complete vs incomplete. The accurate documentation of completeness and the level of injury are of utmost importance since this guides the type of acute treatment, as well as the prognosis of the patient. Always document the type of respiration as well, besides vital signs
■ Bulbocavernosus reflex
■ Different types of incomplete spinal cord syndromes
■ Classification of neurological deficit:
  – Frankel scale
  – American Spinal Injury Association (ASIA) scale

12.1.5 Other Investigations

■ CT:
  – Occult fracture (e.g. lateral masses)
  – Degree of retropulsion
  – Double vertebra sign suggestive of fracture dislocation
  – 3D reconstruction, as well as coronal/sagittal reconstructions
  – The increased use of CT in many trauma centres to clear the cervical spine has just been discussed

- MRI – advantages can assess:
  - Disc
  - Cord (oedema, bleeding)
  - Ligament (integrity)
  - Haematoma (e.g. epidural)

12.2 Spinal Cord Injury (Fig. 12.1)

12.2.1 Introduction

- Epidemiological data indicate that spinal cord injury (SCI) most often occurs in young males, especially between 16 and 30 years of age; there is another smaller peak in the elderly (>65)
- There are 12,000 to 14,000 acute SCIs per year in the US, with a prevalence of 191,000 per year
- The study of SCI is important, especially since it frequently affects individuals in the prime of their life in our society, has devastating consequences and is also costly to society. In the USA, a C4 injury with complete SCI cost US$550,000 in the first year, and US$ 100,000 to maintain the patient per year thereafter

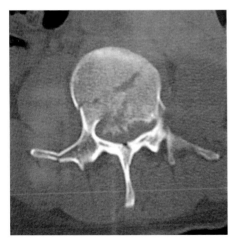

Fig. 12.1 The significantly retropulsed fragment of burst fractures frequently causes neurological damage to the patient

- Most SCIs are the result of high energy trauma such as traffic or falling accidents, or being struck in sport. Up to 50% of SCIs come from injury to the cervical spine
- Despite the initial enthusiasm with hyperacute administration of high-dose steroids, which allegedly have shown some benefit, there is increasing scepticism regarding the original publications from the scientific world, and in some places like Alberta, Canada, surgeons have forsaken the use of steroids for want of better evidence

12.2.2   Key Concept
- Most damage to cord done *at the time of injury*

12.2.3   Concepts of Primary and Secondary Damage to the Spinal Cord
- Primary injury:
  - Sustained at the time of impact
  - From compression and cord contusion
  - Involves neuronal damage, disruption of axonal membrane and blood vessels
- Secondary injury:
  - Involves a cascade of auto-destructive processes lasting hours to days and expanding the injury zone
  - Details of the cascade are discussed under pathophysiology (Sect. 12.2.9)
  - Limiting the extent of secondary injury is part of our goal of management in acute spinal cord injury

12.2.4   Spinal Shock
- Spinal shock mostly occurs after significant cervical cord injury; characterised by a state of flaccid paralysis, hypotonia and areflexia (e.g. absent bulbocavernosus reflex)
- The sensory and motor symptoms usually resolve by 4–6 h, but autonomic symptoms can persist for days or weeks
- Most typical signs include bradycardia despite hypotension, flaccid paralysis and lack of painful sensation to the limbs affected; other

signs that can be present depend on the level of injury. Avoid operation during spinal shock since there is a high risk of mortality

2.2.5 End of Spinal Shock

- Signalled by the return of the bulbocavernosus reflex
- This reflex is elicited by a gentle squeeze of the glans penis in men; and a gentle tug of the Foley catheter in women
- In most cases, this reflex returns within 24 h at the end of spinal shock
- If there is no evidence of sacral sparing or spinal cord function distal to the level of injury when spinal shock is over, we can diagnose complete cord injury with a much graver prognosis. Never comment on the completeness of cord injury during the period of spinal shock

2.2.6 Frankel's Grading of Injury Severity

- Frankel A: complete motor and sensory loss
- Frankel B: motor complete, sensory loss incomplete
- Frankel C: some motor power left, but not useful
- Frankel D: some motor power left, and useful
- Frankel E: normal motor power and sensation

2.2.7 The ASIA Scale

- ASIA A = no motor or sensory preservation, even in the sacral segments S4–S5
- ASIA B = sensory but no motor function preserved below the neurological level including the sacral segments (S4–S5)
- ASIA C = motor function is preserved below the neurological level, and more than half of the key muscles below the neurological level have a muscle grade less than 3 (voluntary sphincter contraction, sparing of motor function more than three segments below)
- ASIA D = motor function is preserved below the neurological level, and at least half of the key muscles below the neurological level have a muscle grade of 3
- ASIA E = motor and sensory functions are normal

12.2.8   Incomplete Spinal Cord Syndrome

12.2.8.1   Central Cord Syndrome

- Mainly affects the upper extremities
- Association with elderly with pre-existing cervical spondylosis
- Hyperextension injury
- Buckling of ligamentum flavum causing compression to medial placed arm fibres in the corticospinal tract
- Subsequent elective laminoplasty or laminectomy with lateral mass plating commonly required

12.2.8.2   Anterior Cord Syndrome

- Aetiology:
  - Anterior spinal artery territory ischemia, e.g. from axial loading or hyperextension injuries, teardrop fractures
- Loss:
  - Motor function and pain, and temperature sensation
- Prognosis:
  - 10–20% muscle recovery, poor muscle power and coordination worst prognosis among the forms of incomplete spinal cord syndrome

12.2.8.3   Posterior Cord Syndrome

- Aetiology
  - Rare
  - Posterior spinal artery damage
  - Diffuse atherosclerosis: deficient collateral perfusion
- Loss: position sense
- Rule out B12 deficiency
- Prognosis:
  - Better than anterior syndrome
  - Poor ambulation prospect: since proprioceptive deficit

12.2.8.4   Brown Sequard Syndrome

- Aetiologies
  - Trauma: penetrating
  - Radiation

Ipsilateral weakness and position sense loss

Contralateral pain and temperature loss

Prognosis:

- — 75–90% ambulate on discharge
- — 70% independent ADL
- — 89% bladder and 82% bowel continent

2.2.8.5 Conus Medullaris Syndrome

Epiconus: L4–S1

- — Sparing of sacral reflex: bulbocavernosus, micturation

Conus: S2–S4

- — Sacral reflex loss
- — Detrusor weakness and overflow incontinence
- — Loss of penile erection and ejaculation
- — If root escapes: ambulatory, ankle jerks normal
- — Symmetric defects: small size of conus
- — Pain: inconstant; perineum and thighs
- — Weakness: sacral
- — Sensory loss: saddle in distribution

Prognosis: limited recovery

2.2.9 Pathophysiology of Spinal Cord Injury in General

Most texts focus on mechanism of secondary injury to the spinal cord

But to think of the body's inflammatory and other responses as purely detrimental is an over-simplification of the state of affairs

There is in fact simultaneous initiation of neuroprotective and injurious mechanisms provoked by the injury

2.2.9.1 Role of the Inflammatory Response: a Blessing or a Curse?

Thanks to well-designed studies by colleagues like Bethea; we now know that there are two sides of the coin

Bethea (2000) pointed out the concept of a "dual-edged sword": thus, the inflammatory process that occurs in response to spinal cord injury can have both deleterious and neuroprotective effects

12.2.9.2 Pathophysiology in Detail

- Pathogenetic mechanisms we know of are based mainly on animal models. They include:
  - Lipid peroxidation and free radical generation
  - Abnormal electrolyte fluxes and excitotoxicity
  - Abnormal vascular perfusion
  - The associated inflammatory and immune response

12.2.9.2.1 Lipid Peroxidation and Free Radicals

- Free radicals are frequently released in spinal cord injuries
- They cause damage by:
  - Disruption of the cell membrane
  - Mediated by oxidation of fatty acids in cellular membrane (lipid peroxidation). This peroxidation process resembles a chain reaction, generating more active lipid-derived radicals
  - Free radicals also damage mitochondrial enzymes inside cells such as ATPase, which produces cell death
- Many therapeutic interventions employ agents that help prevent lipid peroxidation, e.g. methylprednisolone, antioxidants such as tirilazad mesylate (used in a treatment arm in the National Acute Spinal Cord Injury Study [NASCIS])

12.2.9.2.2 Abnormal Electrolyte Fluxes and Excitotoxicity

- Glutamate is a prevalent neurotransmitter in the CNS. Its receptors include NMDA (N-methyl-D-aspartate), among others, which allow ions to pass such as calcium and sodium. (P.S. high cytosolic calcium is lethal to cells)
- Accumulation of glutamate occurs after cord injury, and over-excitation of these receptors can occur, i.e. excitotoxicity, causing abnormal ionic fluxes. Methods to block NMDA receptors have been used as a treatment method to prevent further cellular damage

12.2.9.2.3 Abnormal Vascular Perfusion

- Normal blood flow to the spinal cord is under auto-regulation
- Impaired vascularity of the cord in spinal cord injuries includes:

- Loss of autoregulation
- Spinal shock and hypoperfusion
- Shock due to blood loss from associated injuries

Hypotension and decreased oxygenation need to be avoided at all costs; most patients need ICU care)

2.2.9.2.4 Abnormal Intracellular Sodium Concentration

- Normal intracellular sodium is kept at a low level by ATPase ionic pumps
- Abnormal Na+ fluxes especially affect the white matter glial cells
- Neuroprotection, especially of white matter, can be achieved by blocking abnormal sodium fluxes using pharmacologic agents

2.2.9.2.5 Associated Inflammatory and Immune Response

- Details of interactions between inflammatory mediators are not fully known, but key players include:
  - Tumour necrosis factor: said to have both neuroprotective and neurotoxic properties
  - Arachidonic acid metabolites: these are formed from phospholipase at cell membranes, the accumulation of which is metabolised via cyclo-oxygenase to prostaglandins, which can affect vascular permeability, etc.
- Note that in secondary spinal cord injury, cell death can occur through either cell necrosis or cell apoptosis

2.2.10   Planning of Rn Strategies Based on Pathophysiology

2.2.10.1   Main Strategy Part 1: Pharmacologic Interventions

2.2.10.1.1   Pharmacologic Strategy 1: Steroids

- Steroids mainly act by prevention of lipid peroxidation by free radicals and membrane stabilisation. They may help prevent apoptosis by checking calcium fluxes, improving vascular perfusion, and are thought to help reduce white matter oedema, and enhance Na/K-ATPase activity
- Methylprednisolone was selected from among the different steroids because it is more effective at preventing lipid peroxidation

NASCIS 1 Trial
- Reported in JAMA by Bracken et al. in 1984
- Less often quoted of the NASCIS trials
- This trial showed that late administration within 48 h of relatively lower doses of methylprednisolone (than the high dose used in the NASCIS 2 and 3 trials) showed little significant neurologic recovery

(P.S. Main drawback of NASCIS 1 trial: no control group)

NASCIS 2 Trial
- Found that a higher dose of methylprednisolone given within 8 h causes neurological improvement (not beyond 8 h)
- Paraplegics recovered 21% of lost motor function relative to 8% among controls
- Patients with paraparesis recovered 75% of lost motor function compared with 59% among controls
- Dose of steroid: 30 mg/kg bolus over 1 h, followed by 5.4 mg/kg/h for 23 h

NASCIS 3 Trial
- Further studies based on the findings in NASCIS 2
- Recommend:
  - The dose mentioned in NASCIS 2 for 24 h if patient presents <3 h after injury
  - If between 3 and 8 h, give the above steroid infusion for total of 48 h
  - Tirilazad mesylate (an anti-oxidant) has similar effect to steroid if given in hyperacute phase

Criticism of the NASCIS 2 Trial
- Many criticisms have been lodged against these trials, especially NASCIS 2, e.g. the conclusion of a small but significant statistical benefit in those having steroids within 8 h only occurred in a post hoc analysis – while the primary outcome analysis of neural recovery in all randomised patients was in fact negative
- Functional outcome not measured

- Gives no explanation why only the *right* side motor examination was measured, and not that of the left side (this same criticism holds for NASCIS 3 trial)
- The medical management of study patients was not consistent within the medical centre or among different medical centres
- Statistical methodology used has also been criticised
- The very high dose steroid therapy was not without significant side effects, such as GI bleeds and severe pneumonia

Current Recommendation Concerning Steroid Therapy
- In the USA, the Congress of Neurological Surgeons, in collaboration with the American Association of Neurological Surgeons, published an important statement in Neurosurgery 2002 March: "treatment with methylprednisolone for either 24 to 48 h is recommended as an option in the treatment of acute SCI patients; this should be undertaken only with the knowledge that the evidence suggesting harmful side effects is more consistent than suggestion of clinical benefit"

12.2.10.1.2 Pharmacologic Strategy 2: Naloxone
- Naloxone is an opiate receptor that was included in one treatment arm of the NASCIS studies
- Found to be effective in the subgroup of patients with incomplete spinal cord injuries (J Neurosurg 1993)

12.2.10.1.3 Pharmacologic Strategies 3: Gangliosides
- These are glycosphingolipids at the outer cellular membranes of the central nervous system
- There is some evidence that gangliosides may have neuroprotective action, with more speedy recovery of motor and sensory function in partial cord injuries
- Although a large multi-centre study failed to show obvious beneficial effects of GM 1 ganglioside at 26 weeks compared with placebo

12.2.10.1.4 Pharmacologic Strategies 4: Calcium Channel Blockers
- Thought to work by improvement in blood flow via vessel dilatation

12.2.10.1.5 Pharmacologic Strategies 5: Antagonists of Glutamate Receptors

■ Works by prevention of excitotoxicity as a result of glutamate ac
  cumulation – helps to prevent abnormal sodium and calcium fluxes
  which may prove lethal to cells

12.2.10.1.6 Pharmacologic Strategies 6: Others

■ Inhibition of cyclo-oxygenase
■ Minocycline
■ Sodium channel blockers
■ Erythropoietin
■ Cyclosporin

12.2.10.2 Main Strategy Part 2: Role of Decompression

■ Persistent compression of the cord from whatever structure is a po
  tentially reversible type of secondary injury
■ Abundant animal studies show beneficial effect from early cord de
  compression (J Neurosurg 1999)
■ Clinical studies in the past had varied results:
  – Some showed little benefit of early surgery (Spine 1997)
  – Some showed beneficial effect (Clin Orthop Relat Res 1999)
  – But note wide variation of definition of early between animal and
    clinical studies, and among clinical studies
■ In general, recent papers tend to propose early interventions as the
  adverse results of older studies are now partly circumvented by im
  provements in anaesthesia and critical care, especially in incomplete
  SCIs

12.2.10.2.1 Decompression in Incomplete Spinal Cord Injury

■ Most experts will agree nowadays to aim at either early (< 24 h) or
  urgent decompression of partial cord injuries
■ However, extreme care needs to be exercised in order to achieve
  stable haemodynamics and adequate oxygenation, especially since
  the patient may be suffering from poly-trauma. Do not operate dur
  ing spinal shock since there is a high risk of mortality

- Also, when the spine is stabilised, intensive physical therapy can be initiated to decrease other complications related to spinal cord injury

2.2.10.2.2 Decompression in Complete Spinal Cord Injury

- Despite the fact that the NASCIS studies were not designed to assess timing of surgery, systematic analysis of the raw data did reveal improved outcome from early surgery, which included both complete and incomplete cord injuries (except maybe central cord syndromes)
- Also, even in the face of complete cord injury, early spinal stabilisation (if indicated) eases nursing and prevents complications like decubitus ulcers and pulmonary problems. In summary, the main indication for spinal surgery in the face of complete SCI is for spinal stabilisation and deformity correction

2.2.10.3 Main Strategy Part 3:
Prospects of Spinal Cord Regeneration

- Progress has also been made in this exciting field recently, although there are still obstacles to be surmounted
- Regeneration is difficult and involves:
  - Need to overcome the inhibitory environment inside the CNS
  - Relative lack of regenerative capacity of CNS neurones
  - Neurotropic factors to support axonal sprouts
  - Bridging strategies across the zone of injury
  - Presence of navigation molecules to let the axons grow into proper targets
  - Finally, the re-grown axons must be functional and develop a synapse at the target tissue

2.3 Cervical Spine Injury

2.3.1 Fractured Occipital Condyle

- Most result from direct blow in association with head injury
- Easily missed on X-ray, may need CT for Dx

12.3.1.1   Anderson and Montesano Classification
- Type 1: impacted fracture with comminution
- Type 2: associated with fractured base of skull
- Type 3: avulsion fracture of alar ligament attachment

12.3.1.2   Treatment
- Types 1 and 2: stable, rigid collar ± halo
- Type 3: unstable, needs halo immobilisation

12.3.2   Occipitocervical Instability/Dislocation
- The incidence of occiput–C1 is higher in children, since the lateral masses (articulating with the occipital condyles) are flatter. Important soft tissue supports in this region include: alar ligament, tectorial membrane, joint capsule and apical ligament. True incidence is unknown, many are fatal
- Classification is according to the direction of displacement. Dx depends on index of suspicion, radiologic clues, such as the Power's ratio, and CT scan

12.3.2.1   Classification of Occiput–C1 Instability
- Type I: occiput condyles subluxate anterior to lateral mass of C1
- Type II: vertical displacement of occiput condyles > 2 mm with respect to superior C1 articular process
- Type III: involves the rare posterior dislocation of occiput condyles

12.3.2.2   Treatment
- Acute situation: halo traction contraindicated in type II. In children, use the paediatric halo for acute stabilisation
- Then elective occipital-cervical fusion (mostly by occipito-cervical plating), beware of Cx like vertebral artery injury and that of cranial nerves

12.3.3   Fracture Atlas C1 (Figs. 12.2, 12.3)
- Injury mechanism: axial loading and frequently hyperextension

- Canal is spacious here, neural deficit rare
- But need to rule out associated injuries
- Bilateral posterior arch fracture more common than the real Jefferson (or burst) fracture
- Suspect transverse ligament rupture if overhang ≥ 6.9 mm

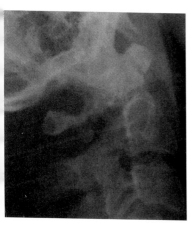

Fig. 12.2 This lateral cervical spine X-ray reveals fracture of the C1 arch

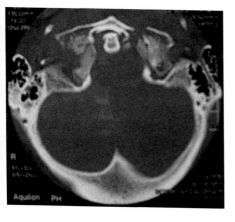

Fig. 12.3 CT is a good assessment of bony injury, in this case the fractured C1 arch

12.3.3.1 Levine Classification of C1 Fractures

- Type 1: fractured posterior arch
- Type 2: fractured lateral mass
- Type 3: classic Jefferson's burst fracture (Levine and Edwards 1985)

12.3.3.2 Treatment

- Types 1 and 2: halo treatment, recheck flexion extension X-ray after halo is removed, consider fusion if unstable
- Type 3: operative fusion
- Cx: include non-union, which is predisposed to transverse ligament rupture

12.3.4 Fractured Odontoid C2

- 20% cervical spine injuries
- More in elderly from simple falls. In younger individuals, may result from a blow to the head ± high speed accidents
- Present with suboccipital pain, neural deficit uncommon, but can vary from neuralgia to quadriparesis

12.3.4.1 Anderson and D'Alonzo Classification

- Type 1: Only the tip is fractured – essentially an avulsion injury of the apical and alar ligaments. Rule out distraction-type injury
- Type 2: Waist fracture – non-union risk increased in: smokers, >5 mm displacement, advanced age; type 2A subtype has basal comminution
- Type 3: Body fracture – union not a problem since large and vascular cancellous surface

12.3.4.2 Risk Factors for Non-union

- >4 mm fracture displacement
- Age >40
- Type 2 fracture
- Posterior displacement (these fractures can cause respiratory difficulties)

12.3.4.3 Treatment

- Type 1: orthosis adequate if no distraction injury
- Type 2: consider halo if undisplaced, displaced cases either anterior odontoid screw (one or two screws), or posterior C1–C2 fusion
- Type 3: depending on the fracture personality, either Minerva or halo, seldom require surgery

12.3.4.4 Surgical Options for C1–C2 Fusion

- Brook's fusion
- Posterior transarticular screw
- Anterior odontoid screw

12.3.4.4.1 Brook's Fusion

- Contraindicated if fractured C1 arch present
- Indication: RA, extreme osteoporosis

12.3.4.4.2 Transarticular Screw

- Contraindications:
  - Anomalous vertebral artery (preoperative CT pick-ups, incidence up to 15%)
  - Extreme osteoporosis
- Indications:
  - C1–C2 non-union
  - Type 2 odontoid and fractured C1 arch
  - Rheumatoid arthritis

12.3.4.4.3 Anterior Odontoid Screw (Fig. 12.4)

- Contraindications:
  - Comminuted C1–C2 articulation
  - Posterosuperior to antero-inferior fracture
  - Irreducible or pathologic fracture
  - Marked osteoporosis
  - Transverse atlas ligament disruption
  - Anterior C2 body fracture (relative)

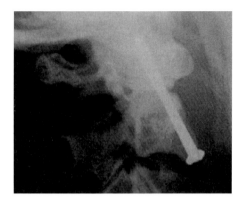

Fig. 12.4 This lateral cervical spine X-ray reveals the position of the anterior odontoid screw for fractured odontoid

- — Short neck and barrel chest
- — Gross obesity
- — Non-union
- — Thoracic kyphosis
- Indications:
  - — Good bone and fracture reducible
  - — One screw has 70% stiffness of two screws, two screws more rotational stability

12.3.4.5 *Rate of Non-union*
- Type 2: 30% non-union with halo, decreases to 4% with posterior fusion
- Type 3: 20% non-union rate with halo

12.3.5 Traumatic Spondylolisthesis of Axis (Hangman's Fracture)
- Normal stress on the pars is great because the axis acts as a transition vertebra between the upper and lower cervical spine
- Usual mechanism: involves hyperextension, flexion ± usually element of axial loading. (P.S. differs from the traditional act of hanging prisoners in which the mechanism involves hyperextension and distraction)

Neurologic deficit rare because canal spacious. Most (70%) injuries belong to Type 1 injury

2.3.5.1 Effendi Classification of C2 Post-traumatic Spondylolisthesis (Fig. 12.5)

- Type I: mainly hyperextension injury, < 3 mm translation, no angulation. Type IA fracture is oblique and Dx may only be certain with CT
- Type II: vertical fracture close to pedicle–body junction. Involves hyperextension, axial loading, then flexion. An element of compression at anterosuperior C3 body common. Also characterised by translation ≥ 3 mm and angulation. Type IIA refers to a subtype characterised by minimal translation but significant angulation. This subtype is caused by flexion/distraction, and is contraindicated to be treated by traction since this will increase the deformity and cause disc widening
- Type III: involves fractured pars with displacement and C2/C3 bilateral facet dislocation. Mechanism involves flexion distraction (causing facet dislocation) followed by hyperextension (causing the pars fracture). Can cause neurologic deficit. OR of the C2/C3 facet dislocation may need to be followed by fusion

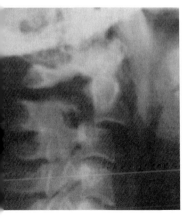

Fig. 12.5 Lateral cervical spine X-ray showing Hangman's fracture

12.3.5.2 Treatment

- Type I: collar
- Type II: halo-vest for 12 weeks
- Type IIA: halo-vest for 12 weeks
- Type III: surgery (C2–C3 fusion, sometimes posterior C1–C3 fusion)

(P.S. Surgery is also occasionally needed in the face of severe angulation > 11° in Effendi type II fractures)

12.3.6 C1–C2 Subluxation: DDx

- Can be seen with ruptured transverse ligament, or rotatory subluxation as described by Fielding and Hawkins (1977)
- C1–C2 subluxation may also be associated with atlas or odontoid fractures

12.3.6.1 Ruptured Transverse Ligament

- Rupture is suggested by ADI > 3–5 mm, all ligaments likely ruptured if ADI > 7 mm, cord compression likely if interval > 10 mm
- Management: halo will suffice in > 3–5 mm group, although recheck flexion/extension X-ray when halo taken off at 3 weeks; C1–C2 fusion if > 5 mm

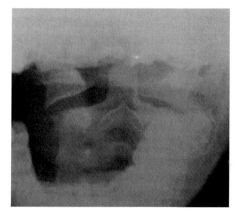

Fig. 12.6 Open mouth X-ray of the cervical spine showing evidence of rotatory subluxation

12.3.6.2 Rotatory Subluxation

- More often seen in children
- Clinically, the head is tilted towards the side of fixation, while the chin is pointed in the opposite direction. Open-mouth X-ray view is useful (Fig. 12.6), while the use of dynamic CT (Figs. 12.7, 12.8) aids in the Dx, especially of more subtle cases

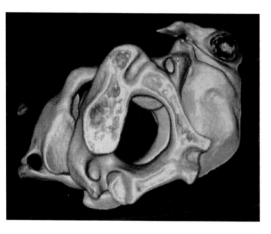

Fig. 12.7 Dynamic CT in the assessment of rotatory subluxation and fixation

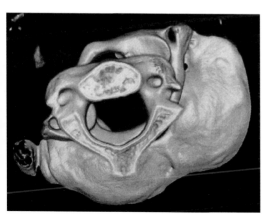

Fig. 12.8 When dynamic CT is used, the patient will be asked to rotate the neck to the right and left

12.3.6.2.1 Hawkins and Fielding Classification
- Type 1: rotational displacement only, no anterior translation
- Type 2: rotational displacement and anterior translation 3–5 mm
- Type 3: rotational displacement and anterior translation >5 mm
- Type 4: posterior translation and rotation (rare)

12.3.7 Injury to the Sub-axial Cervical Spine
12.3.7.1 Normal Structural Constraints
- Most of the flexion/extension movements of the cervical spine occur at the most mobile segment, C3–C7, and injury in this region is common. Incidence of non-contiguous injuries (i.e. at another level of cervical spine or at thoracolumbar region) amounts to near 10%
- Resistance to hyperextension is offered by: anterior longitudinal ligament (ALL), annulus fibrosis, anterior two-thirds of the vertebra
- Resistance to hyperflexion is offered by: facets and capsule, ligamentum flavum, the supraspinous and interspinous ligament
- In this book, Allen's classification of injury to the cervical spine is followed (Allen et al. 1982)

12.3.7.2 Criteria for Cervical Spine Instability (Panjabi and White)
- This was based on biomechanical laboratory experiments on cadavers
- The following parameters are assessed and a score of ≥5 implies instability. However, if the spine is obviously unstable (e.g. fracture dislocation), no need for such calculations
  - Anterior element destroyed or cannot function: 2 points
  - Posterior element destroyed or cannot function: 2 points
  - Sagittal plane translation > 3.5 mm: 2 points
  - Sagittal plane rotation > 11°: 2 points
  - Positive stretch test: 2 points
  - Damage to cord: 2 points
  - Damage to root: 1 point
  - Abnormal disc narrowing: 1 point
  - Anticipate dangerous loading: 1 point

12.3.7.3 Allen's Mechanistic Classification
- Vertical compression
- Compressive flexion
- Distractive flexion
- Lateral flexion
- Compressive extension
- Distractive extension

12.3.7.3.1 Vertical Compression
- Mostly from diving injuries or car accidents
  - Stage 1: affects one vertebral end plate
  - Stage 2: affects both end plates
  - Stage 3: burst fracture

Treatment
- Stage 1: rigid cervical orthosis
- Stage 2: halo immobilisation
- Stage 3: most require operation especially if neural compromise by anterior decompression, grafting and anterior ± posterior instrumentation frequently added

12.3.7.3.2 Compressive Flexion
- There are five stages in Allen's classification, with increasing vertebral compression/comminution, and disruption of the posterior tension band. Constitutes 20% of sub-axial injuries
- The descriptive term flexion "teardrop" fracture depicts complete ligamentous and disc disruption at level of injury (Orthop Clin North Am 1986)
- Caused by axial loading injuries as in diving and vehicle collisions
- Incidence of cord injuries: 25% if stage 3; 38% if stage 4; 91% if stage 5

Treatment
- Stages 1 and 2: cervical orthosis

- Stage 3: halo immobilisation
- Stages 4 and 5: assess need for anterior decompression, bone grafting and instrumentation. (Posterior stabilisation considered if significant disruption of the posterior tension band)

12.3.7.3.3 *Distractive Flexion (Fig. 12.9)*

- Constitutes 10% of sub-axial cervical spine injuries
- There are four stages:
    - Stage 1: facet subluxation only in flexion, may have widening/divergence of spinous processes, Dx not easy, may need flexion/extension views when pain subsides 3 weeks later
    - Stage 2: unilateral facet dislocation ± associated fracture of articular process or pedicle; 25% anterior displacement
    - Stage 3: bilateral facet dislocation with 50% anterior displacement on lateral X-ray
    - Stage 4: bilateral facet dislocation with 100% vertebral body displacement

Treatment of Different Scenarios

- Scenario 1: awake co-operative patient with facet dislocation and neurological deficit

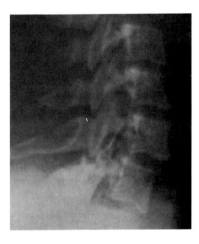

Fig. 12.9 Lateral cervical X-ray showing facet dislocation

- Scenario 2: comatose/semi-comatose patient with facet dislocation and suspected neurology
- Scenario 3: awake co-operative patient with facet dislocation but no neural deficit

Management of Scenario 1

- Emergency axial traction to attempt closed reduction
- Proven successful in 80–90% cases, worsening of neurological deficit uncommon (many experts feel that in this particular clinical scenario, there is no absolute need for MRI, this may be disputed by some who work in specialised centres where MRI is readily available 24 hours a day – but this is the exception rather than the rule for most general hospitals. Thus, if MRI can be quickly arranged, then MRI may be performed). MRI can not only detect disc prolapse, but any compressing haematoma can also be seen
- Starting from around 8–10 lb (3.6–4.5 kg) weight, the in-line traction is increased and expect around 10 lb (4.5 kg) per segment rostral to the level of injury. Weight needed for reduction is frequently higher in unilateral facet dislocation. Notice that the lower the level of facet dislocation, the more difficult it is to obtain CR and the higher the amount of traction that may be required
- After CR, reduce the weight and put in halo
- If CR unsuccessful, carry out urgent MRI and prepare for OR. If there is a need for anterior decompression from a prolapsed disc, anterior discectomy and decompression should be performed before any attempt at posterior procedures
- If MRI does not reveal anterior compression, OR from posterior approach and instrumentation will suffice, e.g. by the use of lateral mass screws. For situations that require anterior decompression discectomy and grafting, biomechanical studies found that for these cases adjunctive posterior instrumentation (rather than anterior) is recommended to confer adequate stability. (This is quite different from corpectomy followed by BG and anterior cervical plating for compressive failure alone of the vertebral body wherein anterior adjunctive plating suffice as far as stability goes)

Management of Scenario 2

- If the patient is not awake, it is strongly advised to carry out urgent MRI to look for any anterior compression, say, from a prolapsed disc before initiation of closed reduction

Management of Scenario 3

- In the neurologically intact patient, situation is less urgent than in scenario 1
- Can consider urgent MRI if facility is available. If MRI not readily available, proceed to CR as described in scenario 1

12.3.7.3.4 Lateral Flexion

- Stage 1: ipsilateral fracture of the centrum and posterior arch
- Stage 2: ipsilateral fracture of the vertebral body and contralateral bone/ligament failure
- Most of these injuries need traction reduction and surgical stabilisation

12.3.7.3.5 Compressive Extension

- Stage 1: posterior arch fracture and anterior disc failure in tension. Many of these injuries need either posterior surgery and/or anterior discectomy and plating
- Stage 2: characterised by bilaminar fracture, sometimes at multiple levels. Mostly treated by halo
- Stages 3–5: increasingly severe circumferential disruption
- Most severe end of the spectrum involves fractured vertebral arch and 100% anterior displacement of the vertebral body. Fracture dislocations need combined anterior and posterior surgery

12.3.7.3.6 Distractive Extension

- Stage 1: Characterised by a spectrum of disruption of anterior constraints (ALL and anterior annulus) to the posterior annulus and posterior longitudinal ligament (PLL). May try halo, especially if bony rather than ligamentous failure is involved. Operative fixation usually involves plating and anterior reconstruction

- Stage 2: as above with added disruption of the posterior ligamentous complex with resultant retrolisthesis. These injuries need a combined anterior and posterior approach. Most occur in ankylosing spondylitis

12.4 Thoracolumbar Fractures

12.4.1 Introduction

- It is commonly mentioned that most thoracolumbar injuries result from high energy trauma
- While this is still true, be aware of the sharp rise in the incidence of wedge compression fractures in the elderly osteoporotic population. To this end, a section on the use of vertebroplasty and kyphoplasty is included in this chapter (Sect. 12.4.13.2.1)
- Although most texts consider thoracolumbar fractures together, it is more useful to divide these into three functional regions

12.4.2 Three Functional Regions

- Thoracic spine: stability enhanced by the rib cage, but has a narrow canal and blood flow watershed near the mid-thoracic spinal cord. Hence, although thoracic fracture is less common than in the other two regions, there is a higher chance of cord injury if fracture occurs. The cord:canal ratio is 40% for the thoracic spine, compared with 25% in the C-spine
- Thoracolumbar junction: region of high stress as there is change in sagittal profile and the spine transitions from the stiff thoracic region to the mobile lumbar region; 50% of fractures occur in this region. Depending on the location of the conus, neural injury can present as upper or lower motor neuron pattern or mixed. The relative incidence of thoracolumbar fractures according to Gertzbein: T1–T10 16%, T11–L1 52%, L1–L5 32%
- Lumbar spine: notice L3–L5 vertebrae lie below the pelvic brim with added stability from the iliolumbar ligament. For this and other reasons, the success rate of non-operative treatment of fractures in this

region is higher than at the TLJ. Neural deficit is seldom complete because of wider spinal canal, and the cauda equina is more resistant to compression than the cord. Finally, beware of the patient with ankylosing spondylitis, these frequently have three-column fractures that are easy to miss on X-ray (Vaccaro 2005) and may require CT. These fractures are difficult to heal owing to the long moment arms

12.4.3 Clinical Assessment

- Assess vital signs and general assessment
- Local spinal assessment of the acute trauma patient follows the ATLS protocol, remember to log roll the patient, check for palpable steps, etc.
- Assess any neurological deficit and carry out per rectum examination
- Associated injuries (of the axial skeleton or otherwise) are common in those suffering from high energy trauma

12.4.4 Radiological Assessment

- X-ray: assess overall coronal and sagittal alignment, soft tissue shadows, amount of vertebral height loss and of translation or rotation. Check the posterior vertebral line or profile to detect any middle column involvement. X-ray of the entire spine in two views recommended in high energy trauma
- CT: good to see bony details, e.g. useful in assessing the middle column in suspected burst fracture, assessing the degree of retropulsion, sometimes used to assess the presence and direction of contrast leakage after vertebroplasties have been performed
- MRI: good to assess ligamentous injuries, e.g. suspected ligamentous chance fractures; and for assessing spinal cord injuries

12.4.5 Denis Concept of Three Columns

- Anterior column: include mainly the ALL, anterior vertebral body, anterior annulus
- Middle column: includes mainly the PLL, the posterior vertebral body and posterior annulus

- Posterior column: includes mainly the posterior capsuloligamentous complex, facet, pedicles

12.4.6 What Constitutes Instability?

- The reader may choose to use the guidelines designed by White and Panjabi obtained as a result of biomechanical experiments on cadavers
- However, it is clinically useful to consider instability being present if:
  - Marked neurological deficit (some spinal fractures or subluxations can spontaneously reduce after injury. If, during the moment of impact, the spine deforms sufficiently to cause significant injury to the neural elements, it is highly likely the spine is unstable)
  - Risk of deformity progression (radiologic clues include: >25° kyphosis, >50% vertebral height loss, >40% canal compromise)
  - ≥ Two Denis's columns disrupted, especially if the middle column is not intact

12.4.7 Goal of Treatment

- Correction or prevention of further deformity
- Restoration of stability
- Neural decompression if necessary
- If fusion anticipated, attempt to achieve stability with fusion of as few as possible motion segments

12.4.8 General Approach

- Classify the fracture
- Can the fracture be treated conservatively?
- If operation required, what approach should we use?
- What are the deforming forces, and how can we go about reducing the fracture?
- What instrumentation is needed, if any?

12.4.9   Classifications

12.4.9.1 Denis Classification (an X-ray Classification)

- Minor injuries: include fracture of transverse process, spinous process, pars, facet articulations, etc.
- Major injuries:
  - Compression fracture
  - Burst fracture
  - Flexion distraction injury
  - Fracture dislocation

12.4.9.2 McAfee Classification (a CT Classification)

- Wedge compression fracture
- Stable burst fracture
- Unstable burst fracture
- Chance fracture
- Flexion distraction injury
- Translational injury

12.4.9.3 Allen's (Mechanistic) Classification

- Compression flexion
- Distraction flexion
- Lateral flexion
- Translational
- Torsional flexion
- Vertical compression
- Distractive extension

12.4.10   Conservative Versus Surgical Treatment

- The previously mentioned concept of instability is very useful here
- Most thoracolumbar fractures can in fact be treated conservatively, especially if there is no significant deformity or neurological deficit
- A recent study in a group of stable burst fracture patients without neural deficit revealed comparable clinical outcome with either conservative or operative treatment (J Bone Joint Surg 2003)

12.4.11 Anterior, Posterior or Combined Approach

■ Indication for anterior approach: logical for dealing with sizable retropulsion fragments causing anterior compression. Also indicated in delayed situations when indirect reduction from posterior approach difficult (thoracolumbar approach for TLJ fractures, retroperitoneal approach for lumbar fractures)

■ Indication for posterior approach: chance fracture, flexion distraction injury, some unstable burst fractures

■ Combined approach: fracture dislocation cases, some ligamentous chance fractures

■ Posterolateral approach: occasionally used if desire instrumentation with recourse to a second anterior operation, and/or to tackle a compressed nerve root

12.4.12 Selection of Instrumentation

12.4.12.1 What Is the Preferred Posterior Lumbar Fixation?

■ Most posterior instrumentation nowadays uses segmental pedicle screw fixation since it has superior stability as it stabilises all three columns, spans fewer segments (e.g. compared with hook-rod constructs), and is easier to restore an element of lordosis. If short segment of the spine is spanned, use of cross-links is recommended to confer torsional stability

12.4.12.2 What About the Thoracic Spine?

■ Use of pedicle screws in the thoracic spine is more controversial, with literature both in support of (Suk 2001) and cautioning (Xu 1998) its use, for fear of decreased safety margin for neurological injury

■ Two possible ways to circumvent the problem:
  − Use of hybrid constructs replacing the upper fixation at the thoracic level by the use of hooks
  − Using a posterior thoracic extrapedicular fixation via the use of a slightly different trajectory of screw insertion to prevent spinal canal penetration (Spine 2003), although clinical results are pending

12.4.12.3 Instruments for Anterior Fixation

- Commonly used constructs for anterior instrumentation include:
  - Plate-style systems (e.g. Sofamor-Danek Z-plate, Depuy Profile systems) and rod-style systems (e.g. Synthes Ventrofix, Kaneda Acromed device)
  - Anterior fusion cages

12.4.12.3.1 Plate-Style and Rod-Style Systems

- In vitro biomechanical studies indicate that these are load-sharing constructs, one-third of the stiffness of the whole construct depends on the graft
- However, the same study did not find a significant difference between different plate-style and rod-style systems (Fig. 12.10). Both systems were able to stabilise a corpectomy reconstruction model with respect to axial load, flexion/extension, axial rotation, and lateral bending

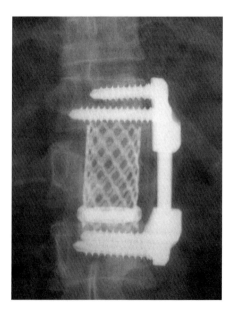

Fig. 12.10 Implants like the AO Ventrofix are useful in neutralisation of deforming forces after ASF

- This stresses the importance of graft preparation and placement. The graft contributed to the overall construct stiffness, especially in lateral bending (Brodke et al. 2003)

12.4.12.3.2 Anterior Fusion Cages
- Anterior grafting is especially indicated if we need direct decompression of a retropulsed fragment, or when the vertebral body is destroyed or non-functional
- Both autograft and allograft (e.g. allograft femur) have been used. Cages (Fig. 12.11) are sometimes needed to provide additional support as when the host bone stock is poor. It acts as a load-sharing device restoring axial stability until fusion occurs
- However, it is not easy to assess healing with the use of metal cages or to scientifically follow the different stages of graft incorporation; we have traditionally relied on clinical parameters, and others like cage migration, change in alignment, flexion/extension films, and CT (artefacts less with Ti cages). But is there more scientific research to tell us about the very basic graft healing and incorporation process in the setting of spinal cages?

Basic Science: Spinal Fusion Cages
- An interesting recent spine injury model in goats with a cage inserted was reported. This made use of bioabsorbable poly L-lactic

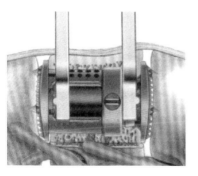

Fig. 12.11 Cage insertion can be useful if the host bone stock is deficient or of poor quality as in extreme osteoporosis

acid fusion cages (instead of Ti cages) and sacrificing the animals at intervals of 3, 6, 12, 24, 30 and 36 months (Smit et al. 2003)

- It was found that:
  - The trabecular bone architecture within a spinal cage changes during the fusion process
  - A more mature interbody fusion is manifested by a more homogenous bone architecture
  - The bone architecture becomes coarser with time
  - The stiffness of the fusion cages can affect the fusion process
  - Excessive cage stiffness had a negative effect on fusion rate

12.4.13 Management of Individual Fractures

- The following clinical fracture types will be discussed:
  - Minor fractures, as defined in the Denis classification (Denis 1984)
  - Simple wedge compression fractures (not burst fractures) and the role of vertebroplasty
  - Stable burst fractures
  - Unstable burst fractures
  - Flexion distraction injuries
  - Translational injuries
  - Distraction extension injuries

12.4.13.1 *Minor Fractures*

- Minor injuries include fracture of transverse process, spinous process, facet articulations, etc.
- According to Denis, most of these are adequately treated by conservative means such as thoracolumbosacral orthosis (TLSO)

12.4.13.2 *Wedge Compression Fractures*

- Mostly occur in osteoporotic elderly, especially females
- Most can be treated conservatively, but a handful with failed conservative treatment may benefit from vertebroplasty or kyphoplasty, provided there is no contraindication

12.4.13.2.1 Vertebroplasty and Kyphoplasty (Fig. 12.12)
Introduction: Osteoporotic Vertebral Fractures

- Vertebral fracture is the most common of the fragility fractures
- It is not without morbidity, which includes:
  - Kyphosis and loss of proper sagittal alignment
  - Pain
  - Loss of height
  - Effect on pulmonary function especially if the thoracic vertebrae are involved
  - Some data to support increased mortality (Am J Epidemiol 1993)

Common Yardstick to Assess Osteoporotic Vertebral Fractures

- A common yardstick does not exist

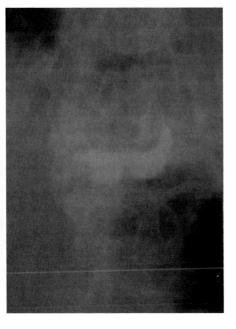

Fig. 12.12 Antero-posterior X-ray of lumbar spine after cement vertebroplasty

- This makes comparison between different papers on this topic difficult
- A more commonly used semi-quantitative assessment is designed by Genant (J Bone Min Res 1993):
  - Mild deformity = 20–25% height reduction (lateral X-ray)
  - Moderate deformity = 25–40% height reduction
  - Severe deformity = >40% height reduction

What is Vertebroplasty?
- Vertebroplasty is a surgical procedure in which bone cement is injected into a usually collapsed, compressed (osteoporotic) vertebral body
- The procedure was first described by French surgeons. The cement is injected at high pressure via an 11-gauge needle through the pedicles under screening by biplanar fluoroscopy

Possible Mechanism of Action
- Heat injury to afferent nerve fibres
- Improved support and force transmission at anterior vertebral body
- Mechanical stabilisation of microfractures
- Fracture reduction – helped to some extent by kyphoplasty (if fracture not too old and can be reduced)

(Most [around 90%] patients had pain relief)

What is Kyphoplasty?
- Essentially similar procedure to vertebroplasty
- The Kyphon Inc. company developed a "bone tamp" that can be inserted through a cortical window via a trans-pedicular route or through the body to attempt reduction of the compressed vertebra
- Reduction is not always straight-forward since conservative treatment is administered for 4–6 weeks before such procedures are underataken, and reduction may not be easy after 6 or more weeks. Most successful cases can thus only effect partial reduction

Indications for Vertebroplasty
- Failed conservative management 4–6 weeks

- Clinical pain location corresponds with radiologic abnormalities
- Pathologies that can be so treated:
  - Osteoporotic vertebral collapse
  - Other pathologies sometimes treated by vertebroplasty: vertebral metastases, vertebral haemangioma, myeloma

Indications for Kyphoplasty

- Same as vertebroplasty
- But here the restoration of vertebral height is attempted

Contraindications

- Coagulopathy
- Pain due to other causes, e.g. referred pain
- Burst fracture or fractured pedicle or level above T5
- Significant vertebral collapse/vertebra plana
- Pre-existing neurological deficit or narrowed canal
- Contrast allergy
- Sepsis
- Unable to lie prone (e.g. chest disease)

Advantages of Vertebroplasty

- Reliable and quick pain relief (within hours)
- Improved force transmission
- Early mobilisation
- Early hospital discharge

Complications of Vertebroplasty

- Neurological Cx: e.g. radiculopathy
- Cement extravasation into spinal canal
- Cement intravasation as pulmonary emboli and hypotension
- Allergic reactions
- Fractured pedicle or rib reported
- Pneumothorax
- Sepsis
- Epidural haematoma in patients with coagulopathy

- Late Cx: compression fracture of adjacent vertebra, since the stiffness of the vertebra after cement vertebroplasty may be higher than for its alternatives

Preoperative Work-up
- Preoperative clinical assessment and neurologic assessment
- Preoperative X-ray and CT to assess posterior cortex
- Selected cases may need bone scan/MRI
- Intraoperative venography found to be useful to identify situations of rapid venous egress, either to the epidural venous plexus, the IVC or paraspinal veins. This may help avoid leakage and pulmonary emboli

Key Difference Between Vertebroplasty and Kyphoplasty
- The only main difference is that in kyphoplasty, we try to restore vertebral height, reduce kyphosis. Since the pressure of injection is less theoretically, the chance of cement extravasation is smaller

Why Do Some Experts Argue that Vertebroplasty Alone Suffices?
- They argue that the dynamic mobility of some vertebral fractures can allow for height restoration even with vertebroplasty
- In one recent report, up to seven vertebral bodies were injected in patient, with good results

Areas of Uncertainty
- It is *not* certain whether:
  - There is a case for performing vertebroplasty for multiple levels of compression collapse of vertebrae, in view of reports of adjacent level vertebral fractures after such procedures, especially if vertebroplasties are performed on non-consecutive levels
  - What is the best material to be injected: is it bone cement, injectable bone substitute or other substances?

12.4.13.3 Stable Burst Fractures
- Feature: besides anterior column compressive failure, there is by definition involvement of the middle column

- Radiologically, increased inter-pedicular distance (Fig. 12.13) is seen on the AP X-ray; look for a contour disruption of the posterior vertebral line on the lateral X-ray. CT is useful in assessing burst fractures (Fig. 12.14)
- There are myths surrounding the topic of burst fracture, which will be discussed. Note that some reports indicate evidence of healing (especially in young patients) and remodelling of the retropulsed fragment, decreasing the severity of canal compromise over time (Spine 1998)

12.4.13.3.1 Myths Concerning Burst Fractures

- There is no evidence of any direct correlation between degree of retropulsion and neurological deficit in burst fractures
- There is no concrete evidence for comments like 40% or 50% canal compromise requiring surgery
- There is no concrete evidence that surgery itself leads to lower DVT or PE rates

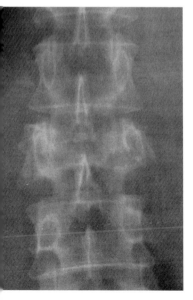

Fig. 12.13 Note the increased inter-pedicular distance in burst fracture

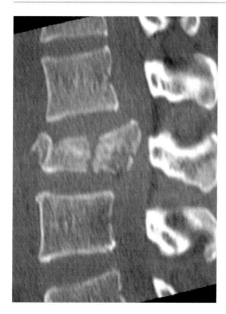

Fig. 12.14 Sagittal CT showing the retropulsed fragment of a burst fractur

- There is no concrete evidence that surgery produces fewer complica
  tions

12.4.13.4 Unstable Burst Fractures
- Feature: besides compressive failure of the anterior and mid
  dle columns, there is also tensile failure of the posterior colum
  (Fig. 12.15)

12.4.13.4.1 Unstable Fractures Without Neurological Deficit
- Burst fractures are caused by flexion and axial loading forces, operat
  ive reduction can be attained posteriorly with reduction and fixatio
  by extension and distraction
- According to experts like Garfin, operative intervention should b
  considered if: >25° kyphosis, >50% loss of vertebral height, >40°
  canal compromise

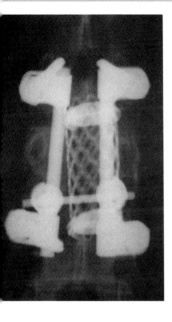

Fig. 12.15 Postoperative X-ray of a burst fracture that involved all three Denis columns and required anterior and posterior surgery

12.4.13.4.2 Surgical Approach

- Posterior instrumentation options include hook-rod systems (these need long moment arm and span more motion segments), pedicle screw systems (more rigid segmental fixation can span fewer segments and provide three-column support); wires are uncommonly but sometimes used as bail out in intraoperative complications or extremely osteoporotic bones. Use of sublaminar wires is contraindicated in patients with neurological deficit
- Overall, posterior surgery alone usually suffices in these injuries, but the occasional patient with significant kyphus and comminution needs longer posterior instrumentation. It is essential to restore the sagittal alignment
- Anterior approach may be needed to retrieve sizable retropulsed fragment or if there has been a delay for several days rendering indirect reduction by posterior approach difficult. Anterior grafting al-

lows the graft to be in compression and available for load sharing
Whether adjunct instrumentation is needed anteriorly or posteriorly
needs to be individualised

12.4.13.4.3 Unstable Fracture with Neurological Deficit

- Anterior approach is logical if feasible to relieve the anterior source
  of neural compression, especially in the presence of a sizable retropulsed fragment, i.e. direct decompression
- Whether to add on anterior instrumentation like AO Ventrofix depends on factors like quality of the graft obtained, number of segments that need surgery, and whether posterior surgery is planned
  for any concomitant posterior injury

12.4.13.4.4 Indirect Reduction and Posterior Surgery

- Indirect reduction from the posterior approach is based on ligamentotaxis. Studies revealed possible reduction of canal compromise by
  up to 50% (Harrington et al. 1993)
- However, it must be noted that the efficacy of indirect reduction decreases after day 5. Neither is ligamentotaxis effective in the face of
  PLL rupture or extensive comminution

12.4.13.5 Flexion Distraction Injuries

- Feature: distraction injury of anterior and middle column, and ten-
  sile failure of the posterior column
- The centre of rotation falls posterior to the ALL sometimes, and in
  such cases the anterior column will have compressive failure
- Level of injury can be either one or two spinal levels
- Injury force can go through bone or ligaments
- Called a "bony chance fracture" if the injury force goes horizontally
  through bone
- Called a " ligamentous chance fracture" if the injury force goes hori-
  zontally through ligaments
- Two-thirds of chance fractures are associated with abdominal inju-
  ries, according to Denis, and may require operative intervention

12.4.13.5.1 Principles of Treatment

- Ligamentous chance fractures treated conservatively will usually fail, although have been tried with some reported success in children. Ligamentous chance fractures in adults all require posterior surgery for stabilisation and frequently anterior surgery as well. Preoperative MRI to check the disc status is advisable
- Not all bony chance fractures require operation. Fractures with <15° kyphosis and no neural deficit have been treated with success by extension casting (Anderson et al. 1991)
- The rest of bony chance fractures require surgery. Most require posterior surgery (the injury had already done the dissection for us), but not infrequently anterior surgery may need to be added

12.4.13.6 Translational Injuries

- This group includes fracture dislocation injuries
- Involve facet dislocation or subluxation, the direction of which depends on the direction of the external force. Possibilities include anterior, posterior translations frequently with a rotational element
- All are treated surgically via a posterior approach usually with segmental pedicle screw fixation. This time, short segment fixation is not adequate, and we should instrument two levels above and below the level of injury
- Intraoperative reduction is necessary before pedicle screw application. Remember to tackle the not infrequent finding of *dural tear*

12.4.13.7 Distraction of Extension Injury

- Rare
- More common in patients with ankylosing spondylitis
- Caused by an extension force striking the lower back, can cause disruption to the anterior tension band (ALL and annulus). In severe cases the posterior elements can be injured as well
- Operative treatment is indicated if the fracture is unstable

12.4.14 Complications

- Iatrogenic neural injury

- Sepsis
- Loss of reduction
- Hardware problem and failure (e.g. when there is inadequate anterior support and the posterior instrumentation is subjected to cyclic loading)
- Failure of healing of the bony fracture or the ligamentous injury

12.5   Spine Fractures in the Elderly

12.5.1   General Features

- Sometimes after minor trauma, some are pathological
- Hx more difficult to obtain
- Pain – note any radiation patterns, DDx referred pain
- P/E – check whether clinical tenderness corresponds to radiological anomaly
- X-ray – most have superimposed degenerative changes
- Role of bone scan – can show occult fracture, metastases, but cannot rely on bone scan to pick up myeloma
- MRI – good to assess soft tissue and any neural compression

12.5.2   Reasons for the Weakened Bone

- Osteoporosis
- Other secondary causes:
  - Osteomalacia
  - Steroids
  - Metastases
  - Myeloma
  - Paget's, etc.

(P.S. Rule out treatable diseases causing osteoporosis like thyroid disorders)

12.5.3   Common Patterns

- Cervical – odontoid fracture, Jefferson fracture ± burst fracture
- T/L spine – collapse ± burst fracture

■ Sacrum – insufficiency fracture (H-shaped appearance on bone scan)

12.5.4 Problems in Management

■ Medical – rest, brace, pain control
■ Surgical – more Cx in the elderly – poor nutrition, more sepsis, bone does not hold implants well, dangers of thoracotomy in elderly, difficulty with intraoperative positioning (stiff joints, previous total joints, kyphosis). Fixation is a big issue (may sometimes need more levels, A + P surgery, delayed union is more common), rehabilitation slow since poor mobility

12.5.4.1 Example 1: Thoracolumbar Spine Fractures

■ Common
■ 60% silent
■ Up to quarter females > 50, 40% > 80
■ Problems: decreased height, deformity, pain, poor mobility
■ Rn: brace (TLSO), drugs (calcium, vitamin D, bisphosphonates, calcitonin, hormones)
■ Role of vertebroplasty and kyphoplasty has been discussed (Sect. 12.4.13.2.1)

12.5.4.2 Example 2: Odontoid Fractures

■ Features:
   - Low energy trauma, can be after minor injury (80%)
   - Index of suspicion
   - Most are posteriorly displaced
   - Most are osteoporotic bones

12.5.4.2.1 Two Main Problems

■ Mechanical – non-union 50% in type 2 odontoid fractures, 90% if posteriorly displaced 4–5 mm
■ Neurologic risk – incidence not high (Webb), but if non-union sets in, incidence may increase with time. Onset of myelopathy can be very gradual

12.5.4.2.2 Treatment
- Undisplaced – collar, halo poorly tolerated, earlier ROM
- Displaced – early posterior fusion

12.5.4.2.3 Fusion Method
- Odontoid screw – not good for the elderly (base of C2 is osteoporotic)
- Transarticular screw – assess feasibility
- Others – e.g. wires

12.6 Principles of Spinal Fixation and Instrumentation

12.6.1 Implants Making Use of the Tension Band Principle
- Tension band principle has already been discussed elsewhere
- This method of fixation works on the principle of dynamic fixation
- Using the cervical spine as an example, the use of posterior cervical hook plates is an example of a tension band device. This cervical hook plate system works only if the anterior load-bearing support of the anterior column is intact

12.6.2 Implants Making Use of the Neutralisation Principle (Figs. 12.16, 12.17)
- This means the use of the implant to minimise the bending, shearing torsional and axial loading forces on, say, a vertebral reconstruction
- In short, it is commonly used to protect the graft or the neural structure before fusion occurs
- This includes different kinds of stabilisation systems placed anteriorly, posteriorly, etc.
- An example will be the use of the AO Ventrofix system for neutralisation after anterior spinal fusion (ASF)

12.6.3 Implants Making Use of the Buttress Principle
- The aim of buttressing is to prevent axial deformity

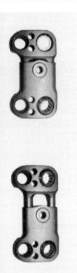

Fig. 12.16 Newer Ventrofix implants allow compression of the nearby anterior bone graft

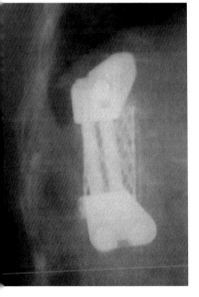

Fig. 12.17 Lateral lumbar spine X-ray showing the AO Ventrofix implant in situ

- In order for buttressing to work, the following points must be heeded:
  - Maximise surface area of contact
  - Begin screw insertion closest to the area that needs buttressing and insert the remaining screws one by one towards the ends of the plate
  - Placement of the buttress plate on the side of the load application to minimise shear and compression forces

12.6.4   Use of Cages

- Popular in some countries as an interbody spacer in anterior spinal surgery
- Titanium is a common material used, and it is MRI-compatible
- Mainly used in anterior interbody spinal fusions from L1–L2 to L5/S1

12.6.4.1   Advantages of Cages

- Offer immediate stability, can be used in conjunction with posterior instrumentation (Fig. 12.18)
- Well-designed cages can help restore the natural lordosis of the lumbar spine
- Large hollow cages allow the use of autografts or allografts, or even newer coralline hydroxyapatite

12.6.4.2   Basic Science of Graft Incorporation in the Presence of Spinal Cages

- An interesting recent spine injury model in goats with cages inserted was reported. This made use of bioabsorbable poly L-lactic acid fusion cages (instead of metal cages) and sacrificing the animal at intervals of 3, 6, 12, 24, 30, and 36 months (Smit et al. 2003)
- It was found that:
  - The trabecular bone architecture within a spinal cage changes during the fusion process
  - A more mature interbody fusion is manifested by a more homogenous bone architecture

- The bone architecture becomes coarser with time
- The stiffness of the fusion cages can affect the fusion process
- Excessive cage stiffness had a negative effect on fusion rate

2.6.4.3 Disadvantages of Cages

- Assessment of bony fusion difficult
- Requires an intact end plate to prevent subsidence into the vertebral body
- If stability is in question, may need adjunctive instrumentation

2.6.4.4 Tackling Cage-Related Problems

- Some possible methods of assessment of fusion include: monitoring of clinical symptoms, serial X-rays to look for any subsidence/migra-

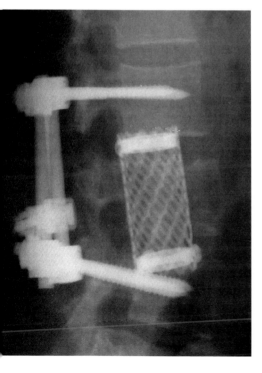

Fig. 12.18 Postoperative lateral lumbar spine X-ray showing anterior fusion cage plus posterior pedicle screw system in situ

tion, sometimes use of flexion/extension X-rays, CT can be used an Ti cages cause less artefacts; exploration is the last resort

- Some new improvements in cage design include: presence of teet on both sides allowing better holding of the end plate and preventin migration; shape follows that of the natural anatomy of the end plate and some can be expanded after insertion to allow a snug fit

General Bibliography

1.   Vaccaro A, Todd A (2001) Master cases in spine surgery. Thieme, New York

Selected Bibliography of Journal Articles

1.   Allen BL, Ferguson RL et al. (1982) A mechanistic classification of closed, indirec fractures and dislocations of the lower cervical spine. Spine 7:1
2.   Anderson PA, Henley MB, Grady MS et al. (1991) Posterior cervical arthrodesis wit AO reconstruction plates and bone graft. Spine 16 [3 Suppl]:S72–S79
3.   Bethea JR (2000) Spinal cord injury-induced inflammation: a dual-edged sword Prog Brain Res 128:33–42
4.   Bracken MB, Collins WF (1984) Efficacy of methylprednisolone in acute spinal cor injury. JAMA 251(1):45–52
5.   Bracken MB, Shepard MJ et al. (1990) A randomized controlled trial of methyl-pred nisolone or naloxone in the treatment of acute spinal cord injury study. N Engl J Me 332:1405–1411
6.   Brodke DS, Gollogly S, Bacchus KN et al. (2003) Anterior thoracolumbar instru mentation: stiffness and load sharing characteristics of plate and rod systems. Spin 28:1794–1801
7.   Cotler JM, Herbison GJ et al. (1993) Close reduction of traumatic cervical spine dis location using traction weights up to 140 pounds. Spine 18:386–390
8.   Denis F (1984) Spinal instability as defined by the three column spine concept i acute spinal trauma. Clin Orthop Relat Res 189:85
9.   Fielding WJ, Hawkins RJ (1977) Atlantoaxial rotatory fixation. J Bone Joint Surg Ar 59:37
10.   Harrington RM, Budorick T, Hoyt J et al. (1993) Biomechanics of indirect reductio of bone retropulsed into the spinal canal in vertebral fracture. Spine 18(6):692–699

1. Levine AM, Edwards CC (1985) The management of traumatic spondylolisthesis of the axis. J Bone Joint Surg 67:217

2. Ryan MD, Taylor TKF (1993) Odontoid fractures in the elderly. J Spinal Disord 6:397–401

3. Smit TH, Muller R, Van Dijk M, Wuisman PI (2003) Changes in bone architecture during spinal fusion: three years follow-up and the role of cage stiffness. Spine 28(16):1802–1808; discussion 1809

4. White AA, Johnson RM et al. (1975) Biomechanical analysis of clinical stability in the cervical spine. Clin Orthop Relat Res 109:85

5. Wood KB, Vaccaro AR et al. (2005) Assessment of two thoracolumbar fracture classification systems as used by multiple surgeons. J Bone Joint Surg 87(7):1423–1429

| 13 | **Paediatric Trauma** |

Contents

13.1   General Features of Fractures in Children

- Children are not just mini-adults; this is true also of fractures in children:
  - Anatomically, there are growth plates and ossification centres that can give rise to special fracture patterns and growth disturbance. It is assumed that the reader is familiar with the Salter–Harris classification of growth plate injuries
  - The long bones of children have a thick periosteum and increased plasticity compared with adults, thus giving rise to other special fracture patterns like plastic deformation
  - The healing rate of childhood fractures is quick, and especially in infants. Follow-up after fracture reduction should be frequent in the first 1–2 weeks, since late reduction is seldom successful because of the rapid rate of healing, and in fact forceful late reduction attempts in peri-articular fractures can damage the growth plate

13.2   Physeal Injury: Basic Concepts

13.2.1   Possible Response of Physeal Plate After Injury
- Stimulated then retarded
- Retarded
- Stimulated
- Arrested
- Premature closure
- One side arrested ± closed, i.e. asymmetrical (no bar)
- Asymmetrical growth with bone bar

13.2.2   Physeal Arrest
- Complete – by definition no angular deformity, complete no growth, no bars
- Partial – *due to bar formation* that can sometimes cause angular deformity (if involve periphery), which sometimes self-corrects after bar excision if mild, but requires osteotomy if severe

- Types of bone bars:
  - Central – requires excision through metaphyseal window – do not touch the perichondral ring of Ranvier
  - Peripheral – commonly causes angular deformity (e.g. recurvatum if at anterior proximal tibia)
  - Longitudinal (said to result from type 5 Salter–Harris injury according to Peterson)

13.2.3 Dx: Physeal Bar
- Best shown on tomogram
- Sometimes CT or MRI useful
- Serial changes possible, e.g. serial X-ray may show tenting of the distal femoral physis
- Early detection is important

13.2.4 Four Major Factors Affecting Prognosis (Decreasing Order of Importance)
- Injury severity – displacement, comminution, open vs closed
- Age
- Physis involved
- Salter-Harris type

13.2.5 Does Bar Excision Work?
- Yes. According to Langenskiold (1967)
- Keys to success:
  - Careful calculation of the area and mapping of the bar
  - Different strategies with different bar locations
  - Careful and correct use of interpositional materials
  - Monitoring of success or failure/Cx
  - Future: use of physeal/apophysis or chondrocyte allograft transplant beyond the laboratory

13.2.6 Goal of Bar Excision Surgery
- Ensure complete bar excision
- Prevent blood recollection in the cavity created by inter-positional materials (and excision of overlying periosteum for peripheral bars)

13.2.7 Technical Pearl 1 – Area and Mapping

- Excision of bar effective if ≤ 50% of area (although some had tried the same for a larger area in a very small child)
- Mapping is difficult since:
  - Seldom able to see the whole physis in one axial cut on CT
  - Experts like Peterson maintain that tomography may still be the best (many subtypes can be detected on tomogram: linear, circular, ellipsoidal, spiral, hypocycloidal)
  - MRI some advantage: no radiation, superior image, thin cuts in any plane, data can be programmed to depict the entire physis with its bar on one plane despite contour irregularities caused by the bar itself or very nature of the growth plate proper (as in plates near the knee – they undulate – the advantage of this design is that it help insulate them from injury, but when injury does occur, the same undulations predispose to damage of the growth layer of the physis)
  - The undulating bars as mentioned before are not easy to map

13.2.8 Technical Pearl 2: Strategies by Location

- Peripheral – direct approach, periosteum over the bar should be excised to prevent bar reforms
- Central – open metaphyseal window to avoid the perichondral ring of Ranvier, and use a small, 5-mm dental mirror in electric burring (Peterson commented that he is not too worried about heat from burr, and he only occasionally uses the curette/osteotome)
- Longitudinal (linear/elongated) variety: these patterns are highly indicated for careful mapping to plan our approach for its proper excision

13.2.9 Pearl 3: Interposition Materials

- Fat – buttock fat used by Langenskiold since inert, but not too helpful in stopping bleeding, can float away, and not load-share – a feature needed if in large bars in weight-bearing areas
- Pure methylmethacrylate – very different from the cement containing barium in total joint – characterised by little exothermic reaction, load-sharing, inert, with little rejection/sepsis/neoplastic trans-

formation – since used by neurosurgeons for decades. Radiolucency allows detection of recurrent bar formation (another name: cranioplast). Other advantages: cheap, easy to mould, the liquid monomer and powder polymer are sterile-packed with no need to take cultures; no second incision as in fat harvest. Can be poured or allowed to set a little and pushed like putty. It provides haemostasis by virtue of occupying the entire desired portion of the cavity

- Silastic – toxic, creates synovitis, withdrawn in US market in 1987
- Cartilage – a logical way and theoretically ideal as it is the tissue damaged; sources:
    - (Iliac crest) apophysis – but may not have the same growth potential as epiphyseal cartilage; and difficulties in procuring and insertion
    - Chondrocyte allograft transplant – requires time for it to develop matrix; possible immune response if transfer between humans

(Also experimental is use of Indocid to prevent bar reforming)

13.2.10   Monitoring Progress

- Metal markers have been used, implanted at metaphyseal cancellous bone (but not in contact with the cavity or may migrate into it) – these markers help DDx overgrowth of physis at other end of bone and helps more accurate X-ray measurements
- Scanograms are the most precise way to measure the increasing distance between the two metal markers

(Ti markers useful if subsequent MRI planned)

13.2.11   Unifocal Versus Multifocal Physeal Injury

- Multifocal more likely in, say, severe trauma to the whole limb
- Causes of injury include: infection (staphylococci – more focal, neiserria – more diffuse); neoplasm (e.g. fibromatosis), endocrine, hemihypertrophy, vascular, idiopathic – e.g. Perthes

13.2.12   When to Intervene

- Mainly depends on amount of growth remaining (age is important):

- The presumption that physeal injuries that occur late have much less effect is only partially true – two main exceptions:
  - Severe trauma – here growth retardation can be clinically significant
  - A growth-retarded child can suddenly speed up growth with, say, endocrine replacement

13.2.13   Pitfalls

- Growth velocity of plate cannot be assessed with current means, nor growth potential despite seeing an open plate on X-ray
- Cannot always predict what behaviour the physis will adopt after injury (not possible at present); the behaviour also changes with time
- Hence, close monitoring important: of LLD, X-ray, tomogram, etc.

13.2.14   Steps in Management

- Assess extent of injury/number of plates affected (or likely to be affected) – sometimes need close monitoring to tell
- Define exact 3D nature of injury and check any bone bar
- Treat any underlying treatable cause
- Get rapport with parents that plate behaviour may change with time
- With established pattern (e.g. plate arrested), likely effect depends on amount of growth remaining, and any treatable cause – bar, endocrine, tumour, etc.
- If no treatable cause, or unresponsive despite Rn, see discussion on LLD correction in the companion volume of this book

13.2.15   The Langenskiold Procedure

- Goal: attempt to restore growth by excision of bone bridge – if < 50% physis affected
- Expected result: some growth at least restored in 80% of cases
- Sometimes need simultaneous corrective osteotomy if angular deformity > 20°
- If central bar → needs approach through metaphysis if peripheral bone wedge → direct approach

Table 13.1 Disadvantages of various materials

Disadvantages	Fat	Cement	Silastic
Toxicity	−	+	+
Infection	−	−	+
Remove	−	+	+
No support	+	−	−

- Fat interposition
- Cx: fractured epiphysis, recurrent bone bridge (Acta Orthop Scand)

13.2.16   Merits and Demerits of Materials for Interposition
- Another method: in animal experiments – transplant of iliac apophysis (Lee et al. 1993)

13.3   Upper Extremity Injuries

13.3.1   Fractured Proximal Humerus
- Metaphyseal fractures: more often seen in pre-adolescents, heal easily because of cancellous bone being involved. There is great remodelling potential (especially in the plane of joint motion) for these fractures, since the proximal humeral physis is capable of rapid growth in children
- Epiphyseal injuries: more commonly seen in adolescence, can be Salter–Harris type 1 or 2, caused by axial loading or an abduction and external rotation mechanism. Owing to the muscle attachments, the distal fragment usually displaces anteriorly and laterally. Displaced fractures in the older child may need reduction and pinning (e.g. angulation $> 45°$, > 3 cm shortening). OR only considered if there is associated vascular injury, soft tissue entrapment, or skin impingement, or in patients with multiple injuries

13.3.2 Supracondylar Humerus Fractures in Children (Figs. 13.1, 13.2)

13.3.2.1 Introduction

■ Second most common child fracture, (first being fracture of the distal forearm), most common fracture around the elbow

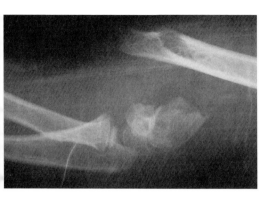

Fig. 13.1 Displaced supracondylar fracture of the distal humerus

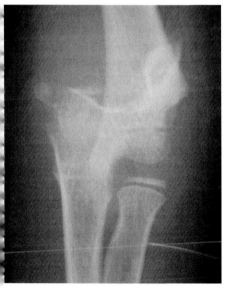

Fig. 13.2 Another view of the same fracture

- Mostly age 1–7 (theoretically, birth to fusion of the distal humeral physis); peak at age 6

13.3.2.2 Relevant Anatomy
- Distal humerus – a 1-mm wafer of bone flanked by larger medial and lateral columns form the distal humeral metaphysis
- The thin bone separates the anterior coronoid fossa from the posterior olecranon fossa
- Fracture tends to rotate, reduction is like balancing two knives on one another (Dameron); hence, easy loss of reduction and angular deformity – anatomic restoration important
- Normally, the brachial artery is protected by the brachialis muscle

13.3.2.3 Mechanism of Extension and Flexion Injuries
- Laxity of ligaments in the child; hyper-extended elbow; thin distal humeral metaphyseal bone
- Result – axial force turned into a bending force
- Extension type in 96% of cases, flexion type uncommon (falling on a flexed elbow)

13.3.2.4 Initial Assessment: History
- Injury mechanics
  - Extension type – child usually holds elbow in extension (some authors say flexion)
  - Look for: associated injuries, especially shoulder and distal forearm, neurovascular compromise

13.3.2.5 Physical Assessment
- Vascular: group 1 – signs of major vessel injury; group 2 – sign of acute compartment syndrome
- Neural exam: incidence of injury 10% (much more than lateral condyle cases) anterior interosseus nerve (AIN) most common; others: radial nerve > median > ulna nerve affected
- Local exam of the elbow: Bucker sign (Fig. 13.3) suggests vascular insult, local swelling, tenderness
- Associated injury: especially distal forearm, proximal humerus, etc.

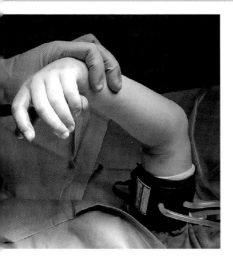

Fig. 13.3 Bucker sign is suggestive of possible underlying vascular injury in this child with supracondylar fracture of the distal humerus

13.3.2.6 Dealing with Suspected Vascular Insult

- Group 1: signs of acute vascular insult
  - Symptoms: pain, aesthesia of nerves of affected compartment
  - Signs = absent/feeble pulse, Bucker sign suggestive of poor limb circulation, can also have pain on passive muscle stretch
- Group 2: signs of acute compartment syndrome (which sometimes rapidly develops in the first 24–48 h) – most important symptom = pain out of proportion; most important sign = tense compartment (whole territory), other signs – pain on passive muscle stretch (also found if there is associated fracture or muscle contusion)

13.3.2.7 Possible Scenarios of Vascular Status After CR and Pinning

- Pulse and pink limb: danger still not over, watch out for delayed compartment syndrome (if there was vascular compromise before CR)
- Pulse – and pink limb: some will observe, others do angiogram. One recent study shows that even if intervention is undertaken if angiogram is abnormal in this group, there is a high chance of re-occlusion. In most cases limb viability can probably be maintained by good collateral circulation (instead of angiogram, can use MRA,

since less invasive; angiogram has a risk of its own, e.g. contrast sensitivity)

- Pulse – and ischaemic limb: always explore

13.3.2.8 Delayed Vascular Problems – Compartment Syndrome

- After reperfusion
- Tight cast – hence, many just give a splint in acute setting if gross swelling
- Rebleeding

(P.S. *total* vascular occlusion rare in children since collaterals at the elbow region)

13.3.2.9 Key Concept

- Arterial injury involves large vessels
- Compartment syndrome affects small vessels and pulse can still be present in compartment syndrome (Rang 1974)

13.3.2.10 CR Manoeuvres

- Need intraoperative X-ray screening in both AP and lateral planes
- After carefully documenting the neurovascular status, start by longitudinal traction
- Then correct any varus/valgus malalignment and any rotational malalignment
- Hyperflexion (while monitoring the pulse) to reduce the hyperextension of the distal fragment (in extension-type injury). Percutaneous pinning can be done at this juncture
- Recheck the alignment after pinning, and decrease flexion of the arm to 90°. In most cases the forearm is kept pronated to help prevent varus deformity. But need to individualise depending on the personality of the fracture

13.3.2.11 Pinning Manoeuvres

- If pinning is deemed necessary, the author finds that two lateral smooth k-wires are usually adequate

- Avoid crossing the k-wires at the site of the fracture since this will defeat the purpose of the anti-rotation effect of using two k-wires
- Crossed k-wires can be considered in very unstable fractures; it is recommended that a mini-incision be opened on the medial side in these situations to avoid ulna nerve injury

13.3.2.12 Complications

13.3.2.12.1 Cubitus Varus – 3D Deformity

- Horizontal plane – varus
- Coronal plane – internal rotation
- Sagittal – extension

(Importance of the Baumann's angle to follow up these fractures cannot be overemphasised)

13.3.2.12.2 Other Complications

- Nerve injury: at presentation, most commonly involved nerve is the AIN portion of the median nerve, followed by radial and ulna nerves. But iatrogenic ulna nerve injury is not uncommon when using crossed pinning of these fractures
- Volkmann ischaemic contracture, as a result of undiagnosed or mistreated vascular injury

13.3.3 Lateral Condyle Fractures (Fig. 13.4)

13.3.3.1 Introduction

- Peak at age 6–10 (range, 3–14 mostly)
- ≥50% of distal humeral physeal fractures in children

13.3.3.2 Why Is There a High Chance of Fracture Non-union?

- Iatrogenic – if the posterior surface was stripped during ORIF
- Bathing the fracture in synovial fluid hinders callus formation (as in untreated displaced fractures)
- Tension of the extensor muscles, especially in late displacement cases in a cast

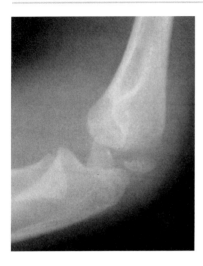

Fig. 13.4 The X-ray depicts a displaced fractured lateral condyle of the distal humerus

13.3.3.3 Pearl
- A fracture seen on X-ray in the lateral portion of the distal humerus in a child <10 most likely a lateral condyle fracture (since lateral epicondyle ossifies at age 11)
- DDx = mainly from transphyseal fracture that sometimes has a metaphyseal fragment in a younger child – may need arthrogram to be sure in these cases (or MRI)

13.3.3.4 Injury Mechanism
- Varus stress on an extended elbow with forearm supinated
- Fracture begins at lateral aspect of distal metaphysis and travels obliquely and medially through the physis

13.3.3.5 Milch Classification
- Type 1 Milch = fracture line through the ossific nucleus to exit at the radiocapitellar groove (Salter–Harris type 2)
- Type 2 Milch = fracture line extends around the entire physis and exits through the trochlear notch, intra-articular and more common (Salter-Harris type 4)

13.3.3.6 How Does Milch View the Two Types in His Original Paper?

■ He differentiates types 1 and 2 *not* by whether the fracture involves the ossific nucleus or not, but by where the fracture line crosses the epiphysis, especially focusing on whether the fracture is associated with ulna dislocation, since a dislocation is more likely with fracture lines lateral to the trochlear groove

13.3.3.7 Rate of Union

■ Notice that the *amount of displacement* is more important than fracture line location (Rutherford)

13.3.3.8 Physical Assessment

■ Lateral elbow swelling, locally tender
■ Look for associated injury, sometimes dislocation or olecranon injury

13.3.3.9 Radiological Assessment

■ Posterior fat pad should be assessed
■ AP/lateral ± oblique views
■ Arthrogram:
  – Useful in DDx of distal humeral physeal separation with a metaphyseal fragment in younger children, especially < 6
  – Checking the amount of displacement and rotation of the fracture
  – Check for an adequate alignment after pinning
  – Some say interpretation best if done < 24 h

13.3.3.10 Role of MRI

■ Useful in atypical fracture patterns
■ Unsure even after arthrogram or if interpretation of arthrogram is less accurate if delayed for a few days

13.3.3.11 Key to Management

■ Displaced 2–4 mm fractures are most difficult to recognise – traditionally and paradoxically have the worst results in these cases, since prone to redisplacement in casts, and healing can be significantly delayed even with a very small amount of displacement

13.3.3.12   Conservative Treatment
- Only for cases < 2 mm displaced and stable
- Monitor closely just in case there is delayed redisplacement – some use tomograms
- Drawback – stiff elbow since >6 weeks in plaster are sometimes needed, if healing is slow

13.3.3.13   Operative Treatment
- All others
- ORIF in many cases – reason even experts say that CRIF quite difficult to achieve anatomic reduction
- Pearl – expose joint anteriorly to help achieve anatomic reduction, avoid posterior stripping to preserve vascularity

13.3.3.14   Importance of Anatomic Reduction
- Avoid bone bridge formation between the two portions of the ossific nucleus, which can lead to growth arrest in that area
- CR seldom successful for >1 cm displaced cases

13.3.3.15   Delayed Fixation for Late Displacements at Around 2 Weeks
- Anatomic reduction getting difficult from bone resorption and early callus in casted cases, use intraoperative arthrogram to assess adequacy of reduction if proceeding to surgery

13.3.3.16   Chronic Cases
- Many avoid taking down the non-union in order to anatomically repair it. (Prefer later osteotomy in non-union cases and sometimes with ulna nerve transposition)
- Proponents of the above concept: the blood supply of the fragment is tenuous, and putting metal across the fragment further endan-

gers the blood flow, leaving the patient with AVN and usually a stiff elbow
- Those opposing the above concept: some surgeons claim they can put screws across with reasonable results, but in fact "capsular releases" are frequently needed in their published results, which may risk further devascularisation

13.3.3.17 Complication: Elbow Deformity
- Overall, since non-union common (and most likely in the subgroup of patients in whom half-hearted treatment of 2–4 mm displaced ones that later displaced had been carried out) → hence cubitus valgus more common
- But if fracture unites, cubitus varus does sometimes occur; this is from growth stimulation – theoretically more likely if more time has elapsed before fracture consolidates
- Rn of varus seldom required; valgus deformity after non-union sometimes treated with a varus osteotomy, especially for late presenters

13.3.3.18 How Does Elbow Deformity Differ from the Sequelae of Supracondylar Fractures
- Here the deformity is mainly in the coronal plane and there is usually little rotation
- Refer to the 3D deformity in supracondylar fractures just discussed (varus, IR, and frequently extension in the sagittal plane)

13.3.3.19 What Is a "Fishtail Deformity"?
- Called a "fishtail deformity" because there is a gap, looks like the tail of a fish
- Incidence unknown
- Type 1: sharp and demarcated – tail formed by a gap of separation between lateral condyle physis and medial crista of the trochlea
- Type 2: smooth and angular – from AVN of lateral aspect of medial crista of the trochlea

- Sequelae of fish-tail: OA, more fracture risk (since stress riser), limited ROM

13.3.3.20   Complication: Lateral Condylar Prominence

- Common – 40% in some series
- Prime parents before operating
- Little functional disability
- No treatment
- Good remodelling ability usually
- Sometimes associated with and exaggerates subsequent cubital varus

13.3.3.21   Complication: Delayed Union

- Also common
- Consider Dx if no healing after 6–8 weeks
- Common causes: untreated/improperly treated fractures, insufficient immobilisation, etc.
- Can continue cast, if no progress sometimes bone graft and fixation proposed by some authors

13.3.3.22   Rare Complications

- Malunion
- Nerve palsy – sometimes tardy ulna nerve palsy, secondary to subsequent elbow deformity

13.3.4   Fractured Medial Condyle

- Much rarer than fractured lateral condyle
- Occurs at age 8–14 years
- Mechanism: falling on a flexed elbow
- Types:
  - Fracture line crosses apex of trochlea
  - Fracture line crosses capitulotrochlear groove
- Not easy to diagnose since does not ossify early
- Cx: occasional varus or valgus instability
- Rn: posteromedial exposure with open reduction and fixation usually required

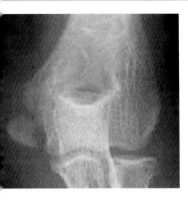

Fig. 13.5 The X-ray showing fractured medial epicondyle of the distal humerus with displacement

3.3.5 Fractured Medial Epicondyle (Fig. 13.5)

- Mostly at age 9–14
- Half associated elbow dislocation (some may have reduced spontaneously)
- Rn: < 5 mm (some say < 10 mm) conservative. Consider operation if > 5 mm displaced (or entrapped fragment)/or large valgus stress expected in sporty children
- Cx – late valgus instability ± sometimes growth disturbance reported

3.3.6 Fractured Lateral Epicondyle

- Very rare
- Peaks at age 12–14
- Most conservative Rn
- Open reduction only carried out if varus unstable

3.3.7 Distal Humeral Physeal Fracture

- Only in infants and toddlers
- Dx needs ultrasound/MRI/arthrogram
- Rn:
  - CR – correct the *medial* displacement in extension, then stabilise by flexion and pronation

- – If OR – fixation: by two pins – needed since not easy to assess reassess
- ▪ Cx: cubitus varus

13.3.8   T-Condylar-like Fracture Patterns

- ▪ Fracture line through central groove of trochlea extending to olecranon and coronoid fossa (hence divides the medial and lateral humerus of distal humerus)
- ▪ Rare in children
- ▪ Occasionally seen in near mature child
- ▪ Mechanism: wedge (or hammer-like) effect of olecranon on distal humerus
- ▪ Rn:
  - – If aged near adult – two plates in two planes
  - – If young – k-wire
- ▪ Cx: stiffness/non-union/AVN/partial growth arrest

13.3.9   Elbow Joint Dislocation

- ▪ Peaks at age 11–20, more in males
- ▪ Most are posterior
- ▪ Associated fracture: medial epicondyle, radial head fracture
- ▪ Rn:
  - – CR posterior dislocation: longitudinal traction to unlock coronoid, flexion to stabilise, occasionally supinate to unlock radial head
  - – Cx: entrapped fracture medial epicondyle can go undetected; heterotopic ossification (HO); recurrent dislocation – from, say, medial instability

13.3.10   Pulled Elbow

- ▪ Peaks at age 2–3 years
- ▪ Mechanism: longitudinal traction with extended elbow, and supination (some experts think the common mechanism involved sudden traction of the hand with the elbow extended and the forearm pronated)

- Dx – clinical, does not need X-ray
- Rn – flex the elbow, supinate the forearm with a thumb pressing on the subluxated radial head. (Sometimes reduction is spontaneous or after elbow flexion and adds pronation or supination motions to the forearm)

13.3.11 Fractured Olecranon

- Not too common in children
- Mechanism: direct blow, on outstretched hand
- Many possible associated fractures:
  - Monteggia fracture dislocation
  - Others: lateral (medial) condyle, distal radius, supracondylar fractures, etc.
- Rn:
  - < 3 mm cast
  - > 3 mm ORIF

13.3.12 Fractured Radial Neck

- ≥ 4 years old (much less common in the pure cartilaginous head in the very young child)
- Mechanism: fall on outstretched hand
- Feature: most are metaphyseal (± intra-articular only after physis closed)
- CR method:
  - Patterson method: longitudinal traction/supinate/with thumb pressure
  - Percutaneous Steinmann pin as joy-stick
  - IM wire insertion via the distal radius to hook proximal radius piece; casted in flexion and pronation
- Rn:
  - Cast if < 5 mm displaced and 30° angulation
  - CR and cast: 30–60° angulation
  - > 60° angulation: most need OR (lateral approach)
- Cx: ↓ROM, AVN, radio-ulna synostosis

(Pitfall: avoid transcapitellar pin – can break)

13.3.13   Forearm Fractures (Fig. 13.6)

- Third most common site of children's fractures
- Most important principle is to aim at restoration of pronation and supination. Normal radial bow restoration is needed. Proper reduction in three dimensions is needed to avoid complications
- Minimal remodelling is possible if healed in malrotation. As little as 10° of angulation can cause limitation of rotation of 20°

13.3.13.1   Subtypes and Their Management

- Greenstick fractures: should not be regarded lightly as recurrence of deformity can occur if the intact side cortex is not broken, proper moulding of the plaster after reduction into an oval cross-section of the normal forearm shape is essential
- Plastic deformity: never underestimate these fractures, as great force and three-point fixation principle may sometimes be required for reduction. Untreated, these injuries can cause limitation of motion and ugly deformity

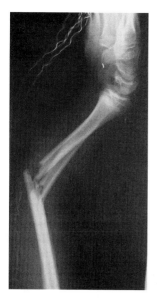

Fig. 13.6 The X-ray showing displaced fracture of both forearm bones

- Completely displaced forearm fractures: unstable as the periosteum of both bones is ruptured, CR can be tried if the fracture can be brought end-to-end, many do require fixation by IM k-wires of one or both bones depending on alignment; or plating of both bones in older children

3.3.13.2   Forearm Fractures: Acceptable Limits

- < 8 years, can accept 15–20° angulation
- > 8 years, only < 10° can be accepted
- Rotational alignment does not remodel (previous claims that significant angulation like 30° rotation malalignment can be accepted should be heeded)

3.3.13.3   When to Operate and How

- Operate if:
  - CR does not reach the acceptable limits mentioned
  - Very important to assess fracture stability; irreducible or unstable fractures should be treated surgically regardless of age or fracture alignment

3.3.13.4   Fixation Methods in Forearm Fractures

- IM fixation – as an internal splint, maintains both length and alignment; application: needs a gentle curve throughout the entire radius and ulna, three-point contact to give stability. Casting needed since little rotational stability. In younger children a bent k-wire can be used, in older ones a flexible Ti rod

3.3.13.5   IM Fixation: Do We Fix One or Both Bones?

- After ulna has been fixed by IM method, may reduce the radius fracture: if a stable anatomic reduction can be obtained; single bone fixation employed
- Otherwise fix both (if need to fix the radius, dorsal incision just proximal to Lister tubercle, dissect between second and third extensor compartments; for radius passage, a 20° bend in the rod/k-wire will make passage easier)

13.3.13.6 Other Fixation Choices

- Plate and screw: in older children (especially if only 1 year of skeletal growth remains); other indications: comminuted fracture, open fracture, vascular injury, re-fracture after displacement or failed IM method
- Issue of removal of plates:
  - Pros: metal corrosion, late infection, stress shield, long-term bone overgrowth makes later removal very difficult
  - Cons: neurovascular injury during dissection and chance of re-fracture

13.3.13.7 Forearm Fracture Dislocations
(Especially Monteggia Fracture Dislocation)

- Definition of Monteggia: a fracture of the ulna with an associated PRUJ dislocation – although the original description is proximal one-third of ulna fracture, now includes any ulna fracture
- Monteggia not very common, but easily missed
- If missed, causes chronic functional loss
- Monteggia > Galeazzi fracture dislocation in children
- *Need to rule out Monteggia in all skeletally immature patients with forearm injuries*
- Pitfall: DDx from chronic congenitally dislocated radial head: suggested by small, convex radial head and hypoplastic capitellum

13.3.13.7.1 Monteggia Fracture Dislocation Rn

- Associated plastic deformation/incompletely fractured ulna: careful CR then plaster casting (POP) in 90–100° flexion and supination
- Associated complete ulna fracture: operation needed to avoid late redisplacement in most cases
- Chronic and very chronic lesions:
  - Up to 3–4 weeks: can still consider OR and annular ligament reconstruction ± ulna correction osteotomy
  - >6 weeks, debatable, some leave alone – decision depends on symptoms, ROM, alignment, and surgeon's experience

13.3.13.7.2 Prognosis: Chronic Monteggia

- Long-term prognosis of chronic neglected Monteggia is uncertain, but in chronic injury it is not uncommon to develop pain, stiffness, deformity, instability, even degeneration

13.3.13.8 Forearm Fracture Cx

- Non-union – associated with open fracture, infection, impaired vascularity. Rn by restoring vascularity, BG, rigid fixation
- Malunion – normal supination range (80–120°), normal pronation (60–80°). Malunion can decrease rotation range ± ADL impairment – in severe cases consider corrective osteotomy
- Compartment syndrome: can occur after forearm fracture – early Dx and release and remove the source, e.g. tight bandage
- Neurovascular injury – e.g. posterior interosseus nerve (PIN) in posterior radial head dislocation/associated Monteggia fracture; anterior interosseus nerve (AIN) sometimes in fractured proximal radius ± Galeazzi
- Re-fracture after removal of plate
- Altered growth: overgrow – most only 6 mm and may not be of functional significance; growth arrest: commoner in distal physeal injury, can cause abnormal wrist mechanics, ulna impaction. May need epiphysiodesis and osteotomy ± physeal bar excisions

13.3.14 Fractured Distal Radius (Fig. 13.7)

- Features:
  - Great remodelling potential, especially if young
  - Another important factor in considering whether patient will need operation is fracture stability (proportional to the amount of initial fracture displacement) – here, fracture healing can be considered as a race between remodelling and instability. In unstable fractures, loss of reduction is common, and if there is significant fracture instability, an operation must be considered

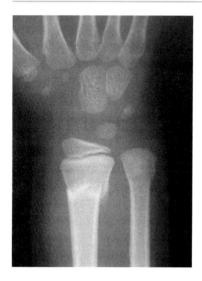

Fig. 13.7 Fractures around the distal radius are the most common fractures in the upper extremities of children

13.3.14.1 Common Clinical Types

- Types:
  - Distal metaphyseal fracture
  - Distal physeal fracture

13.3.14.2 Distal Metaphyseal Fractures

- Bicortical fractures: more prone to displacement than unicortical – in recent years, more advocates of percutaneous pinning after CR besides POP
- Drawback of percutaneous pinning: pin-track problems, radial sensory nerve damage, and extensor tendon irritation
- Open reduction only if failed CR, such as by soft tissue interposition

13.3.14.3 Acceptable Limits

- < 12 years, accept up to 20–25° in sagittal plane
- > 12 years, only accept up to 10–15° in sagittal plane, and ≤ 10° RD

13.3.14.4 Distal Physeal Fractures

- CR needed in the often displaced Salter-Harris type 1 and 2 injuries
- Avoid forceful and repeated CR, and avoid CR for delayed cases
- CR and percutaneous pinning recommended for unstable injury and patients with neurovascular compromise

13.4 Lower Extremity Paediatric Fractures

13.4.1 Fractured Hip (Fig. 13.8)

- Rare, but danger of AVN, mostly high energy trauma
- Type 1: trans-physeal (association with hip dislocation)
- Type 2: transcervical (commonest)
- Type 3: cervicotrochanteric (varus tendency)
- Type 4: trochanteric (fewest complications)

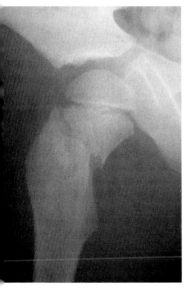

Fig. 13.8 An example of a fractured hip in a child, a relatively uncommon injury

13.4.1.1 Hip Fracture Cx

- AVN in types 1–3, Rn usually observe ± rarely osteotomy
- Varus (coxa vara): from inadequate reduction, type 3 drift to varus if casted. If severe can cause limping – Rn by valgus osteotomy
- Premature physeal closure – 2° to pinning/screw (2–4 mm/year loss of growth) ± contralateral epiphysiodesis, but not always required

13.4.1.2 Hip Fracture Rn

- Type 1: CR (prefer the term "gentle positioning" in exam setting) and pinning ± OR
- Type 2: CR and pinning (or cannulated screw in older child)
- Type 3: undisplaced = screw; displaced = CR/screw
- Type 4: if young = traction then cast; if older/poly-trauma sometimes plate and screw

13.4.2   Hip Subtrochanteric Fractures

- In younger child: cast
- In older child: many choices – EF/plate/IM device if near skeletal maturity

13.4.3   Fractured Femur Shaft

- Management is based on age:
  - < 6 years: early spica (can be with prior traction) in most cases (< 6 months spica also in flexed position, some tried Pavlik for up to 4 months) – think of child abuse if occurring in non-ambulating child
  - From 6 up to near skeletal maturity (age 12): many options → previously mostly used 2 weeks 90/90 traction, followed by cast; current trend flexible IM nail; EF (if open fracture), avoid reamed nail
  - Skeletal maturity: antegrade IM nail ± flexible nail, EF (open fracture)
- Consider possibility of abuse in infants
- Adolescents do better with operative Rn

■ Most do heal, beware of Cx (especially malunion, in varus and IR of distal fragment)

3.4.3.1 Acceptable Alignment

Table 13.2 Acceptable alignment in children < and > 10 years

	< 10 years	> 10 years
Varus/valgus	< 15°	5–10°
Anterior/posterior	< 20°	< 10°
Malrotation	25–30°	25–30°

3.4.3.2 Acceptable Shortening

■ < 10 years: < 1.5–2 cm
■ > 10 years: < 1 cm
■ 2–10 years average overgrowth: 1 cm (range, 1–2.5 cm)

3.4.3.3 Fractured Femoral Shaft Cx

■ Refracture – 10% of EF cases
■ Delayed union – usually open fracture, EF cases
■ LLD – more in ages 2–10
■ Rotational deformity
■ Angular deformity – varus common
■ AVN – avoid piriformis fossa in pre-teens if IM nailing, use the GT (e.g. AO AFN, long Gamma)

3.4.3.4 Summary of Major Operative Options

■ Immediate spica – almost anyone <6 years
■ Traction, spica – < 6 years, those that fail the telescope test upon EUA
■ Flexible nail: 6 to near 12, mid-shaft transverse especially good ± occasional case of proximal and distal third
■ EF: > 6 years, unstable fracture, open fracture, etc.

- Antegrade IM nail: now recommend use after proximal physis closed
- ORIF: consider in vascular injury cases, open fracture

13.4.3.4.1 Appendix 1: Cast/Traction Method

- Pros: effective in < 6, good long term
- Cons: cast Cx, difficult for family
- Contraindication for cast: multiple trauma, fracture very distal floating fracture, gross obesity
- During traction: if legs kept straight – danger of shortening; if 90/90 method used – danger of angulation
- Cast Cx: skin, shortening, angulation, re-fracture, stiffness

13.4.3.4.2 Appendix 2: Role of EF

- Works by getting fracture to length, maintains alignment, but may stress shield
- Indication: open fracture, severe soft tissue injury
- Pros: minimal blood loss, physis injury unlikely, pain lessens quickly small incision
- Cons: pin-track sepsis, re-fracture, stiff knee, scar
- Timing of removal: either wait until callus is mature, or early removal at 8 weeks
- Tip: pin not too near fracture, prevent stress shield, pin care, skin care ± weight-bearing (depends on fracture pattern)

13.4.3.4.3 Appendix 3: Flexible IM Nail

- As internal splint – sufficient motion to allow callus, holds length and alignment, early motion
- Old method like Enders – stability depended on canal fill principle and the bend placed in the nail
- Current Ti flexible nails – work by *symmetrical placement*: balanced force of two opposing nails (proper entry site, nail size and length)
- Drawback: nail back-out, re-fracture, malalignment, nail bending soft tissue irritation

- When to remove – wait until fracture line not seen (6–9 months)
- Contraindication: very proximal/distal, long spiral fracture, very comminuted fracture
- Tip: size – 0.4 of isthmus, distal start point 2.5 cm above physis, bend the nail with gentle bend, leave 1–1.5-cm nail out, check rotation and avoid over-distraction

13.4.3.4.4 Appendix 4: Antegrade IM Nail
- Pros: load share (less stress shielding), stability, good alignment commonly obtained
- Cons: AVN femoral head, growth plate injury
- Indication: more mature adolescent – if in doubt check bone age
- Pearl: better use trochanteric start point (such as the case of some newer nailing systems like AFN), avoid piriformis fossa

13.4.3.4.5 Appendix 5: Plate and OR
- Pros: rigid, early motion, well known technique
- Cons: soft tissue stripping, re-fracture
- Indication: vascular injury, open fracture, multiple injury sometimes, HO, too proximal and distal fracture

13.4.4 Supracondylar Fractures of Femur
- Problem: distal fragment flexed from gastrocnemius pull
- Previous Rn: 90/90 traction/casting; (but not easy to assess varus/valgus alignment with knee flexed)
- Current trend: CR/OR and pinning, then cast in extension to ease assessment of varus/valgus

13.4.5 Fractured Distal Femur Physis
- Key point: although some say the undulating physis makes it less prone to injury), but once injured, danger of partial or complete physeal arrest (30+%)
- Mechanism: extension (sometimes flexion) injury – danger of vascular injury in extension type

- Current trend: anatomic reduction (rationale partly because we hope that, like the case of distal tibia fractures in children, may decrease chance of growth disturbance. But not yet proven for this region)
- Types and Rn:
  - Salter-Harris type 1: extension type CR/smooth pin/cast; cast in relative extension
  - Salter-Harris type 2: if metaphyseal fragment small – pin; if large, screw
  - Salter-Harris type 3: ORIF with screw, then cast
  - Salter-Harris type 4: ORIF with screw in epiphysis and metaphysis

13.4.6   Fractured Patella

- Rather uncommon, ORIF if:
  - >2 mm displaced
  - Sleeve fracture (significant articular surface attached)

13.4.7   Fractured Tibia – Intercondylar Eminence

- 8–14 years
- Mechanism: hyper-extension (associated ACL stretch sometimes gives residual ACL clinical laxity after healing)
- Feature: a common cause of haemarthrosis in pre-adolescence ± afraid to weigh bear, later cannot extend fully
- Classification: (McKeever and Meyers)
  - Minimal displaced fragment
  - Hinged posteriorly (i.e. anteriorly displaced)
  - Completely separated fragment
- Rn:
  - (Near full) extension casting – 6 weeks
  - Attempt CR (OR if not successful)
  - Fixation (arthroscopic or open) – pull-through suture/screw; immobilise in extension (prevent flexion contracture)
- Cx: lack full extension (e.g. from inadequate reduction); mild ACL laxity

13.4.8   Fractured Tibia – Proximal Physis

- Mechanism: hyperextension (and valgus) injury
- Danger: vascular injury (and peroneal nerve) and compartment syndrome
- Rn:
  - Anatomic reduction (CR vs OR) and pin/cast
  - Arteriogram: if any question about vascular status

13.4.9   Fractured Tibial Tubercle

- Age 14–16, jumping sports (more in boys)
- Rn:
  - CR only if not displaced (and intact extensor mechanism)
  - ORIF – suture, screw if fragment is large

13.4.10   Fractured Tibia – Proximal Metaphyseal

- Toddler's fracture, 2–8 years old
- Tendency for valgus angulation (although its development is unpredictable)
- Occasional soft tissue jamming making correction difficult
- Rn: CR – long leg cast moulded in varus (helps prevent valgus tendency)
- Rn of valgus cases:
  - Observation – can resolve in 3 years
  - If not, consider proximal tibial hemi-epiphysiodesis and proximal tibial osteotomy

13.4.11   Fractured Tibia Shaft

- Most common for the tibia
- Rn:
  - Mostly caste (child less prone to ankle stiffness with casting) 6–12 weeks
  - Consider fixation in – open fracture, poly-trauma, soft tissue injury (operation also needed if compartment syndrome)
- Open fracture – better prognosis than adults mostly (healing better, and less sepsis) choices: (pin/cast reported)/EF/ IM rod in older child (Cx – delayed union, non-union, stress shield/pin if EF)

- Accepted alignment of tibial shaft fractures
  - < 7–10 mm shortening
  - < 10° varus/valgus/recurvatum
  - No malrotation

13.4.11.1   Fractured Tibia – Distal Physeal

- Medial malleolus fracture – Salter-Harris type 3 or 4, Rn aggressively with ORIF – danger of physeal arrest. Fixation – cannulated screws
- Tillaux fracture – Salter-Harris type 3 – epiphyseal avulsion at the attachment of ATFL. OR if > 2 mm displaced
- Triplane fracture (Fig. 13.9) – involves three planes (sagittal, coronal and transverse). Investigation: → CT needed. CR seldom successful in three- to four-part triplane (as opposed to two-part/fragmentary triplane fracture). ORIF if articular step-off > 2 mm or a fracture gap > 2–4 mm
- Fixation may cross the physis if needed, articular congruity is most important

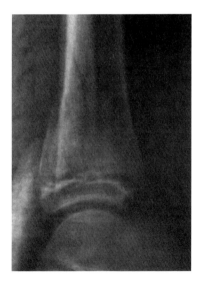

Fig. 13.9 The triplane fracture is sometimes much better seen on a CT scan, which can reveal the fracture in multiple planes

- Direction of closure of distal tibial physis: initially central, then medially and then laterally

(P.S. At this older age, less concern regarding growth disturbance)

13.4.11.2 *Other Types of Distal Physeal Injuries*
- Salter-Harris type 2 – CR and cast (OR if irreducible)
- Salter-Harris type 3 – ORIF > 2 mm displaced
- Salter-Harris type 4 – ORIF mostly (if displaced)

(Take note of open, e.g. lawnmower injuries with severe soft tissue injury – all open injuries are treated with irrigation, debridement and stabilisation, e.g. by spanning EF)

13.4.11.3 *Floating Knee*
- <10 years: higher risk of tibia malunion and LLD
- Principle: in order to improve these outcomes – fixation of ≥1 fracture is needed

13.5 Paediatric Spinal Injury

13.5.1 Different Spectrum of Injuries from Adults
- Injuries mostly concentrated at the upper cervical spine
- Reason = the atlanto-axial joints have not yet developed a "saddle shape" and thus there is a greater likelihood of subluxation than in adults
- Increased elasticity of the tissues is contributory to making the C2/C3 level the fulcrum of movement. Mild degree of C2/C3 subluxation is commonly seen in young infants

13.5.2 Reason for the Difference in Injury Pattern from That of Adults
- Ligamentous laxity
- Relatively large head with respect to body
- Neck muscles not well developed
- Facet joints are more horizontally oriented

- Vertebral bodies do not assume rectangular shape, but tend to be wedged anteriorly

13.5.3 Spinal Cord Injury
- Uncommon
- 10% of all spinal cord injuries
- Vertebral column of the infant can extend significantly while returning to normal, but the spinal cord itself is excessively intolerant of axial distraction
- SCIWORA (spinal cord injury without obvious radiological abnormality) can occur. Constitute 60% of all cord injuries in the child. Most cases occur are < 10 years of age

13.5.4 Other Injury Patterns
- Disrupted transverse atlantal component of the cruciate ligament
- Atlanto-axial rotatory subluxation/fixation – see Chap. 12
- Os odontoideum – now believed to be due to unrecognised odontoid fracture in childhood

General Bibliography

1. Benson M, Fixsen J, Macnicol M, Parsch K (2002) Children's orthopaedics and fractures, 2nd edn. Churchill Livingstone, London
2. Green NE, Swiontkowski MF (2003) Skeletal trauma in children. Saunders, Philadelphia
3. Rang M (1974) Children's fractures. Lippincott Williams Wilkins, Philadelphia

Selected Bibliography of Journal Articles

1. Badelon O, Bensahel H, et al. (1988) Lateral humeral condylar fractures in children a report of 47 cases. J Pediatr Orthop 8:31–34
2. Bado JL (1967) The Monteggia lesion. Clin Orthop Relat Res 50:71–86

3. Bede WB, Lefevre AR, et al. (1975) Fractures of the medial humeral epicondyle in children. Can J Surg 18:137–142

4. Buess-Watson E, Exner GU, et al. (1994) Fractures about the knee: growth disturbances and problems of stability at long term follow up. Eur J Paediatr Surg 4:218–224

5. Dal Monte A, Manes E, et al. (1983) Post-traumatic genu valgum in children. Ital J Orthop Traumatol 9:5–11

6. Grant HW, Wilson WH, et al. (1993) A long term follow up study of children with supracondylar fractures of the humerus. Eur J Paediatr Surg 3:284–286

7. Jeffrey CC (1972) Fractures of the neck of the radius in children. J Bone Joint Surg 54(B):717–719

8. Jones S, Philips N, et al. (2003) Triplane fractures of the distal tibia requiring open reduction and internal fixation. Pre-operative planning using computed tomography. Injury 34:293–298

9. Langenskiold A (1967) Pseudarthrosis of the fibula and progressive valgus deformity of the ankle in children: treatment by fusion of the distal tibial and fibular metaphyses. Review of three cases. J Bone Joint Surg Am 49(3):463–470

10. Lee EH, Gao GX, Bose K (1993) Management of partial growth arrest: physis, fat, or silastic? J Pediatr Orthop 13(3):368–372

11. Vittas D, Larsen E, et al. (1991) Angular remodeling of midshaft forearm fractures in children. Clin Orthop Relat Res 265:261–264

Modern Protocol for Geriatric Hip Fracture Rehabilitation

Contents

14.1   Introductory Comment

- The fracture hip rehabilitation protocol used by the author is divided into three stages. The highlights of the protocol include tackling the immediate direct cause of the fall and its prevention, with emphasis on functional rehabilitation, retraining of the usually weak ankle strategy (discussed in detail in the companion text by the same author) and osteoporosis management, administration of high intensity muscular retraining introduced at a strategic time when the period of negative nitrogen balance is over, then followed by long-term exercises supervised by non-government organisations

14.2   The Three Main Stages of a Rational Hip Fracture Rehabilitation Programme (Fig. 14.1)

- Stage 1: conventional physiotherapy, occupational therapy, adequate nutrition (to tide over a period of negative nitrogen balance), education (time line, first 2–4 weeks)
- Stage 2: concomitant introduction of fall prevention and osteoporosis Mn by FDP, via the PPI network (time line, 4–8 weeks)
- Stage 3: high intensity neuromuscular training and circuit training. Commenced usually at around 2–3 months postoperatively (period of negative nitrogen balance is mostly over; time line, after around the 8th week)

14.3   Rundown of Stage 1 Training

14.3.1   Overview

- Adequate nutrition important since previous research, such as that performed at HSC (Hospital for Special Surgery, USA) found a significant period of negative nitrogen balance after hip fracture. In fact, it was pointed out by the author in this book that the impact of hip fracture on an elderly person is not unlike that of high energy

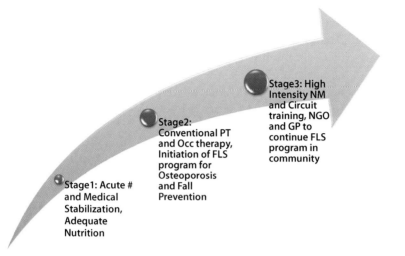

Fig. 14.1 Three main stages of a rational hip fracture rehabilitation programme

trauma in a young patient. The 1-year mortality rate reaches 15–25% due to fracture-related complications

- Absolute fracture risk assessment under the guidelines of the latest WHO criteria as mentioned in Chap. 6 on osteoporosis
- Careful physical examination, both general and local. Local examination involves special emphasis on the frequently weak ankle muscles. Documentation of the power of ankle muscles, especially the tibialis anterior, and other relevant parameters like joint ROM, ankle and foot proprioception and sensation, circulation, skin conditions (like corns, etc.) may need referral for podiatry management as necessary
- Ensure adequate calcium and vitamin D intake. The importance of having a calcium- and vitamin D-replete skeleton is underlined in Chap. 6 on osteoporosis treatment. The elderly, especially those living in nursing homes or living alone, frequently have calcium and vitamin D insufficiency
- Occupational therapy to retrain activities of daily living

- Physiotherapy at this stage involves the following:
  - Adequate pain relief, walking training, use of walking aids, gentle muscle exercises – should not be overdone initially because immediately after hip fracture, the old and frail are in a state of negative nitrogen balance
  - Retraining the ankle, besides a hip strategy to prevent further falls, educate on manoeuvres to mitigate the impact of falls on the hip should a fall occur
  - Education on good posture and the need to walk on a wide base so that the centre of mass will not fall outside the boundaries of the lower limb base of support. Other general advice includes avoidance of double-tasking, especially during walking. Patients with special problems arising from balance will be checked using the SOT (Sensory Organisation Test)
  - Early full weight-bearing is always recommended. If the postoperative radiologic alignment is poor, re-fixation will be ordered. It is unrealistic to expect the elderly to tolerate touch-down or partial weight-bearing
  - Finding out the exact cause of fall and tackling it accordingly. For details see the following discussion

14.3.2 Details of Physiotherapy Training According to the Reason for Falling

- If falls occur during initiation of gait: make a rule of using either the right or left leg during start-up and re-training of the ankle strategy helps
  - The elderly display several striking differences compared with younger individuals during gait initiation: weight-bearing during initial standing is considerably more unequal and reaction time 46% longer. A gradually decreasing anticipatory activation of the ankle muscles is part of the compensatory strategy in the preparatory postural adjustment in elderly people
  - Older adults appear to initiate walking with less TA (tendo Achilles) anticipation and there is evidence in the literature that deficient TA anticipation is accompanied by less anticipatory back-

ward displacement of the centre of foot pressure. One way to circumvent this would be to initiate walking by swaying forward. This type of compensatory modification is in line with previous observations by researchers, revealing that older adults often develop an anterior shift of the centre of gravity within the base of support, thereby improving stability. In practice, this anterior shift of the CG in the elderly is predisposed by the frequently stooped posture that they adopt with an element of thoracic kyphosis and with hips partially flexed

— In the author's institution, the therapists will accordingly place emphasis on the re-training of the ankle strategy, hopefully improving the firing pattern of the triceps surae. The elderly are also advised to always choose either the right or the left leg during start-up in gait; this is because research indicates that the abovementioned deficiency in TA activation will be minimised (Henriksson and Hirschfeld 2005)

■ Falls occurring during negotiation of obstacles: proper hip and ankle strategy, maintain good hip ROM

— In general, studies found that older adults demonstrated greater relative activation levels compared with younger adults. Gluteus medius activity, in particular, was significantly increased in the elderly compared with the young during periods of double-support (weight transfer)

— Increase in obstacle height resulted in greater relative activation in all muscles, confirming the increased challenge to the musculoskeletal system. While healthy elderly adults were found to be able to successfully negotiate obstacles of different heights during walking, their muscular strength capacity was significantly lower than that of young adults, resulting in relatively higher muscular demands. The resulting potential for muscular fatigue during locomotion may place individuals at higher risk of trips and/or falls. In practice, therapists will concentrate on the retraining of gluteus medius strength, on ensuring good hip ROM, on retraining of all the anti-gravity muscles in the kinetic chain of both legs, and on emphasising the retraining of the ankle strategy

- Falls occurring during the act of "turning"
  - Emphasis on proper co-ordination of the "in" leg and "out" leg and training of turning under supervision. Training of walking in both clockwise and counter-clockwise directions during functional rehabilitation is practised by the therapists in the author's institutions
- Falls occurring during gait termination: emphasis on functional reach and on the use of the correct strategy
  - Gait termination is a challenge to stability and the process by which the centre of mass is maintained within the base of support is common to other gait tasks in which the walker is destabilised either by obstructions or changes in direction
  - Another general phenomenon of interest is the realisation of how quantitative changes in one parameter may precipitate qualitatively different responses, either one short or long step or two steps prior to termination. The short-step response in termination is a particularly interesting feature of human gait that is infrequently reported in traditional accounts of symmetrical phases of the stride cycle (Sparrow and Tirosh 2005). In general, patients will be taught to stop at a preferred or comfortable speed, not suddenly stopping when walking faster or accelerating, such as in real life when running to catch a bus or to cross the road. In practice, the author has found that in order to improve stability in gait termination, training by therapists should include functional reach as well as the muscle groups involved in deceleration in normal gait such as the hamstrings and the hip extensors
- Falls occurring during descent of stairs: emphasis on eccentric exercise
  - Descent of stairs mainly involves eccentric exercise instead of concentric strength. A recent study found that training using eccentric ergometers improved stair descent speed in frail older adults whilst training using conventional resistance machines did not (Lastayo et al. 2003)
  - Resistance training of frontal and transverse plane hip muscles may be key factors in improving negotiation of stairs

- The implication here is that merely prescribing exercises involving relatively lightweight elastic resistance bands targeting the hip abductors and external rotators produces inadequate muscle loading to induce significant strength improvements in these muscles – one further reason for higher intensity muscle strengthening exercises in frequent fallers and after hip fractures. Furthermore, performing exercises whilst changing levels, such as with the use of a stepping box, may be more beneficial for future stair negotiation
- The aerobic component of our training programme (part of circuit training, which will be discussed later) should also include exercises designed to challenge dynamic balance maintenance

14.4   Details of Stage 2 Training

14.4.1   The Overall Protocol

- This stage involves concomitant training of fall prevention and osteoporosis management. Fall prevention will be discussed in Chap. 15, while details of the run-down of osteoporosis management are illustrated in the protocol in Fig. 14.2

14.4.2   Qualifier Concerning the Protocol

- The protocol depicted is one deemed suitable for the local circumstances of the catchment area of the author with due regard to local resources
- Notice it has no direct dependence on the use of T-scores as used in the original Glasgow FLS program, and in other UK/European centres

14.4.3   Elaboration of Protocol

- Selection of patients:
  - Our aim is to select patients at high absolute risk of further fragility fractures to ensure the highest cost-effectiveness in a highly cost-conscious health-care environment. The reader is free to de-

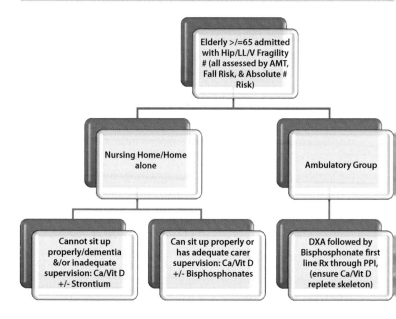

Fig. 14.2 Protocol for the run-down of osteoporosis management

velop his/her protocol to suit his/her local health-care needs and environment

- Why select older patients instead of the original ≥50 years old guideline used in Glasgow FLS program?
    - This is partly due to the relative lack of manpower and resources of the author's institution, and partly because since age is very important and one of the three major factors contributing to the absolute risk of future fractures (see discussion in Chap. 6)
- Why is AMT important?
    - Acts as a good screening measure for dementia. Significantly demented patients (as well as those who are unfit to sit up properly) may not be suitable for the frequently used first-line bisphos-

phonate therapy. They therefore may be offered alternative treatments instead

- Why and by what means do we calculate absolute risks?
  - This point was taken in Chap. 6 on the topic of osteoporosis. To put it simply, the worldwide tendency nowadays is to use absolute risk calculation to help decide the osteoporosis management of patients. In the current scheme, by selecting patients with a mean age much older than the original FLS program, coupled with a documented history of fragility fracture of the hip/lower limb/vertebral fractures, most of the patients will already be included in the high absolute risk category. Thus, our tendency to treat will depend mainly on the score according to the latest WHO-FRAT calculator (see Chap. 6, mainly a standardised fracture risk assessment tool designed by WHO to compute the 10-year fracture risk)

- Why is the T-score not included in the decision-making process as in the original FLS scheme?
  - Inclusion of BMD data in the decision-making process (just like in the original FLS program) is ideal if DXA scanning is readily available. In the author's institutions, many DXA need to be financed by patients themselves; thus, the scheme was modified accordingly to take this into account

- We can see from the protocol that the next level of decision-making depends mainly on the patient's mobility and ambulatory status. What is the rationale?
  - Since bisphosphonate therapy is the usual first-line treatment in most medical centres (assuming a calcium- and vitamin D-replete skeleton), and the mean age of patients with hip fractures is significantly above 65 with the possible element of early dementia, and the safe administration of bisphosphonates frequently requires the patient to sit up for quite a lengthy period with an empty stomach (to avoid the pills sticking and causing irritation to the oesophagus, and the empty stomach is needed as bisphosphonates are quite poorly absorbed), patients' suitability depends a lot on the ready availability of carers

- With the above discussion in mind, the rationale of the last tier of decision-making is easy to understand:
  - For the ambulatory group with reasonable mobility, most of the time DXA is recommended, and, in the author's institutions, patients will be referred to private surgeons or private practitioners via the PPI (public private interface) platform to have osteoporosis medications, as the local health-care system stipulates that bisphosphonates represent a self-financing item to be purchased by patients themselves
  - For the nursing home group, most patients have rather limited mobility, which itself adds to the risk of bone loss. The author will sometimes commence strontium therapy in those nursing home patients with difficulty in sitting up, those harbouring contraindications to bisphosphonates treatment such as history of oesophagitis/renal impairment, and those at high absolute risk – with or without DXA – if the calculated risk is high

14.5   Details of Stage 3 Training

14.5.1   Highlights of this Stage

- This period represents a stage we wait for, i.e. when the period of negative nitrogen balance is over after hip fractures in the elderly. We feel this is the most opportune and most fruitful time to introduce high intensity neuromuscular training (described in detail in the author's companion text: *Orthopedic Rehabilitation, Assessment and Enablement*), as well as the use of the now popular circuit training (Fig. 14.3)

14.5.2   Fall Prevention

- Techniques and concepts of fall prevention will be inculcated into the elderly during all three stages, but are especially important at Stages 2 and 3. This is because it was found and published by the author that even those elderly who initially forgot the mechanism of falling will frequently remember the exact cause upon return to

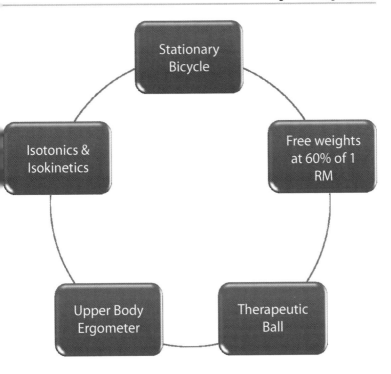

Fig. 14.3 High intensity neuromuscular training, as well as the use of the now popular circuit training

the friendly atmosphere of their home environment. Identification of the exact cause of falls (divided into intrinsic vs extrinsic factors – see next chapter) is important since the cause tends to repeat itself (Ip and Ip 2006). What is more, the author has come up with a new fall scale, now known as the "Simplified Fall Scale", which incorporates four major factors in predicting the tendency of an elderly person with fragility hip fracture to suffer another fall upon discharge: the four factors include age, cause of fall (recorded simply as intrinsic vs extrinsic factors), and ability to arise from sitting to standing independently from a high chair with no arms, and whether the "ankle strategy" is intact or not. The term "Simplified Fall Scale" is used to coin this assessment tool since it can be readily learned by volunteers, carers in nursing homes, carers of the patient at home, without the need for doctors and physiotherapists to spend a lot of time teaching them (see Table 14.1). One should note that many fall scales are more demanding and the details easy to forget even if the carers remember the components initially. More complex fall scales are best reserved for professional medical and nursing staff, as well as therapists. Details of the scale and initial promising results will soon be published separately, for instance comparison of the new scale side-by-side with other scales such as the Berg Balance scale. Further discussion on fall prevention is found in the last chapter of this book

14.5.3 The Importance of NGO, General Practitioners and Volunteers in Health-Care Systems

Many elderly fallers, particularly those whose cause of fall is due to intrinsic factors, need to have long-term maintenance exercise therapy. As most health authorities cannot extend the duration of exercise therapy indefinitely owing to cost concerns, this underlines the importance of non-government organisations (NGO) and the services of volunteers and sometimes community nurses (CNS). Last, but not least, the regional hospital to which the author belongs has started to refer patients with recent fragility fractures to be followed up by general practitioners with regard to osteoporosis management in accordance with the idea and principle laid down by the FLS program, as mentioned previously. This is done via the so-called PPI or public-private interface network, which is so essential for the continued care of our patients. Another very important role played by the general practitioners will be to periodically assess the "fall risk" of our patients when they monitor aspects like drug compliance with the anti-osteoporotic agents. This is performed through the use of the newly described Simplified Fall Scale, which they have found to be user-friendly, does not need special instruments, can be performed in less than 1 min, and as will be reported by the author, has good intra- and inter-observer reliability, besides most importantly

Table 14.1 Scoring form for the Simplified Fall Scale

Parameter	Score
Age of patient: 65–79	1
≥80	2
Cause of fall (divided into "Intrinsic" vs "Extrinsic")	
Extrinsic factor involved	1
Intrinsic factor involved (or if mechanism forgotten)	2
Use of ankle strategy (stress on the function of tibialis anterior) – right ankle	
Diminished power of TA (grade 3–4)	1
Loss of functional power of TA (grade 0–2)	2
Ankle in fixed equinus	2
Use of ankle strategy – left ankle	
Diminished power of TA (grade 3–4)	1
Loss of power of TA (grade 0–2)	2
Ankle in fixed equinus	2
Sit-to-stand functionality (using a standardised high chair with arms)	
Can perform the manoeuvre but unsteady	1
Perform the manoeuvre with one assistant	2
Cannot perform manoeuvre despite one assistant	3
Forward bending with straight knees and spine, and then back (function reach)	
Can perform the manoeuvre but unsteady	1
Cannot perform manoeuvre since cannot stand	2
Cannot perform the manoeuvre starting from standing	2
Romberg's test and assess sensation of both ankles and feet	
Slightly unsteady on Romberg's test	1
Cannot perform Romberg's test and/or sensory loss ankle/feet	2

Interpretation:
— Low fall risk: if total score ≤ 5
— Medium fall risk: if score 6 – 10
— High fall risk: if score 11 – 15

being sensitive to changes in the patient's level of fall risk, thus acting as an early warning system of possible de-conditioning of the elderly patient

Selected Bibliography of Journal Articles

1.   Hatzitaki V, Amiridis IG, et al. (2005) Aging effects on postural responses to selfimposed balance perturbations. Gait Posture 22(3):250–257
2.   Henriksson M, Hirschfeld H (2005) Physically active older adults display alterations in gait initiation. Gait Posture 21(3):289–296
3.   Ip D, Ip FK (2006) Elderly patients with two episodes of fragility hip fractures form a special subgroup. J Orthop Surg 14(3):245–248
4.   Mickelborough J, van der Linden ML (2004) Muscle activity during gait initiation in normal elderly people. Gait Posture 19(1):50–57
5.   Patterson BM, Cornell CN, et al. (1992) Protein depletion and metabolic stress in elderly patients who have a fracture of the hip. J Bone Joint Surg Am 74A:251–259
6.   Petersen SR, Haennel RG, et al. (1989) The influence of high velocity circuit resistance training on VO2max and cardiac output. Can J Sport Sci 14(3):158–163
7.   Peterson GE, Ganz SB, et al. (2004) High intensity exercise training following hip fracture. Top Geriatr Rehabil 20(4):273–284
8.   Sheridan PL, Solomont J, et al. (2003) Influence of executive function on locomotor function: divided attention increases gait variability in Alzheimer's disease. J Am Geriatr Soc 51(11):1633–1637
9.   Sparrow WA, Tirosh O (2005) Gait termination: a review of experimental methods and the effects of ageing and gait pathologies. Gait Posture 22(4):362–371
10.   Thurmon E, Lockhart TF (2006) Relationship between hamstring activation rate and heel contact velocity: factors influencing age-related slip-induced falls. Gait Posture 24(1):23–34
11.   Wallman HW (2001) Comparison of elderly nonfallers and fallers on performance measures of functional reach, sensory organization, and limits of stability. J Gerontol A Biol Sci Med Sci 56:M580–M583
12.   Wolfson L, Judge J, et al. (1995) Strength is a major factor in balance, gait, and the occurrence of falls. J Gerontol A Biol Sci Med Sci 50 Spec No:64–67

Contents

15.1   Why Prevent Falls?

- From an orthopaedist's point of view, we are especially eager to prevent hip fractures since they are expensive fractures and carry the risk of significant morbidity and mortality

15.2   Importance of Preventing Hip Fractures

- The 1 year mortality for fractured hip ranges from 20 to 35% as reported in the literature; not a benign fracture at all
- Morbidity also common
- Cost implications tremendous in view of the aging population, especially in Asia
- Studies have shown an exponential increase in hip fractures after the 5th decade.

15.3   The Basic Question: Why Do the Elderly Fall?

15.3.1   Examples of Extrinsic Causes
- Slippery floor, and/or presence of obstacles
- Slippery bathroom
- Lack of night lights
- Improper shoe wear, etc.

15.3.2   Examples of Intrinsic Causes
- Musculoskeletal problems, e.g. pain and deformity of LL, cervical myelopathy
- Problems of vision, vestibular function, etc.
- Neurological and cardiovascular causes, and psychiatric disturbance
- Acute illness, e.g. delirium from a febrile illness
- Urinary-related problems, e.g. fell while rushing to the bathroom
- Malnutrition
- Medication-related, e.g. psychiatric medications

5.4   Cascade of the Act of Falling Leading to Hip Fractures (After Cummings)

Not all falls result in hip fracture in the elderly, but a model of the cascade from the act of falling leading to hip fracture in the elderly consists of the following (Fig. 15.1) (Cummings et al. 1989):

— Position of impact
— Local protective response
— Local protective soft tissue structures
— Bone mineral density
— Other factors, e.g. local geometry of the femur

5.4.1   Position of Impact

Notice that owing to the difference in the body's response to a fall, the effect of the position of impact is such that a hip fracture is much

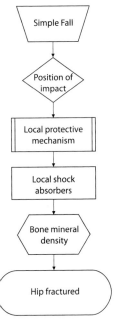

Fig. 15.1 Flow chart diagram of the model of the cascade of events of fall culminating in a fractured hip in the elderly

more likely to result after a fall in a patient in their 80s rather tha
one in their 60s

- This is because when the elderly (say, in their 80s) fall, they usu
ally tend to fall *backwards*, landing on the hip/buttock region. Whe
younger people (say, in their 60s) fall, there is a higher tendency t
have more protective response like using the upper extremities t
blunt the impact of the fall or reach out for supports

15.4.2   Local Protective Response

- The therapist looking after a patient after hip fracture can help b
teaching the patient better protective mechanisms in case of an im
pending fall
- Home modification, training with the use of aids and upper an
lower limb muscle strengthening are also important
- Community Nursing Service (CNS) nurses can help to reinforc
those techniques learned during the hospital stay after the patien
has been discharged from the hospital

15.4.3   Local Protective Soft Tissue Structures

- The adequacy of the soft tissue envelope around the hip, and the bul
and tone of the musculature around the hips of the elderly are im
portant to damp down the energy of impact (e.g. gluteus maximus
gluteus medius and minimus, vastus lateralis)
- Thus, an emaciated and thin patient in their 80s with atrophied hip
muscle is more likely to have a hip fracture after a fall
- The CNS can help teach and supervise the elderly wearing, say, hip
protectors (if the family had purchased one). Advice on nutrition
can also be provided

15.4.4   Bone Mineral Density

- Patients with osteoporosis (BMD – 2.5 SD) are more prone to hip
fractures
- Prevention and management of osteoporosis is most important. Thi
was discussed in detail in the companion volume of this book, and
the FLS (Fragility fracture liaison service)

- CNS nurses can also see whether elderly patients living alone have difficulty in taking medications and help ensure proper administration of medication, e.g. of bisphosphonates. Dietary calcium and vitamin D as supplements are often needed, especially in the institutionalised elderly living in nursing homes. Previous studies by MGH reviewed that silent osteomalacia is not uncommon. General practitioners, and NGO (non government organizations) on the other hand can help to oversee the follow up of the bone health of the patients since family physician were trained to deliver holistic care, and both NGO and family physicians can consider using the user-friendly 'Simplified Fall Scale' as described in the last chapter to monitor the risk of fall of the patient, and consider referring the patient back to the hospital or other fall-prevention clinics/services if de-conditioning sets in.

5.5 What Is the First Step in a Fall Prevention Programme?

- The first step in the right direction in preventing falls is the setting up of a "panel of fall prevention" consisting of trained persons from multiple disciplines
- A multi-disciplinary approach is needed to tackle the complicated long-term rehabilitation of the elderly patient with a hip fracture

5.6 Panel for Fall Prevention

- Rehabilitation specialist
- Traumatologist
- Physiotherapist
- Occupational therapist
- Medical social worker
- Patient relation officer
- Community nurses

15.7   Role of Community Nursing Service

- Community Nursing Service (CNS) nurses, as the name implies, are nurses who actually go to the community and provide nursing care to the discharged patients
- CNS nurses can help identify extrinsic factors (that predispose an elderly person to fall) after a patient with a hip fracture has been discharged from hospital
- Also, CNS nurses may be able to pick up intrinsic factors regarding falls in an elderly person that have not yet been picked up during hospitalisation

15.8   What About Long-Term Care?

- Even CNS nursing service cannot provide indefinite long-term care so who will be caring for our elderly in the long term and reinforcing the methods of fall prevention?
- The answer probably lies in the use of non-government organisations (NGO) and other volunteer charitable organizations, as well as enlisting the help from an elaborate network of family physicians

15.8.1   Non-government Organisations and Other Related Discipline

- NGO
- Home helper
- Carers at nursing homes
- Volunteers
- Home care teams
- General Practitioners

15.8.2   Role of Non-governments Organisations

- The CNS nurses are important as they act as a continuation of the line of care for the elderly with hip fractures after hospital discharge i.e. in the subacute period

- After the initial period of stabilisation, non-government organisations can help take over this vital role in the chronic rehabilitation period
- Before the patient is discharged from the fall prevention programme, the CNS plays a pivotal role in referring suitable patients to the care of an NGO

5.8.3 Role of NGO in Both Primary and Secondary Prevention

- It is expected that the NGO can play an important role in identifying the elderly at risk of falling and/or teaching the elderly about the fall prevention programme (primary prevention)
- In addition, they take over the continuous care of our elderly patients at risk of falling who had entered our fall prevention programme (secondary prevention)

5.8.4 Conclusion

- The expected exponential rise in the incidence of hip fractures in the coming decades underlines the importance of a long awaited fall prevention programme
- Concomitant early detection and treatment of osteoporosis is important
- Although the programme just described was used in the author's home country; it is expected that a similar programme tailored to the local resources will also be of benefit to any country with an aging population

General Bibliography

. Ip D (2005) Orthopaedic principles – a resident's guide. Springer, Berlin Heidelberg New York

. NHS Centre for Reviews and Dissemination, University of York (1996) Effective health care, preventing falls and subsequent injury in old people, vol 2, no. 4

Selected Bibliography of Journal Articles

1. Cummings SR, Nevitt MC, et al. (1989) Factors implicated in the aetiology of a hip fracture. J Gerontol 44:107–111
2. Dolan P, Togerson DJ (1998) The cost of treating osteoporotic fractures in the United Kingdom female population. Osteoporos Int 8:611–617
3. Jarnlo GB, Ceder L, et al. (1984) Early rehabilitation at home of elderly patients with hip fractures and consumption of resources in primary care. Scand J Prim Health Care 2:105–112
4. Seagger R, Howell J (2004) Prevention of secondary osteoporotic fractures – why are we ignoring the evidence? Injury 35:986–988
5. Sheehan J, Mohamed F, et al. (2000) Secondary prevention following fractured neck of femur: a survey of orthopaedic surgeons practice. Ir Med J 93:105–107

Subject Index

A

AAOS
  (American Academy
  of Orthopaedic Surgeon) 198
abdominal compartment
  syndrome 28
abnormal vascular
  perfusion 538
absolute fragility
  fracture risk 199
acceptable radiologic
  alignment 304
acetabular fracture 366, 368,
  510, 515, 517, 526
acetabulum 3, 5
acetabulum fracture 522
acidosis 26
ACJ 259
ACJ dislocation 251
ACJ injury 263
AC ligament 264
acromioclavicular
  joint dislocation 250
acromion 117, 231
ACS guidelines
  (American College
  of Surgeons) 19

active axial
  EF dynamisation 131
active LED
  (light-emitting diodes) 215
active optical localiser 215
acute compartment
  syndrome 232
acute femoral neck fracture 379
acute patella dislocation 411
acute scaphoid fractures 337
adequate circulating volume 242
adequate debridement 150
adequate fluid resuscitation 398
adequate nutrition 622
adequate pain relief 624
adial sensory nerve damage 608
adjunctive fibula fixation 210
adjunctive stabilisers 500
ADL 164
adult respiratory
  distress (ARDS) 18, 22, 34,
  36, 123, 241
advanced trauma life support
  (ATLS) 20, 37, 531, 558
AIN. *see* anterior interosseus
  nerve
alcohol 182